The Practice of

PATIENT EDUCATION

503 -943 - 7362

The Practice of
PATIENT EDUCATION

Barbara Klug Redman, RN, PhD, FAAN

Dean and Professor
University of Connecticut
 School of Nursing
Storrs, Connecticut

EIGHTH EDITION

Illustrated

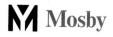 Mosby

St. Louis Baltimore Boston Carlsbad Chicago Naples New York Philadelphia Portland
London Madrid Mexico City Singapore Sydney Tokyo Toronto Wiesbaden

Vice President and Publisher: Nancy L. Coon
Editor: Barry Bowlus
Senior Developmental Editor: Nancy C. Baker
Associate Developmental Editor: Cynthia Anderson
Project Manager: Patricia Tannian
Editing and Production: Top Graphics
Book Design Manager: Gail Morey Hudson
Manufacturing Supervisor: Karen Lewis
Cover Designer: Teresa Breckwoldt

EIGHTH EDITION

Printed in the United States of America
Composition by Top Graphics
Printing/binding by Maple-Vail Book Mfg. Group

Mosby–Year Book, Inc.
11830 Westline Industrial Drive
St. Louis, Missouri 63146

Library of Congress Cataloging in Publication Data

Redman, Barbara Klug.
   The practice of patient education / Barbara Klug Redman.—8th
ed.
      p. cm.
   Rev. ed. of: The process of patient education. 7th ed. c1993.
   Includes bibliographical references and index.
   ISBN 0-8151-9357-2
   1. Patient education. 2. Nurse and patient.   I. Redman, Barbara
Klug. Process of patient education. II. Title.
   [DNLM: 1. Nurse-Patient Relations. 2. Patient Education.
3. Nursing Care. WY 87 R318p 1996]
RT90.R43 1996
615.5′07—dc20
DNLM/DLC
for Library of Congress   96-20571
                                                                CIP

96 97 98 99 00 / 9 8 7 6 5 4 3 2 1

To
Darlien and Harlan Klug
In grateful appreciation
for years of sustenance of various kinds

Preface

This book is written for all health care providers who want to know more about how to teach patients and families. Because the book began as a text in nursing and because nursing has such a rich philosophic and conceptual heritage in patient education, much of the background is still drawn from that field. Students should be ready to use the book when they recognize in their patients the need for learning, when they have enough knowledge to be able to teach the subject matter, and when they are competent in their interactions with patients.

The book was inspired by students who were interested in and excited about teaching patients. It has been nourished over the years by extensive contact with providers who develop and manage programs of patient education.

To reflect the development of the field, the book is entirely reorganized into two basic sections—the first describing the process of learning and teaching and the second reflecting the development of the major fields of patient education practice in place today. Examples given are not meant to be exhaustive; they are only illustrative of the teaching-learning process. It will be advantageous if the student already has a basic understanding of the psychology of learning because this complex subject must be abbreviated in a book of this size.

Barbara Klug Redman

Contents

I THE PRACTICE OF PATIENT EDUCATION

1 The Practice of Patient Education: Overview

Patient education is now well accepted as an essential part of the practice of all health professionals. It seems odd to remember that it was not always so and that the modern movement of patient education into health care is only about 30 years old. Standards of expected practice in this field are still developing, and a procedure-oriented reimbursement system has not provided incentives for incorporating patient education into one's professional practice.

Because learning is at the center of humans' ability to adapt, all social institutions, including health care, make provision for teaching and learning. Much learning (a persistent change in human performance or performance potential) is incidental to experience. Instruction is the deliberate arrangement of conditions to promote attainment of some intentional goal.[1] Patient and public education programs are among the fastest growing components of the health care system, expanding from 50 hospitals with a patient education program in 1970 to the present, when virtually every health care center has some type of patient education activity.[2]

This chapter provides an introductory overview of patient education practice, which will be expanded and developed in subsequent chapters. Patient education is both a practice and a movement. Its *practice* is based on a set of theories, on research findings, and on skills that must be learned and practiced. In addition to general theories of learning and instruction, each area of practice (e.g., diabetes, cardiac, parenting) has evolved with a tradition and a set of goals particular to that area. Patient education is also a *movement* because its acceptance as an essential aspect

of professional practice is relatively recent and still evolving. It is replacing a paternalistic view that held that professionals knew what was best for patients, made decisions for them, and did not share information with them.

Three other aspects of patient education are an organizational form, an evolving set of standards, and an ethical and legal base.

Through its *organizational form,* services are delivered, frequently integrated with other care and across settings (e.g., home, hospital, nursing home) but also in separate programs such as a diabetes self-management program. One of the weaknesses of the field is lack of practitioner responsibility for assessing the need for education and delivering it, as well as its vague organizational accountability for providing the materials and time necessary to teach. Very little economic analysis is available to guide practitioners in decisions about when and how resources are best invested in patient education.

An *evolving set of standards* has emerged, which has been accepted formally in some fields such as diabetes education. Frequently the focus is on ensuring that processes of teaching have been carried out, even though the desired outcomes may not always be achieved.

The *legal* base has been developed through case law and regulations governing professional practice and most especially through the doctrine of informed consent. The *ethical* base is virtually undeveloped. Ideally it requires the competent practice of patient education by professionals, avoidance of the harms that this intervention can induce (such as debilitating confusion), and serious examination of the reasons one is asking the patient or family members to change beliefs and practices, frequently at great cost to themselves. In general, patient education has not been a patient-centered field but rather a practice developed for the convenience of "the system."

Perhaps the field to which patient education is most closely related conceptually is health education. Table 1-1 describes my views of the differences between these two fields.

THE PROCESS OF PATIENT EDUCATION

Patient education is practiced by use of a process of diagnosis and intervention. The needs-assessment phase determines the nature of a need and motivation to learn, and goals are mutually set with the patient. The intervention is constructed to provide instructional stimulation for the exact learning needs the patients have. Evaluation occurs throughout instruction, summarized at periodic intervals to determine whether the outcome goals are being met. Reteaching is frequently necessary because it is not possible to ac-

curately predict what instructional intervention will yield the desired learning by a particular patient.

The process of teaching can be summarized as follows:

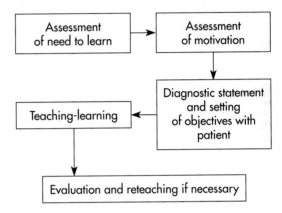

Little is known about how process is actually used by practitioners, but what seems clearest is that it does not flow in an orderly, sequential fashion, as shown in the preceding diagram.

Table 1-1   Comparison of patient education and health education

FOCUS	PATIENT EDUCATION	HEALTH EDUCATION
Philosophy	Patient use of information and skills for whatever purpose is desired	Behavior change for health promotion and compliance with medical regimen
Unit of service	Individuals, families, and other groups	Specific populations
Delivery system	Part of clinical care by all direct-care providers in any setting	Campaigns that include mass media and work through community institutions
Content	Patient experiences, coping, helping patient develop self-management skills, decisional support	Risk factors, health behaviors
Theory base	Direction from field's theory of practice, learning, and instructional theory	Behavioral science, epidemiology
Ethical concerns	Scientific stability and cultural bias of what patients are asked to learn; subtle manipulation possible in provider-patient relationship; inadvertent side effects (e.g., loss of self-confidence)	Scientific stability and cultural bias of what patients are asked to learn; manipulation by government, under which many programs are carried out; inadvertent side effects such as "blaming the victim"
Literature	Integration of literature of disease entity or health problem	Public health literature and certain specialized health education journals
Challenges	Reliable delivery system, including outcome measurement	Accessing very powerful provider-patient relationship

One starts at the beginning of the process but subsequently skips from step to step; however, the elements do serve as checkpoints to ensure that the relevant variables that affect the teaching-learning activity have been considered. Although teaching does not have a complete set of commonly used diagnostic categories, the objectives can serve such a purpose. In addition, as nursing diagnostic categories have been refined and expanded, they are useful but incomplete in categorizing patient learning needs.

The teaching process can be seen as parallel to the nursing process in that each has an assessment, diagnosis, goals, intervention, and evaluation phase (Table 1-2). Because learning about health is pertinent to nursing practice, some general screening questions should be part of the general nursing assessment; for example, what do patients know and how do they see their present problems? If at any time during care the ongoing assessment indicates a patient learning problem that teaching can alleviate, a more refined assessment of need and readiness is made and that problem is dealt with through the teaching process.

Of course, the most cogent question concerns the quality of use of either the nursing process or the teaching process and whether (at least in the psychosocial realm) fine points used in the process make any difference in patient outcome. I believe that there are gross errors in the practice of patient education that make a difference. Errors in practice are probably made in this order: (1) omission of assessment of the patient's need to learn, so that no activity in patient education is initiated; and (2) omission of any given step: for example, omitting the assessment of readiness, the setting of goals, or the systematic evaluation, but not omitting the actual intervention. Of course, it is impossible not to have at least implicit goals when one teaches, but the goals may not be related to a particular patient's readiness and the instruction may not be constructed to meet those goals.

With adequate practice, providers can become proficient in thinking through the required steps of the teaching process. They can become sensitive to expressions of readiness that may be part of an ordinary conversation with the patient and can learn to organize care to elicit measurements of readiness. The teaching that many patients require can be accomplished in the same amount of time that the nursing process takes if it is done at the proper level of proficiency.

Table 1-2   Relationship of teaching process to nursing process

ASSESSMENT	DIAGNOSIS	GOALS	INTERVENTION	EVALUATION
Nursing process				
General screening questions to detect patient's need to learn	One of problem statements may be a need to learn or a nursing diagnosis	Learning goals are a subset of goals	Teaching intervention may be delivered with other intervention	Evaluating whether nursing care outcome was met
Teaching process				
Refined assessment of need and readiness to learn	Learning diagnosis	Setting of learning goals	Teaching	Evaluating learning

SUMMARY

Patient education is an expanding and evolving field, now seen as central to achieving adequate outcomes of care. It is integrated throughout care to individuals and groups in all settings. A diagnostic-intervention-evaluation process model is used to practice patient education.

? STUDY QUESTIONS/ACTIVITIES

1. During a few days of clinical practice, keep a log of instances of paternalism on the part of staff members toward patients. Did these instances occur because the patients involved could not understand the decisions about their care, or did they occur for other reasons? Are these reasons justifiable?
2. T. Berry Brazelton has written: "Demonstrating the behavior of a newborn baby to an inexperienced mother can be both exciting and revealing. The mother's comments as the baby performs are likely to be meaningful in terms of her past experience and present expectations. As her baby goes from sleep to crying in an all-too-short period, the examiner might describe the speed of the state change without labeling it with a value judgment. The mother may then feel it safe to say: 'I just get frantic when he cries and I don't know how to stop him.' The pediatrician or nurse practitioner can then join her, recognizing her anguish and offering to participate with her by saying, 'Well, I don't know how either yet but we can work on it together.' A tacit but powerful alliance between the two is struck, with the baby's behavior a common ground for open communication."*

Label the parts of the teaching-learning process, as discussed in this chapter: assessment of need and readiness to learn, diagnoses and goal setting, intervention, and evaluation.

REFERENCES

1. Driscoll MP: *Psychology of learning for instruction*, Boston, 1994, Allyn & Bacon.
2. Roccella EJ, Lenfant C: Considerations regarding the cost and effectiveness of public and patient education programmes, *J Hum Hypertens* 6:463-467, 1992.

---

*Brazelton TB: Demonstrating infants' behavior, *Children Today* 10(4):5, 1981.

2 Motivation and Learning

MOTIVATION

Motivation is a term that describes forces acting on or within an organism that initiate, direct, and maintain behavior. Motivation also explains differences in the intensity and direction of behavior. In the teaching-learning situation, motivation addresses the willingness of the learner to embrace learning. The term *readiness* describes evidence of motivation at a particular time. This chapter discusses theories of motivation in general, with specific application to health. It also describes assessment of motivation as part of the teaching-learning process and presents teaching practices that stimulate and develop motivation.

Six general theories of motivation can be used to direct learning in a variety of situations.[30]

Reinforcers. In behavioral learning theory the concept of motivation is tied closely to reinforcement of repeated behaviors. For example, behaviors that have been reinforced in the past are more likely to be repeated than are behaviors that have not been reinforced or that have been punished. Reinforcement histories and schedules of reinforcement help explain why some individuals learn better than others.

Needs. Satisfaction of needs for food, shelter, love, and maintenance of positive self-esteem explains the concept of motivation for other theorists. Persons differ in the degree of importance they attach to each of these needs.

Cognitive dissonance. Cognitive dissonance theory holds that individuals experience tension or discomfort when a deeply held value or belief is challenged by a psychologically inconsistent belief or behavior. To resolve the discomfort, patients may change a behavior or a belief or they may develop justifications or excuses that resolve the inconsistency.

Attribution. To make sense of the world, individuals will often try to identify causes to explain why something has happened to them. Persons are particularly motivated to conduct attributional searches in ambiguous, extraordinary, unpredictable, or uncontrollable situations. Attributions may occur after a diagnosis, an exacerbation of chronic illness, an accidental injury, or the relief or cure of a symptom or illness. We know that attributions can have powerful effects on psychological adjustment, behavior, and morbidity. In a study of patients with myocardial infarctions, attributions of patients and their spouses (Why did this happen to me?) significantly predicted whether the family considered itself rehabilitated. Individuals make attributions about disease severity and treatment efficacy. They use these ideas to regulate self-management of their diseases.[17] Thus it is always important to know patients' beliefs about the cause of their present situation because their actions are guided by these attributions.

A concept central to attribution theory is locus of control. Those with an internal locus of control in a situation attribute success or failure to their own efforts or abilities. Those with an external locus of control believe that success or failure depends on luck, task difficulty, or other persons' actions.

Personality. Motivation in personality theory describes a general tendency to strive toward certain types of goals such as affiliation or achievement. An extreme motivation to avoid failure is learned helplessness, which causes persons to believe that they are doomed to failure no matter what. This behavior can arise from an inconsistent and unpredictable use of rewards and punishments by teachers. The problem can be avoided or alleviated by giving learners opportunities to realize success in small steps and by giving them immediate, positive feedback with consistent expectations and follow-through. Coping styles may also be part of personality. Some individuals are vigilant and seek information from all available sources. If these persons find discrepancies in the information they receive, they will feel anxious. Others use a coping style of avoidance. They want little information because it constitutes a source of stress.

Expectancy. Expectancy theories of motivation hold that a person's motivation to realize a goal depends on the perceived chance of success, as well as how much value that person places on success. The theory of reasoned action posits that volitional behavior is predicted by the person's intention to perform the behavior. Intention is, in turn, a function of beliefs about the consequences of the behavior and norms about the behavior that are held by significant others.[22]

Summaries of research have shown a powerful relationship between perceived self-efficacy and adequate performance. How individuals judge their capabilities to produce and regulate events in their lives affects their motivation, their thought patterns, their behavior, and their emotions. Those who believe that they will not be able to cope well dwell on their personal deficiencies and imagine that potential difficulties will be more formidable than they really are. Self-efficacy increases notably when persons' experiences contradict their fears and when they gain new skills in managing threatening activities. Repeated failures lower self-efficacy, especially if failure occurs early in the course of events and does not reflect lack of effort or adverse external circumstances.[2]

Judgments about self-efficacy are based on the following sources of information: performance attainments (the most influential), vicarious experiences of observing performance of others, verbal persuasion and other social influences, and physiological states. Self-efficacy probes during the course of treatment can provide helpful guides for implementing a program of personal change. Adopting attainable subgoals that lead to more impressive future goals can provide the patient with clear markers of progress to verify a growing sense of self-efficacy.[2]

Finally, humanistic interpretations of motivation emphasize personal freedom, choice, self-determination, and a striving for personal growth. Although generally not expressed as a theory in the scientific sense, important assumptions made by humanists cause us to reflect on learners' resolutions to become motivated and to make their own decisions about whether to pursue a course of action.

Two theoretical models used to assess and stimulate motivation in patients follow. Seeking care and adapting to illness are examples of tasks that require motivation on the part of patients and may well be the focus of educational programs.

Health Belief Model

The health belief model[28] affirms that individuals are not likely to take a health action unless (1) they believe that they are susceptible to the ill-health condition in question; (2) they believe that it would have serious effects on their lives if they should contract it; (3) they believe that the benefits of action outweigh the barriers to action; and (4) they are confident that they can perform the action (self-efficacy). Cues, such as an interpersonal crisis or the nature and severity of symptoms, trigger action. This model, which is depicted in Figure 2-1, is an example of the value-expectancy approach, developed to explain an individual's health actions under conditions of uncertainty.

In patient education practice, the health belief model has been used to assess whether an individual holds these beliefs and if not, to direct teaching at missing skills or information. The breast self-examination (BSE) questionnaire

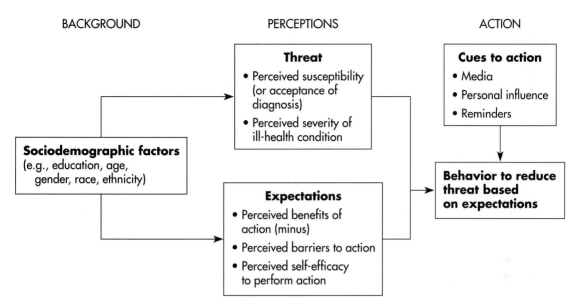

BACKGROUND PERCEPTIONS ACTION

Threat
- Perceived susceptibility (or acceptance of diagnosis)
- Perceived severity of ill-health condition

Cues to action
- Media
- Personal influence
- Reminders

Sociodemographic factors
(e.g., education, age, gender, race, ethnicity)

Expectations
- Perceived benefits of action (minus)
- Perceived barriers to action
- Perceived self-efficacy to perform action

Behavior to reduce threat based on expectations

Figure 2-1 Schematic diagram of components of health belief model. (From Rosenstock IM, Strecher VJ, Becker MH: The health belief model and HIV risk behavior change. In Di Clemente RJ, Peterson JL, editors: *Preventing AIDS: theories and methods of behavioral interventions,* New York, 1994, Plenum Press.)

items (see box, p. 10) provide an example of questions to assess the various elements of the health belief model; item 23 is meant to measure self-efficacy.

A summary of 16 studies found that use of the health belief model did not predict very well the individual's actions in seeking screening, taking risk-reduction action, or adhering to a medical regimen. Difficulty with measurement of the constructs in the model and the lack of clarity about how they interact affected this outcome.[13]

Transtheoretical Model

A second model relevant to motivation is the transtheoretical model of change. It holds that intentional change requires movement through discrete motivational stages over time, the active use of different processes of change at different stages, and modifications of cognitions, affect, and behaviors. Although it has been most thoroughly studied with addictive behaviors such as smoking, it is also useful in prediction and intervention with

behaviors more open to the effects of patient education, such as exercise, diet change, and mammography screening. Progression through the stages is not usually linear; for most health-behavior problems the majority of individuals relapse and return to earlier stages of the model before eventually succeeding in maintaining change.

The stages of change are as follows[26]:

1. *Precontemplation.* Individuals are not considering change within the next 6 months. They may be resistant, have lack of knowledge, or be overwhelmed by the problem.
2. *Contemplation.* Individuals are seriously thinking about changing within the next 6 months, but because of ambivalence, they may remain in this stage for years.
3. *Preparation.* Individuals are seriously planning to change within the next month and have already taken some steps toward action.
4. *Action.* This stage, which involves overt modification of the problem behavior, can last from 3 to 6 months.

■ BREAST SELF-EXAMINATION QUESTIONNAIRE ITEMS

Perceived seriousness

Q1. When you go to your physician for examination, about how often does *the doctor* examine your breasts?

_____ never _____ most of the time
_____ sometimes _____ always

Q2. One of the reasons I don't do self-exams is I'm not concerned about breast cancer.

___ yes ___ no

Q3. How serious would it be to get breast cancer?

serious ___: ___: ___: ___: ___: ___:
___ not serious

Perceived susceptibility

Q4. If I had to think about the possibility that I might someday get breast cancer, I would rate my chances as compared with other women as: (circle one)

a. average b. above average c. below average
(more likely I   (less likely I
would get it)   would get it)

Q5. Whenever I hear of a friend or relative (or public figure) getting breast cancer, it makes me realize that I could get it too.

agree ___: ___: ___: ___: ___: ___: disagree

Q6. Do you have a *family* history of *breast* cancer?

___ yes ___ no ___ I don't know

Q7. I know a close friend/relative who has had breast cancer:

___ yes ___ no

Q8. Have you had any *personal* history of breast *lumps?*

___ yes ___ no

Perceived benefit of action

Q9. If a woman gets breast cancer and it is detected and treated early, what are the chances that it can be cured? (circle one)

15% chance 33% 50% 67% 85% 99%

Q10. Even though breast tumors can be discovered, they seldom can be totally removed. (circle one)

disagree 1 2 3 4 agree

Q11. After a doctor finds out that a woman actually has breast cancer, what do you think is done to treat the disease? (NOTE: This item was scored "has" or "does not have" knowledge of treatment.)

Q12. If you found a breast lump, do you know where to turn for help?

___ yes ___ no

Barriers to action

Q13. Even though it's a good idea, I find having to examine my breasts an embarrassing thing to do. (circle one)

disagree 1 2 3 4 agree

Q14. Examining my breasts often makes/would make me worry unnecessarily about breast cancer. (circle one)

disagree 1 2 3 4 agree

Q15. The BSE is too complex to remember. (circle one)

disagree 1 2 3 4 agree

Q16. If I lost a breast, I would feel less feminine. (circle one)

disagree 1 2 3 4 agree

Q17. Is it possible to surgically *replace* a breast removed because of cancer?

____ yes ____ no ____ I don't know

General health motivation

Which of the following things do you do to take care of your health?

                                regularly   seldom

Q18. Have Pap smear

___: ___: ___: ___: ___:

Q19. Have blood pressure checked

___: ___: ___: ___: ___:

Q20. How many times during the past year did you go to a doctor for a general checkup—that is, *not* because of a specific illness or condition? Don't include eye doctors or dentists. How many times? ____

Modifying variables

Q21. Socioeconomic status (Green's index based on income, education, occupation).

From Rutledge DN, Davis GT: *Oncol Nurs Forum* 15:175-179, 1988.

■ BREAST SELF-EXAMINATION QUESTIONNAIRE ITEMS—cont'd

Q22. Do you have any method of reminding yourself to do breast self-exams?
___ no ___ yes (please list your method)

Q23. How confident are you in your own ability to do a breast self-examination? (place a check)
confident ___: ___: ___: ___: ___: ___: ___ not confident

Q24. Were you taught BSE:
_____ individually (you and an instructor only)
_____ in a group setting (with other women)
_____ impersonally (you alone, no instructor present)
_____ not at all

Q25. In learning BSE, did you practice on yourself or on a breast model?
_____ yes _____ no

Q26. Does your doctor ask you if you are doing monthly BSE?
_____ yes _____ no

Q27. Are you encouraged to do BSE?
_____ yes _____ no
If yes, by: ____ friends ____ spouse ____ other relative

Q28. Age _____

---

5. *Maintenance*. This period begins after 6 months of continuous successful behavior change. Individuals can remain in maintenance from 3 to 5 years and yet still experience temptations to relapse.

In early stages the decisional balance is stronger for the cons—that is, against taking the action—than for the pros—that is, for taking it. Before action occurs, the balance must have swung so that the pros outweigh the cons. For example, in adoption of exercise behavior, the pros might include helping relieve tension, liking my body better, helping me have a more positive outlook on life, sleeping more soundly, and having more energy. The cons might include being too exhausted to exercise, taking too much time, and feeling uncomfortable from getting out of breath.[19] Predictably, perceived self-efficacy (confidence that I can succeed in taking this action) is lowest during the early stages and rises as one progresses.

Typically, about 50% of populations at risk are in the precontemplation stage and only 10% to 20% are in the preparation stage. It is essential that the instructional strategy be matched to the stage; many educational programs are implicitly designed for individuals who are ready to take ac-

tion. The boxes on pages 12 and 13 provide examples of staging questions to determine what stage an individual is in and intervention approaches appropriate for the various stages.

Seeking Care

Available evidence indicates that seeking health care is influenced by many factors and by the interplay among them. A single factor, such as ignorance, is often not solely responsible for delay or promptness in seeking health care. Denial may play a part. Economic need for care is bound up with health beliefs and with values about the priority of health among many motivations. The individual's, the family's, and the culture's answers to the following questions help to determine whether care will be sought: What is the meaning attached to a symptom located at a particular body site? How are hospitals, health care personnel, surgery, and the body itself viewed? Does the family support the health action psychologically and financially? How do individuals view their responsibility for their own health? How important is the individual? What kinds of care facilities are acceptable for use? All these factors influence the way in which persons select, perceive, and interpret information and services available to them.

■ STAGING QUESTIONS FOR DIETARY FAT REDUCTION

Note, the item in brackets was asked of Sample B but not of Sample A. This item was not included in the staging algorithms for either sample.

1. Have you ever changed your eating habits to decrease the amount of fat in your diet?

Yes	1
No	2 (Skip to #2)

1A. IF YES, Are you currently limiting the amount of fat in your diet?

Yes	1
No	2 (Skip to #2)

1B1. IF YES, How long have you been limiting the amount of fat in your diet?

Less than 30 days	1
1-6 months	2
7-12 months	3
Over 1 year	4

[1B2. IF YES, Would you say you are now eating a low-fat diet?]

Yes	1
No	2

2. In the past month, have you thought about changes you could make to decrease the amount of fat in your diet?

Yes	1
No	2

2A. How confident are you that you will make some of these changes during the next month?

Very confident	1
Somewhat confident	2
Mildly confident	3
Not at all confident	4

Staging algorithm

Stage	Question(s)	Answer(s)
Precontemplation	1 or 1A	No
	2	No
Contemplation	1 or 1A	No
	2	Yes
	2A	Mildly or not at all confident
Decision	1 or 1A	No
	2	Yes
	2A	Somewhat or very confident
Action	1 and 1A	Yes
	1B1	6 months or less
Maintenance	1 and 1A	Yes
	1B1	7 months or more

From Curry SJ, Kristal AR, Bowen DJ: *Health Educ Res* 7:97-105, 1992.

Certainly the development of anxiety helps to determine action in seeking health care. Mild anxiety is useful because it causes the individual to act. However, greater degrees of anxiety interfere with adaptive action. Fear of negative reactions from high-status medical personnel may prevent some individuals from going to the provider with an "insignificant" symptom. Often, persons have no clear understanding of their disorder and will wait for symptoms that they consider worthy of medical attention and treatment and that they are no longer willing to tolerate.

Providers have assumed that the physical symptoms of those patients seeking care accurately reflect the extent of tissue abnormality.

However, recent evidence indicates that the symptoms of organic disease vary widely among patients with the same tissue abnormality. For example, myocardial ischemia may not generate a report of chest pain for the following reasons: (1) the patient is hyposensitive to visceral sensation; (2) the patient is coping with the threat of heart disease by denying pain; or (3) the patient misunderstands the cause and significance of a vague or ambiguous cardiac sensation. Also, many patients with symptoms have no demonstrable electrocardiographic findings, and numerous patients with arrhythmias do not report symptoms. Between 10% and 30% of patients with angina-like pain that is severe enough to warrant coronary

■ STAGES OF CHANGE

	Precontemplator (unaware)	Contemplator (not quite ready yet)	Preparation (intention soon)	Action (modifying target behavior)	Maintenance (stabilizing new behavior)
Assess	Cognitive insights Attitudes Beliefs	Coping skills Risk status	Instrumental skills Social support	Self-management skills	Positive momentum Role of relapse
Advise	Messages that raise pros and lower cons	Personalize risk messages	Multiple cognitive and behavioral strategies	Criterion for altered behavior	Upward spiral may regress temporarily
Agree	Think seriously about target behavior	Build commitment Optimism	Small steps toward action	Alter target behavior	Anticipate relapse situations
Assist	Tailor information to educational needs Provide consistent message that health is important	Insight Clarification Cognitive restructuring	Therapeutic alliance Self-monitoring Goal setting	Stimulus control Positive reinforcement Life change counseling	Positive reinforcement Substitute behaviors
Arrange	Create awareness of need for change Provide patient education material Note in medical record that patient not ready (labeling) Reassess readiness to change at next appropriate opportunity	Environmental context Evaluation Risk assessment	Self-help materials Define role of medication Cue sheets	Follow-up Social support Skills training Group programs Linkage with community resources	Relapse prevention training

From Elford RW and others: *Patient Educ Couns* 24:175-183, 1994.

angiography are without significant coronary stenosis. Similarly, the existence of a peptic ulcer is only weakly related to symptoms; arthritic pain cannot be predicted from x-ray studies of the spine; dyspnea reported by asthmatic patients corresponds poorly to objective measures of airway obstruction; and symptoms of diabetes correlate better with depression levels than with glycosylated hemoglobin levels. Do these patterns occur because patients acknowledge and selectively attend to only those symptoms that alert them to an aberration in health and body? Or is something additional occurring?[5]

One conceptual model of how individuals decide to seek health care, shown in Figure 2-2, builds on the self-regulatory theory of health and illness behavior.[6] According to the model, symptoms are key factors in the cognitive representation of health threats. These somatic changes are compared with memories of prior episodes of symptoms, thus generating a notion of identity, duration, consequences, causes, and expectations of controllability. Failure to cope either with the symptom episode or with the distress induced by the episode can motivate health care use. A person's interpretation of a symptom and ways in which the individual is coping with it can, of course, be elicited in a patient assessment. This model acknowledges that other factors, such as inability to perform social roles, may also affect care-seeking.

Adapting to Illness

The experience of illness carries with it certain adaptive tasks that occur in stages and that very much focus motivation. Table 2-1 describes one

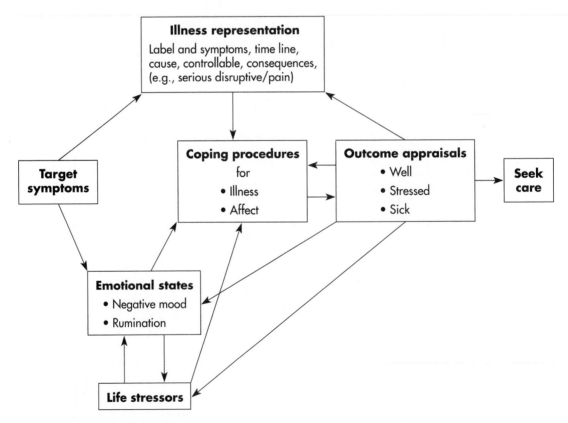

Figure 2-2   Self-regulatory model of health and illness behavior. (From Cameron L, Leventhal EA, Leventhal H: *Health Psychol* 12:171-179, 1993.)

Table 2-1   Fredette model for improving cancer patient education: summary

PERIOD	ADAPTATION STAGE	CONTENT	STRATEGIES
1	Existential plight: impact distress, disbelief, shock	Talk about the cancer as it relates to: harms, threats, resources. Discuss disease: personal aspects, family, social concerns.	Be present whenever diagnosis and therapy are discussed by physician. Move out of denial/avoidance. Use one-on-one approach, pamphlets, discussion—short frequent sessions; provide what is asked for.
2	Existential plight proper, developing awareness	Correct misinformation. Expand knowledge base. Reexplain concepts formerly blocked. Explain treatment plan. Teach self-care. Teach about coping strategies, especially information seeking.	Continue one-on-one. Be accepting of anger and crying. Watch for a "teachable moment." Have short frequent sessions. Toward end of period, use simple audiovisuals always followed by discussion.
3	Mitigation, reorganization, restitution	Strengthen coping. Introduce new ideas and options about disease, treatment side effects, and treatments for side effects. Reteach facts presented in earlier period. Teach anxiety reduction methods. Model expression of feelings. Use "I Can Cope" program.	Use pamphlets, videotapes, films, self-learning packages, longer sessions, group education. Continue to reserve time for questions/discussion. Include family.
4	Accommodation, resolution and identity change	Discuss new identity, further therapy, treatment of side effects, second opinions, work, sexuality, interpersonal issues, fear of recurrences, coping with a chronic illness, living as a cancer survivor. Teach stress reduction. Use "Living With Cancer" program.	Use group teaching, support groups, all other methods. Encourage all free expression.
5	Decline and deterioration, stages of dying	Answer questions asked. Interpret what is happening in the illness. Explain/discuss options. Validate patient's right of choice. Stress hope for comfort rather than cure.	Use one-on-one. Take cues from patient as to when and what to teach.
6	Preterminality and terminality, stages of dying	The dying process. The grieving process. Spiritual-existential concerns. Physical symptom management. Psychologic symptom management. Interpersonal/communication problems. Need for open, honest communication.	Use one-on-one. Include family. Use short verbal explanations. Use periods of acceptance and physical comfort. Take cues from patient. Have patience with "middle knowledge phenomenon."

From Fredette SL: *Cancer Nurs* 13:207-215, 1990.

such model specific to adapting to cancer, with suggestions for content and teaching strategies appropriate to the stage the patient is experiencing. Assessments and interventions are designed to assist the patient and family to move forward through the grieving and adaptation process, including decision making and self-management.[10]

General Principles of Motivation

Basic principles of motivation exist that are applicable to learning in any situation.

The environment can be used to focus the patient's attention on what needs to be learned. It should provide an atmosphere in which the patient is encouraged to practice what is to be learned, with feedback for correction.

Internal motivation is longer lasting and more self-directive than is external motivation, which must be repeatedly reinforced by praise or concrete rewards. Individuals who want to learn are internally motivated, as are those who become absorbed in the task and achieve a sense of accomplishment from it. Some individuals have little capacity for internal motivation and must be guided and reinforced constantly.

Learning is most effective when an individual is ready to learn, that is, when he or she wants to do something. Sometimes the patient's readiness to learn comes with time, and the caregiver's role is to encourage its development. If the need for behavior change is urgent, a teacher will need to stimulate motivation.

Motivation is enhanced by the way in which the instructional material is organized. In general, the best organized material makes the information meaningful to the individual. One method of organization includes relating new tasks to those already known.

None of these techniques will produce sustained motivation unless the goals are realistic for the learner. The basic learning principle involved is that *success is more predictably motivating than is failure.* Ordinarily, individuals will choose activities of intermediate uncertainty rather than those that are difficult (little likelihood of success) or easy (high probability of success). For goals of high value there is less tendency to choose more difficult conditions. Having learners assist in defining goals increases the probability that they will understand them and want to reach them.

Because learning requires change in beliefs and behavior, it normally produces a mild level of anxiety, which is useful in motivating the individual; however, severe anxiety is incapacitating. During an emergency, teaching-learning is at a minimum because other goals are more important and because anxiety is high. Individuals with less severe health crises may also react with intense anxiety because they feel threatened by what has occurred. If anxiety is severe, the individuals' perception of what is going on around them is limited. They are oriented more toward gaining relief than toward attending to learning, and they show physical signs and symptoms of anxiety. For this reason, mothers who are highly distressed because of their children's illness may be unable to learn skills with which to care for them.

It is important to help each learner set goals and to provide informative feedback regarding progress toward those goals. Setting a goal demonstrates an intention to achieve and activates learning from one day to the next. It also directs the learner's activities toward the goal and offers an opportunity to experience success.

Both affiliation and approval are strong motivators. Individuals seek out others with whom to compare their abilities, opinions, and emotions; they also may seek acknowledgment that they are doing well.

Many behaviors result from a combination of motives.

These general principles of motivation are interrelated. A single teaching action can use many of them simultaneously. For example, having a display of teaching pamphlets available in the patient lounge of a maternity clinic may focus the patients' attention on things to be learned, taking advantage of their natural curiosity about subjects such as breastfeeding or postpartum exercises. The content of these pamphlets is aimed at helping patients set and attain realistic goals and often is organized to relate new material to that which most women know. A display of teaching pamphlets can encourage questions as well as convey the staff's interest in the patients' learning.

Finally, it should be noted that an enormous gap exists between knowing that health behavior is motivated and identifying the specific motivational components of any particular act. Providers must focus on learning patterns of motivation for an individual or group, with the realization that errors will be common.

Assessment of Motivation

It is important to begin with a needs assessment, which can be used to establish what a patient needs to learn. For example, while conducting an admission assessment, a provider might ask these questions: What do you know about your disease and treatment? How do you cope with symptoms? How do you manage stressful situations? How do you prefer to learn new information? What concerns you the most right now?[32]

Assessments should also be done to tailor an educational program to the particular needs of a specific group of persons who will receive it. For example, a "community needs" assessment structured by the health belief model was used to assess women who needed mammograms. The women in this particular community believed they were susceptible to breast cancer and were cognizant of the benefits of mammography. Fear of pain and radiation, as well as embarrassment, proved to be significant barriers for some of the women. Also, women over 65 rarely had physicians who recommended mammography; therefore the intervention included educating physicians and using senior citizen groups to encourage older women to be more assertive in asking for referrals. Because the assessment also found a need to reach Spanish-speaking Hispanics, a bilingual mammography facility guide was developed.[21] The intervention was of course validated by an increase in the number of women obtaining mammograms.

Two examples follow of specialized measuring tools that may be used to assess the patient's need for education and his or her ability to learn. The self-efficacy scale (Figure 2-3) measures cardiac patients' perceived ability to perform various physical tasks. The value of the method re-

10	20	30	40	50	60	70	80	90	100
Quite uncertain				Moderately certain					Certain

Walk (distance)	Can Do	Confidence
Walk one block	_____	_____
Walk two blocks	_____	_____
Walk one mile	_____	_____
Walk two miles	_____	_____
Walk three miles	_____	_____

Figure 2-3   Self-efficacy scale. (From Houston-Miller N: *J Cardiac Rehabil* 4:104-106, 1984.)

sults from the close relationship that exists between self-efficacy and the probability that a given activity will be attempted. These scores can also be used to evaluate interventions, such as exercise testing when it is followed by explanation of test results by staff members. This scale measures perceived self-efficacy for walking. Results likely would not hold true for dissimilar tasks.[14] Also, a brief test to assess the baseline knowledge of pregnant women with overt diabetes is shown in the accompanying box; it could also be used to evaluate the outcomes of instruction.[31] This test should be used with other assessment devices. Although knowledge is necessary, it alone is not sufficient to achieve most positive health outcomes.

Finally, tools for assessment of motivation and readiness to learn exist within the context of the patient-provider relationship. Rapport within this relationship is necessary to obtain evidence about motivation, and data from tools must be synthesized with data from interactions with the patient. In addition, teachers frequently stimulate motivation by questioning, by caring, and by

---

■ Diabetes in Pregnancy Knowledge Screen

Below are questions about diabetes during pregnancy. Answering these questions will help us determine your current knowledge about diabetes during pregnancy and enable us to provide the best care possible during your pregnancy. Many questions have more than one answer; therefore circle "I don't know" rather than guessing. By answering to the best of your knowledge, we will be able to counsel you most effectively about diabetes during your pregnancy.

1. Which of the following feelings may result from a reaction? (Circle all that might happen, not just those that have happened to you)
   a. Difficulty thinking
   b. Blurred vision
   c. Nervousness or shaky
   d. Numbness
   e. Sweating
   f. I don't know

2. What should you do if you have a reaction? (Circle all that apply)
   a. Walk it off
   b. Sit down and rest
   c. Eat crackers or cheese
   d. Drink milk
   e. I don't know

3. Glycosylated hemoglobin levels are drawn about once per month during pregnancy. Why are these levels taken?
   a. They measure previous blood sugar control
   b. They measure the amount of iron in your blood
   c. They measure how helpful your diet is in controlling your blood sugar
   d. I don't know

4. When planning vigorous exercise (e.g., swimming, playing tennis), what changes should you make in your daily diabetes routine? (Circle all that apply)
   a. Decrease insulin
   b. Carefully time when to do your exercising
   c. Increase the amount of carbohydrates (e.g., bread, fruits) you eat
   d. Increase the amount of protein (e.g., meat, cheese) you eat
   e. I don't know

5. On days when you are sick, what steps should you take to control your diabetes?
   a. Increase the amount of water or other fluids
   b. Stop your insulin
   c. Call your doctor
   d. I don't know

6. The normal range for blood sugar during pregnancy is:
   a. 40-150 mg/dl
   b. 60-120 mg/dl
   c. 100-200 mg/dl
   d. I don't know

From Spirito A and others: *Diabetes Care* 13:712-718, 1990.

■ DIABETES IN PREGNANCY KNOWLEDGE SCREEN—cont'd

7. A specific meal plan has been devised for you by the dietitian. Which of the following statements about your meal plan are correct? (Circle all that apply)
   a. You should eat everything on your meal plan
   b. You can reduce the amount of food you eat if you're not hungry
   c. You should control the amount of food you eat all the time
   d. You can eat your meals any time during the day as long as you eat everything on your plan
   e. I don't know

8. Bedtime snacks are an important part of your meal plan because they help you avoid having reactions overnight. (Circle one)
   True or false

9. Margarine is mainly:
   a. Protein
   b. Carbohydrate
   c. Fat
   d. Mineral and vitamin
   e. I don't know

10. Rice is mainly:
    a. Protein
    b. Carbohydrate
    c. Fat
    d. Mineral and vitamin
    e. I don't know

11. If you don't feel like having the egg on your diet for breakfast, you can: (Circle two)
    a. Have extra toast
    b. Substitute one small chop
    c. Have an ounce of cheese instead
    d. Skip the egg, and don't eat anything else
    e. I don't know

12. If you have problems controlling your blood sugar during pregnancy, what are some of the possible effects on your baby after birth? (Circle all that apply)
    a. Could be born with low blood sugar (hypoglycemia)
    b. Could be a large baby making delivery more difficult
    c. Could have breathing problems after birth
    d. I don't know

13. What does glucagon do?
    a. Helps liver release more sugar into blood
    b. Makes liver stop releasing sugar into blood
    c. Helps pancreas release more insulin
    d. Stops pancreas from releasing insulin
    e. I don't know

14. After using glucagon, it's most important to:
    a. Drink plenty of fluids
    b. Get plenty of rest
    c. Eat a meal so your blood sugar doesn't drop
    d. None of the above
    e. I don't know

helping the patient reach a learning goal, as well as by encouraging the sense of commitment a patient develops toward a caregiver.

Teachers must consciously activate motivation before learning and help the patient maintain it during learning. The construction of goals is important, especially ones that are specific, moderately difficult, and attained quickly. Such goals enhance motivation and encourage persistence because they provide clear standards for judging performance. Teachers also must provide clear feedback on the quality of the learners' performances, help them feel pride and satisfaction in their achievements, and assist as the learners try to maintain manageable levels of anxiety.

LEARNING

Instructional practices are also based on the psychology of learning and on material that has produced results for practitioners in the past. Although bright and motivated individuals can learn a great deal without a teacher, their efforts to learn can be quite inefficient. Individuals who need to learn health information and skills, even if they are motivated, often do not have sufficient orientation to health matters to attain the goal alone.

Theories of Learning

Learning involves changing to a new state; it is a state that persists. What can be learned? New thinking strategies, new motor skills, and new attitudes are learned in complex patterns that can promote a new performance. General conditions exist (such as reinforcement and transfer) that are applicable to all kinds of learning and learners. Particular conditions that facilitate particular kinds of learning are also present.

Twentieth century learning theories may be classified into two broad categories: *behavioral* and *cognitive,* with Bandura's social cognitive theory containing many key elements of both.[3]

Behavioral learning theory

The most important principle of behavioral learning theory is that behavior changes according to its immediate consequences. Pleasurable consequences strengthen behavior (reinforce it), whereas unpleasant consequences weaken it. Reinforcers may be food, water, warmth, praise, recognition, grades, or paychecks, varying from one individual to another. Extinction is a process used to decrease a previously reinforced behavior by ceasing reinforcement. Also, punishment delivered immediately in response to a particular behavior may decrease that behavior; however, the results of punishment are unpredictable. The Premack principle theorizes that a particular behavior performed by a person frequently can be used to reinforce a low-frequency behavior. Shaping involves applying reinforcements in accordance with gradually changing criteria. As the performer begins to roughly approximate the target behavior, closer approximations of the final response are needed before reinforcement can be delivered.[30]

In teaching, one must be sure that effective reinforcement is applied to a well-defined behavior so that learners will understand what they did to warrant the reward. As new behaviors are learned, reinforcement is frequent; however, after behaviors are established, reinforcement is given at random to encourage persistence of the behavior.

Cognitive learning theory

In cognitive theory, learning is the development of insights or understandings that provide a potential guide for behavior. New insights lead to a reorganization of the individual's cognitive structure, which is stored internally in visual images and in propositional networks and schemata. Within this framework, learning makes change in behavior possible, although not necessary. Motivation to take action results from a need to make sense of the world and solve problems.

Teachers using this theory would determine the schemata of the learner and would organize content so that it could be assimilated easily into the existing schema. Some learning can be described as an accumulation of new information in memory; however, the basic goal is to direct a longitudinal development of increasingly sophisticated mental models. Each level of learning addresses a larger set of problems. Novices can relate only superficially to the problem area or to the subject matter and must use preexisting schemata to interpret these isolated pieces of data. Experts, on the other hand, quickly identify the problem and know how to approach it, consolidate information in meaningful ways, and monitor and accurately predict the outcome of their performance.[11] In contrast to general learning skills, expertise is increasingly viewed as specific to a particular domain of knowledge or thought.

Social cognitive theory

Social cognitive theory as developed by Bandura[3] is largely a cognitive theory but incorporates principles of behaviorism. According to this theory, humans respond primarily to cognitive representations of the environment rather than to the environment itself.

Individuals acquire information, values, attitudes, moral judgments, standards of behavior, and new behaviors through observing others. Infants who are several months old model behavior with competency and continue to do so throughout their lives. Individuals can learn and formulate rules of behavior by observing persons, films or videotapes of models, symbolic models (written accounts of a performance), or sets of instructions (compressed accounts of a performance). This coded information serves as a guide for future action. The learner also gets information about the probable consequences of modeled action. Individuals visualize themselves executing the correct sequence of actions; therefore cognitive rehearsals and actual performances increase the proficiency of individuals, give them a sense of efficacy, and reduce the tendency to forget learned behaviors.

In social cognitive theory, behavior is regulated by expectations for similar outcomes on future occasions. Individuals will persist for some time in actions that go unrewarded on the expectation that their efforts will eventually produce rewarding results. Extrinsic incentives are especially necessary in early stages of developing competencies (such as playing the piano) until competency becomes self-rewarding. The natural social environment is often inconsistent, contradictory, and inattentive. To ensure that the individual's newly acquired skills generalize and endure under these less than favorable circumstances, transitional practices must gradually approximate those of the natural social environment.

Much behavior is motivated and regulated by internal standards and self-evaluative reactions to the individual's own actions, including self-incentives and self-concepts of efficacy. To function competently requires skills and perceived self-efficacy. Perceived self-efficacy is a belief in one's ability to realize a certain level of performance. It must be distinguished from outcome efficacy, which judges the likely consequence certain such behaviors will produce. Judgments of self-efficacy are based on four principal sources of information: (1) performance attainments, the strongest of the sources, which involve acting out the desired behavior, with repeated failures lowering self-efficacy, (2) vicarious experiences through observing the performances of others, especially if the model is similar to the learner in ability, age, sex, and experiences, (3) verbal persuasion, and (4) perceived physiological states from which individuals partly judge their capability, strength, and vulnerability. For example, cardiac rehabilitation programs are structured to provide information from these four sources, and the patient's perceived self-efficacy to perform various tasks is closely related to whether he or she will attempt those activities.

Types of Learning

Transfer of learning

Transfer of learning, the effect of prior learning on subsequent learning, is one of the most important products of education, inasmuch as no learner can practice for all situations that will arise. It is more efficient for an individual to learn general information, skills, and ways of thinking and apply them to a variety of situations instead of learning specifically for each situation. Teaching for transfer is based on evidence that individuals forget nonsense material and isolated facts. However, individuals remember general ideas, attitudes, ways of thinking, and skills that are meaningful to them and that they have thoroughly learned and applied.

For the transfer of learning to occur, the individual must also recognize that the new situation is similar to previously learned situations and he or she must remember which specific thoughts or behaviors are appropriate. In behavioral learning theory, transfer has an increased probability for responses occurring in the future because of past performance or because of the appearance of identical stimuli. In cognitive learning theory, transfer is not automatic; when it occurs, it is in the form of generalizations, concepts, or insights that have been developed in one situation and are being used in other situations.

Many studies provide evidence that generally positive transfer increases when overall training and application conditions coincide. Practice in a variety of contexts enhances transfer (less like the original learning). Indeed, extensive, varied practice based on imitating a model and driven by reinforcers can lead to the automatic triggering of a well-learned behavior in a new context. Use of examples aids transfer, especially if one extracts the rule from the present example and uses it in new situations.[29] Instruction must be planned to ensure that transfer will occur.

Memory

Forgetting learned material is one of the banes of our existence. Not using learned material, interference of other learning, loss during reorganization of ideas, and motivated forgetting (which may be subconscious) constitutes an explanation for not remembering learned materials. Nevertheless, ideas are remembered for a long time, whereas facts are not.

The cognitive process involves the following: (1) selective perception of stimuli from the environment; (2) storage in short-term memory persisting for as long as 20 seconds; (3) encoding (leaves short-term memory and enters long-term memory); (4) storage in a meaningful mode as concepts, propositions, schema, and imagery in long-term memory; (5) retrieval; (6) response generation; (7) performance (patterns of activity that can be observed); and (8) feedback. Instruction can aid each of these steps by providing, for example, differentiation of features facilitating selective perception, verbal instruction or pictures that suggest encoding schemes, or cues that aid retrieval. Retrieval time is slow except for the short-term memory, which holds only about six items. Forgetting is characteristically a progressive loss of precise information about an event rather than the total loss of a stored item and usually occurs because of the ineffectiveness of search and retrieval processes.

Ways to increase memory retention include fostering intent to learn and to remember, finding meaning in material to be learned, applying newly learned material to a practical situation (practicing), rehearsing remembering, using organizing strategies and visual imagery, and learning over a period of time.

Ley completed a series of studies on patient memory of clinical advice, which is summarized in an excellent article.[18] Neither age nor intelligence showed any consistent relationship with recall. Diagnostic statements were best recalled and those concerned with instructions and advice most poorly recalled. These findings seemed to result from perceived "importance" effects. Four methods were found to increase recall: use of shorter words and sentences, explicit categorization, repetition, and use of concrete-specific rather than general-abstract statements (general: "You must lose weight"; specific: "You must lose 7 pounds"). Using these tactics plus giving instructions and advice and stressing their importance resulted in significant differences in the amount of information recalled by patients.

Professionals have been shocked and dismayed at patient recall of informed-consent conversations that generally include explanation of diagnosis, the nature of the illness, proposed surgery, risk of death or complications, benefits, and alternate methods of management, with the chances for failure or success. Patients frequently remember fewer than half the items covered, as verified against recordings of the initial conversation. Certainly use of the approaches just outlined would improve retention.

Problem solving

Problem solving is frequently a desired goal in learning situations. Problem tasks are more complex if they have one or more of the following characteristics: (1) incompletely defined alternatives, (2) existence of a number of subproblems, (3) several ways to reach the goal, (4) need for a large number of information sources to solve the problem, or (5) a rapidly changing problem situation.[7] Problem solving can be broken into a series of steps: (1) identification of the problems, (2) determination of possible actions and their probable results, (3) selection of one action, (4) implementation of it, and (5) evaluation of problem-solving effectiveness. Frequently, breaking the problem into parts is helpful. Learners may need help at any of the stages of problem solving.

The following is an example of a nurse helping the patient solve his problem: An elderly man who lives alone has had heart damage and is about to be discharged from the hospital with permanent limitation of activity. He will therefore have a problem in caring for himself as he did before his illness. Although he recognizes the situation as a problem, he needs help in defining its breadth—the extent to which this restriction will affect his daily pattern.

The nurse is a source of information to clarify the meaning of activity restriction. She also knows the amount of energy the patient will expend in different activities and can help him to consider how he can economize in the use of his resources. The patient, with the help of the nurse, concludes that he can meet the restrictions and remain living alone by having his groceries delivered and by allowing a daughter to do his cleaning, washing, and ironing. It is agreed that these new living arrangements will be judged by the amount of energy he must expend, by how tired or how contented he is, and by his and the provider's opinion about his state of health.

The patient then goes home and tries out the hypothesized solutions, evaluating them as determined. At this stage he again needs the nurse's help, best given in his home, in assessing his subjective feelings of tiredness and the total amount of energy he expends. By visiting the home, the nurse is able to think of new solutions that need to be tried. Of course, the situation in this example may be altered slightly or considerably by such factors as the patient's ability to understand the situation, his emotional readiness to deal with it, a decrease in income, the daughter's moving away, or a change in his health status. This example is not meant to imply that each patient has only a single problem, but such difficulties are often interrelated.

Attitude learning

Attitudes pervade all spheres of learning. They may be defined as learned, emotionally toned predispositions to react in particular ways toward an object, an idea, or a person. *Values,* which are similar but more permanent, are expressions of how individuals believe an object or relationship affects them. Over the years feelings are developed, become well established, and are reflected in behavior. Often we do not realize that we are acquiring attitudes. Membership in groups, particularly primary ones, seems to influence acquisition of attitudes.

Suggestions for teaching attitudes follow directly from knowledge about how they are learned and include employing someone to teach whose attitudes the learner can view and imitate. This model may not be a health care professional but possibly another patient with whom the learner can identify, which is the reason for establishing colostomy and ileostomy clubs and other such groups. Another way of influencing attitudes is to provide satisfying experiences, so that the person develops a positive response to ideas or feelings associated with the experiences. For example, personnel in a health care clinic should try to provide experiences of the sort that help the patient have positive feelings about the clinic.

Psychomotor learning

Anyone recalling the awkwardness of a puppy or a child or the unsteadiness of an old man and comparing it with the sure coordination of a skilled artist can observe a variation in motor skills. These skills can vary with strength, reaction time, speed, balance, precision, and flexibility of tissues. Motor skills are usually composed of an ordered sequence of movement that must be learned. Separate parts of a motor act can be learned and practiced separately as part-skills.

To execute a particular skill, a person must possess a neuromuscular system that is capable of performing the skill and must have an ability to form a mental image of the act. A mental image is created when the learner watches a demonstration that shows the skill and points out relevant cues for a successful performance. Relevant cues often involve muscular cues of balance and pull; cues may also be seen or heard. When learning to walk with crutches, a person must see the floor or objects that might get in the way, hear persons approach from behind, and feel whether he or she is balanced. The cues must be obvious to the beginner and often are not noticed much in advance of the action. The person experienced in using the motor skill can use many cues rather than just the obvious ones. He or she is not confused by irrelevant cues, attending to them with less conscious concentration. Also, the person experienced in certain motor skills reacts faster and can take advantage of cues far in advance of action. The goal is a smooth, coordinated sequence of action with a minimum expenditure of energy.

The learner practices to develop a proficient performance. The mental image is a guide. At first, however, the teacher may need to guide the person's body so that he or she experiences the physical sensations that accompany correct motions. For example, one might guide a child's hands as she learns to drink from a cup. It is best for the learner to practice in a situation that provides cues similar to those in the environment where the skill will be used. For example, the person with a colostomy is taught in a setting that simulates a bathroom at home. During the crucial early stages of practice, information about the patient's progress, or lack of it, is important. Learners often need help in judging their own performances, even though they can judge someone else's. Eventually, learners receive messages from their own physical sensations and can decide if their objectives have been accomplished.

It is generally recommended that practice periods be short and infrequent enough to avoid fatigue. If intervals between practices are too long, the learner may forget. Once a motor skill has been learned, it can be quickly recaptured even after an interval of many years.

Developmental Phases

Adult learning

The dominant current theory of adult learning builds on the cognitive tradition, and the kind of learning most characteristic of the adult phase is transformative learning. The challenges of adulthood involve a process of traveling through an uncertain number of changes that transform the individual. A disorienting dilemma usually motivates reflection about one's perspectives and assumptions. Although the learner does not return to an old perspective once a transformation occurs, the passage involves difficult negotiation and compromise, stalling, and backsliding. Self-deception and failure are common. The crucial difference between the transformation lag and that of primary socialization (child) is that adults are capable of being critically reflective. Assistance with perspective change involves helping the person see the problem and providing access to alternate-meaning perspectives to help the individual interpret his or her reality. Adult learners then can examine their assumptions critically by using stories and pictures that pose hypothetical dilemmas, with conflicting rules and assumptions in the areas of critical concern.

Indeed, support groups often involve adults who come together in response to the same life dilemma. These groups foster critical reflection. They help the participants gain and apply insights to their own lives. One can study the outcomes of this kind of education by interviewing and by comparing movement in problem awareness, expectations, and goals.[20] Health-threatening situations frequently cause individuals to feel disoriented and precipitate self-reflection.

Learning in children

Ability to learn depends on maturation, and a great deal of maturation occurs in childhood. Readiness to learn in childhood changes considerably, beginning with visual, auditory, and motion stimulation of infants. The primary dimension of children's development is the degree of differentiation they make between the self and others. Children move toward a clearer distinction between the internal and the external self. The general principles and comments about learning outlined in previous sections of this chapter are applicable to children within their readiness level.

Intellectual development moves from concrete to abstract. During the preschool years, children can use language to represent objects or experiences and can solve problems by direct manipulation of physical objects. Young children are egocentric and interested in only what affects them. They want explanations for everything but are not concerned with supplying reasons for their questions. If children have a background of direct nonverbal experience during the elementary school years, they can verbally manipulate relationships between ideas without having the objects present. As they grow toward adolescence and then adulthood, they gradually come to understand and manipulate relationships between abstractions without any reference to the concrete. Eventually, they can formulate and test hypotheses based on the possible combinations of several ideas.

Children must develop motor skills and feelings, as well as grow intellectually. Developing trust in the first 2 years is crucial. At that point children become more autonomous, learning to walk, run, jump, and feed themselves. Between the ages of 3½ and 7, children develop imagination and learn to take the initiative. During the early school years they become industrious, turning their attention to the outside world. As adolescents they develop their identities.

Knowledge of growth and development suggests that teachers should determine realistic objectives and explain them in a way that children can understand. Allowing children to handle equipment, such as a breathing mask, seems to encourage acceptance of the treatment. This is especially true during the years when direct nonverbal experience is important. Because children younger than 5 years experience egocentricity and fear of injury, they need to know how procedures will affect them. For example, it may be explained to children that during a chest x-ray examination they will just have to stand still, to hold their breath for a few seconds, and not to worry because they will not feel anything.

Research has consistently reported limited periods of behavioral upset followed by rapid recovery after discharge from the hospital. (Children between 6 months and 4 years are the most vulnerable.) Young children, in particular, consider illness to be self-caused and punitive. It has been suggested that if a child is younger than 4 years, explanation of anatomy and physiology is not useful because the child does not have the necessary understanding and is prone to develop undesirable fantasies. Separation anxiety in this age-group is a primary problem. Therefore teaching should stress that the same provider needs to care for the child, and the parents should be encouraged to help.

For children older than 7 years, more sophisticated language and drawings can be used. Children of school age also benefit from tours of hospital playrooms and wards and from discussion in which they can learn about their illness, its origins, and proposed plans of treatment. Because school-age children have a more mature concept of causality, they have the capacity to understand that neither illness nor treatment is imposed on them because of their own misdeeds. These children are able to cooperate with treatment because they can think before they act. Inasmuch as they can express their feelings in words and have a greater grasp of time sequences, they can better tolerate a separation from their parents.

Children's health attitudes and behaviors show a critical period of change around the time they enter the third grade. Third graders are able to decide whether to report illness or injury. They have developed cognitive abilities, and they have learned the social rules that govern illness and when to seek care. By the sixth grade these abilities are refined.

Adolescents must master the ability to think in abstractions and to imagine the possibilities that are inherent in a variety of situations. Many adolescents need help in thinking through behavioral alternatives. They may need guidance through steps of problem solving and planning. Role playing in peer groups can help illustrate appropriate norms of behavior. It can also translate abstract information into stories that are easier to remember.

Chronically ill children become increasingly able to understand their illnesses as they develop intellectually. Cognitive development brings with it the ability to grasp the meaning of a poor prognosis or of functional limitations.

Adolescents frequently display particular thought patterns involving an imaginary audience or a personal fable, consistent with a stage of intense preoccupation with themselves. They believe that if everyone is watching them and thinking about them, thanks to the imaginary audience, they must be something special, unique, or different. Teenagers with chronic illness may stop taking medications because they believe they are special and different and can manage without the medications. Believing that they are immune to the natural laws that other persons must obey can also cause them not to use contraceptives. Unprotected intercourse is not viewed as a risk by the adolescent.[9] Pestrak and Martin[24] believe that many adolescents are functioning at a cognitive level that renders them unable to practice most forms of birth control effectively. The authors conclude that the effective practice of birth control requires that individuals accept their sexuality and acknowledge that they are sexually active, anticipate the present, and view potential future sexual encounters realistically.

Pridham, Adelson, and Hansen[25] have developed a useful tool (Table 2-2) describing how features of development are pertinent in helping children deal with procedures.

Application of Learning Theories

All of the theories described in the early part of this chapter are frequently used in health situations. In this section clinical examples of learning theory application are provided.

Behavioral learning theory suggests use of a patient-provider contingency contract. Desired behaviors, rewards, punishments, and time frames are discussed, written, and signed by the patient. An example of such a contract may be seen in Figure 2-4. Research shows that the patient-provider contingency contracts yield at least short-term, positive effects across a variety of medication conditions and health-related behaviors. However, long-term results show considerable recidivism.[15]

Parents have been taught to use behavior modification with their children and can learn how to modify any class of overt child behaviors. Behavioral management skills that parents frequently need to learn include (1) obtaining the child's attention before issuing a request, (2) issuing one request at a time, (3) waiting after each request for 8 to 15 seconds without talking, (4) helping the child, (5) assuming a threatening or cajoling expression until the requested action is completed, (6) issuing discipline when the child is noncompliant after the first repetition of the request, (7) praising the child's compliance, and (8) requiring time-out when appropriate.[27]

Cognitive learning theory suggests a focus on attributions (a form of cognitive interpretation about why something happened) and schemata. A persuasive theory suggests that individuals tend to attribute the cause of serious illness to their emotional state, their health behaviors, confidence in their ability to control the outcome of the problem, or the ability to contend with uncertainty regarding their condition. This may explain why attributions predict morbidity in some serious illness.[1]

Some examples may be helpful. Bar-On and Cristal[4] report a study of male patients younger than 60 years who had had their first myocardial infarction. Their attributions about the cause and outcome of the infarction formed five clusters: (1) some of the patients attributed the myocardial infarction to fate, luck, or the pressures of life; (2) some denied the problem and said that the infarction was a matter of chance and that they would continue to do what they had been doing; (3) some wanted to control the future by building their bodies and following their physicians' advice; (4) some believed that their anger had caused the attack and that with the help of physician and family, they would be able to cope; and (5) some believed that their bodies were vulnerable because of inherited tendencies, smok-

Text continued on p. 31.

Table 2-2   Features of development that are pertinent to helping children deal with procedures

	BIRTH-2 YEARS	2-7 YEARS	7-12 YEARS	ADOLESCENCE
How the child thinks and problem-solves	Sensory-motor experience develops schema (well-defined and repeated sequences of actions and perceptions). Memory is obvious by 3-4 months and is demonstrated in second year by child's imitations of parents' activities. Between about 18 and 24 months, use of symbols for thought-reasoning communication appears.	Preoperational stage (thinking is dominated by the child's perceptions rather than logic). Verbally communicated information is increasingly important in learning; exploratory manipulation of objects also helps the child to learn. Child watches, listens, asks questions (why? how?). Child can (a) label (classify) familiar things; perception is often limited to a single, salient feature, making it difficult for child to see things in a context or differentiate unessential from essential properties of an experience; (b) use memory to reconstruct past events; (c) use imagination to deal with events, people, objects; (d) about age 4, begin to infer outcomes; (e) define objects/events in terms of their use/function. Thinking relies on the child's own point of view (egocentricity), since children do not have the capacity to identify a point of view other than their own. As the child gets older, he or she begins to be able to think in terms of quantities (e.g., to	Concrete operational phase. Child learns from observing/interacting with peers as well as from own experiences. Can use symbols to organize thoughts and represent experience. Features of thinking include increasing capacity to (a) understand viewpoints of others; (b) see the relative nature of things (e.g., this hurts a little; that hurts a lot); (c) use deductive logic in respect to tangible (concrete) experiences (if this, then that); (d) classify things in terms of several characteristics, implying that the child can view things in context, for example, "The shot hurt, but it will make me feel better"; (e) evaluate painful intrusive actions in terms of logical function rather than in terms of punishment; and (f) understand unseen body mechanics/functions. Child can make use of sensory as well as procedural information.	Stage of formal operations. At this point, there is use of reason and logical thinking and interest in theoretically possible problems and questions. The adolescent can engage in self-reflection and think about own thinking and can learn from verbally presented ideas and arguments.

Continued.

From Pridham KF, Adelson F, Hansen MF: *J Pediatr Nurs* 2:13-22, 1987.

Table 2-2 Features of development that are pertinent to helping children deal with procedures—cont'd

	BIRTH-2 YEARS	2-7 YEARS	7-12 YEARS	ADOLESCENCE
		recognize variation in quantity; to use numbers to count). Attention is increasingly selective as the child's schema or perceptual sets become more refined.		
Major fears and worries	After about 6 months: separation from parents; unfamiliar people/experiences/places, especially when not accompanied by parent.	Separation from parents; harm to body, including fears of castration after about age 3; punishment for wrongdoing.	Body injury; disability (loss of body functions); loss of control; loss of status.	Uncertainty about selves as persons (especially early and middle adolescence); concern about whether or not body, thoughts, and feelings are "normal."
Understanding cause and effect	By about 3 months, may associate an action with a result. In second year: magical thinking: belief that what is wished for happens.	Beliefs: (a) everything happens by intention; (b) imminent justice—misbehavior is followed by punishment; (c) belief that events that in fact are associated only by happenstance are connected.	Child 6-8: conclusions are based on perceptions. Child 9-12: applies logical operations (deductive thinking) to concrete (immediately experienced) circumstances. Prior to about 9 years, children are likely to view their illness as a consequence of transgressions of rules. (Rules exist in their own right and misdeeds have their own inherent punishment.) Prior to about 9 years, children are likely to believe that illness is caused by germs whose presence is sufficient for illness. At about 9 years, children begin to understand that (a)	Can use formal rules of logic and evidence to assess cause and effect.

(continued from previous page)	an illness may have multiple causes; (b) the body's response to an agent or a combination of agents may vary; and (c) host factors interact with agent(s) to cause illness.			
Concept of time	By about 3 months, shows anticipation for feedings. Can wait as a consequence of perceiving clues of a familiar and desired activity.	Organized around familiar/routine activities of daily living. By about age 4, has concept of time and day and knows days of week.	Has a concept of the past and future as well as of the present. Can understand time intervals between events and can tell time by a clock. Sense of time is thus more independent of perceptual data, e.g., activities of daily living.	Can synthesize the past, present, and future in thinking.
Intentions, goals, and plans	By about 4 months, may show signs of intention/a sense of making an effort to get a result. In second year, child can make a choice of two options.	About age 4, begins to plan and anticipate actions in the near future; has objectives for activities.	Plans more elaborate projects that involve others to a greater extent.	By midadolescence (about age 15), makes future plans for self. Can think in terms of tasks as well as responsibilities in relation to them.
Handling emotion	By about 7 months, the child cries for attention, help, or when distressed. By about 9 months, begins to express fears (e.g., separation) in play.	Expresses emotion motorically and through play. Learns to label feelings. Needs trusted adult to reassure, set limits, prevent loss of self-control.	Has a greater capacity to express emotion in verbal terms; can describe fears. Can use projective methods to describe fears (e.g., explain how another child might feel or respond in a specific situation).	May use a range of modalities, from relatively sophisticated verbal or written expression to motoric activity and, perhaps, regressed ways of behaving. Thoughts, feelings, and fears may be shared with friends, especially peers.

Continued.

Table 2-2 Features of development that are pertinent to helping children deal with procedures—cont'd

	BIRTH-2 YEARS	2-7 YEARS	7-12 YEARS	ADOLESCENCE
Relationship with parent/clinicians	Developing a sense of self/others. In latter half of first year, beginning to sustain the memory of parent in parent's absence, at least for a short time. Depends on adult to know child's wants/needs.	Child is likely to have had experience in relating needs and worries to day-care or church school teachers or clinicians. Children may not expect clinicians to perceive/understand how they feel about things until about the age of 10 years.	May test limits set by caretaker/clinician.	By midadolescence, has begun to learn how to negotiate a relationship with a clinician.
Self-evaluation	Feelings about self are derived from feeling tones communicated by others and perceived by the child.	Develops expectations of self; learns to inhibit own actions. Begins to use other children as models.	Evaluates self in terms of performance relative to that of peers and in relation to the set of norms that children believe to be predetermined for them.	May use a set of criteria consciously adopted to evaluate self.

Date _____

Health-care contract

Contract goal: (Specific outcome to be attained)

I, (client's name), agree to (detailed description of required behaviors, time and frequency limitations)

in return for (positive reinforcements contingent upon completion of required behaviors; timing and mode of delivery of reinforcements)

I, (provider's name), agree to (detailed description of required behaviors, time and frequency limitations)

(Optional) I, (significant other's name), agree to (detailed description of required behaviors, time and frequency limitations)

(Optional) Aversive consequences: (Negative reinforcements for failure to meet minimum behavioral requirements)

(Optional) Bonuses: (Additional positive reinforcements for exceeding minimum contract requirements)

We will review the terms of this agreement and will make any desired modifications, on (date). We hereby agree to abide by the terms of the contract described above.

Signed: (Client) _____
Signed: (Significant other, if relevant) _____

_____
Signed: (Provider) _____
Contract effective from (Date) _____
to (Date) _____

Figure 2-4   Patient-provider contingency contract. (From Janz NK, Becker MH, Hartman PE: *Patient Educ Couns* 5[4]:165-178, 1984.)

---

ing, or bad habits; however, they believed that medication would help. Those with the fourth pattern of attribution were more likely to recover and return to work.

Likewise, a study of parents who cared for their adult children with schizophrenia discovered four patterns of attribution for the cause of the illness and for appropriate caretaking: (1) schizophrenia was caused by chemical imbalance, and care should be oriented to monitoring and limiting the ill member's intake of chemicals; (2) the adult children could be persuaded to respond to reason; (3) symptoms were largely out of the individual's control but could be reduced if he or she avoided certain environments that exacerbated symptoms; and (4) because the symptoms

were the patient's way of coping with the confusion, the appropriate model of care was gentle support.[8]

Finally, Gray[12] studied parents' explanatory models of autism, a condition in which both etiology and prognosis are poorly understood, effectiveness of treatment is limited, and the disabling nature of the disorder presents serious difficulties for parenting. There is no confirming biological test, and families reported that diagnosis frequently took up to a year. This kind of situation means that lay conceptions of the situation are essential to coping because they make sense of the illness, its cause, and course. The most common explanation offered by parents was trauma related to a difficult birth.

SUMMARY

Motivation and learning theory provide the base that is needed to plan and be successful in teaching. Learners are motivated by helping them set their own goals, expressing clear feedback about what they did right, and providing effective praise. Individual differences in self-directedness, failure tolerance, attributional style, past experience with the task, and expectation of success influence choices to engage and persist in learning. Learning theory, research about kinds of learning, and developmental phases describe conditions understood to be necessary in changing to a new state of understanding or behavior that persists.

? STUDY QUESTIONS

1. It has been said that patients seek help when they are no longer able to cope with their problems at their current level of understanding. If this statement is at least partly true, what are the implications for health care services?
2. List the questions that you would ask to assess need and motivation to learn in each of the following nursing situations?
   a. You are to teach breast self-examination to groups of women in the waiting room of a gynecology clinic.
   b. You are to teach a 10-year-old boy, who is mentally disabled, blind, and suffering from cerebral palsy, how to feed himself.
3. Because an increasing number of high-risk infants are discharged to home with complex medical needs, parents are receiving instruction in cardiopulmonary resuscitation (CPR). One study[16] showed that parents lost information over time and that those who were regularly reinforced with hands-on demonstration during clinic visits retained the most skills. Are you surprised by the findings? What learning principles were used?
4. Pelco and others[23] describe an approach to teaching a 4-year-old girl how to take a capsule, using behavioral learning principles. Label the behavioral approaches being used.

Teaching action	Behavioral approach
a. The child refused to accept any capsules.	
b. Therapist showed child how to swallow by putting capsule between his fingers, placing it on back of his tongue, taking a sip of juice, tilting his head, and swallowing.	
c. Explain to child that by doing what therapist asked, she could earn pennies to buy toys displayed in the room.	
d. When the child refused to swallow, therapist placed his hand over the child's and guided it through the steps, until she successfully swallowed capsule.	
e. Pennies and praise were given even if physical guidance was used and the child swallowed smaller capsule. These steps were followed until the child could consistently swallow prescription-sized capsules. The parent was trained how to maintain routine capsule acceptance postintervention.	

REFERENCES

1. Affleck G and others: Attributional processes in rheumatoid arthritis patients, *Arthritis Rheum* 30:927-931, 1987.
2. Bandura A: Self-efficacy mechanism in human agency, *Am Psychol* 37:122-147, 1982.
3. Bandura A: *Foundations of thought and action: a social cognitive theory,* Englewood Cliffs, NJ, 1986, Prentice-Hall.
4. Bar-On D, Cristal N: Causal attributions of patients, their spouses and physicians, and the rehabilitation of the patients after their first myocardial infarction, *J Cardiopulm Rehabil* 7:285-298, 1987.
5. Barsky AJ and others: Silent myocardial ischemia, *JAMA* 264:1132-1135, 1990.
6. Cameron L, Leventhal EA, Leventhal H: Symptom representations and affect as determinants of care seeking in a community-dwelling, adult sample population, *Health Psychol* 12:171-179, 1993.
7. Campbell DJ: Task complexity: a review and analysis, *Acad Manag Rev* 13:40-52, 1988.
8. Chesla CA: Parents' illness models of schizophrenia, *Arch Psychiatr Nurs* 3:218-225, 1989.
9. Elkind, D: Teenage thinking: implications for health care, *Pediatr Nurs* 10:383-385, 1984.
10. Fredette SL: A model for improving cancer patient education, *Cancer Nurs* 13:207-215, 1990.
11. Glaser R, Bassok M: Learning theory and the study of instruction, *Annu Rev Psychol* 40:631-666, 1989.
12. Gray DE: Lay conceptions of autism: parents' explanatory models, *Med Anthropol* 16:99-118, 1995.
13. Harrison JA, Mullen PD, Green LW: A meta-analysis of studies of the health belief model with adults, *Health Educ Res* 7:107-116, 1992.
14. Houston-Miller N: Questions and answers, *J Cardiac Rehabil* 4:104-106, 1984.
15. Janz NK, Becker MH, Hartman PE: Contingency contracting to enhance patient compliance: a review, *Patient Educ Couns* 5:164-178, 1984.
16. Komelasky AL, Bond BS: The effect of two forms of learning reinforcement upon parental retention of CPR skills, *Pediatr Nurs* 19:96-98, 1993.
17. Lewis FM, Daltroy LH: How causal explanations influence health behavior: attribution theory. In Glanz K, Lewis FM, Rimer BK, editors: *Health behavior and health education,* San Francisco, 1990, Jossey-Bass.
18. Ley P: Memory for medical information, *Br J Soc Clin Psychol* 18:245-255, 1979.
19. Marcus BH, Rakowski W, Rossi JS: Assessing motivational readiness and decision making for exercise, *Health Psychol* 11:257-261, 1992.
20. Mezirow J: *Transformative learning,* San Francisco, 1991, Jossey-Bass.
21. Morisky DE and others: The role of needs assessment in designing a community-based mammography education program for urban women, *Health Educ Res* 4:469-478, 1989.
22. Mullen PD, Hersey JC, Iverson DC: Health behavior models compared, *Soc Sci Med* 24:973-981, 1987.
23. Pelco LE and others: Behavioral management of oral medication administration difficulties among children: a review of literature with case illustrations, *J Dev Behav Pediatr* 8:90-96, 1987.
24. Pestrak VA, Martin D: Cognitive development and aspects of adolescent sexuality, *Adolescence* 20:981-987, 1985.
25. Pridham KF, Adelson F, Hansen MF: Helping children deal with procedures in a clinic setting: a developmental approach, *J Pediatr Nurs* 2:13-22, 1987.
26. Prochaska JO and others: The transtheoretical model of change and HIV prevention: a review, *Health Educ Q* 21:471-486, 1994.
27. Rickert VI and others: Training parents to become better behavior managers, *Behav Modif* 12:475-496, 1988.
28. Rosenstock IM, Strecher VJ, Becker MH: The health belief model and HIV risk behavior change. In Di Clemente RJ, Peterson JL, editors: *Preventing AIDS: theories and methods of behavioral interventions,* New York, 1994, Plenum Press.
29. Salomon G, Perkins DN: Rocky roads to transfer: rethinking mechanisms of a neglected phenomenon, *Educ Psychol* 24:113-142, 1989.
30. Slavin RE: *Educational psychology: theory into practice,* Englewood Cliffs, NJ, 1994, Prentice-Hall.
31. Spirito A and others: Screening measures to assess knowledge of diabetes in pregnancy, *Diabetes Care* 13:712-718, 1990.
32. Volker, DL: Needs assessment and resource identification, *Oncol Nurs Forum* 18:119-123, 1991.

3 Educational Objectives and Instruction

Statements of goals and objectives provide direction for instructional activities, that create conditions of learning. Together they constitute a plan for instruction, with use of interpersonal relationships and instructional materials and experiences to stimulate specific learning activities. Thus, making knowledgeable decisions about objectives and stating them precisely is a crucial first step toward effective teaching.

EDUCATIONAL OBJECTIVES

The kinds of learning goals to be reached are frequently well-developed by consensus and based on a body of research within various areas of patient education practice. Part II of this book describes a number of such areas of practice, some well-established and others just becoming established. Against this set of common expectations, a needs assessment is completed for a particular patient or group, with whom learning objectives are negotiated.

A statement of objectives requires the use of terms with precise meanings, a statement of both a behavior and a content, and the classification of objectives in established taxonomies (classification systems), which helps one know what kind of instructional strategies are necessary to meet the objective. The objectives flowing from the situation described in the accompanying box demonstrate these characteristics.

■ STATEMENT OF OBJECTIVES

Situation

A home health nurse is teaching a wife and a daughter how to care for a bedfast elderly father and husband. The patient moves little but has not been incontinent. He has had no skin breakdown to the present but, according to the wife, has been allowed to lie in one position for 4 hours. The main objective is part of the more encompassing objective, to avoid harmful consequences of bed rest.

Main objective

To avoid decubitus ulcer formation (psychomotor, cognitive, affective)

Subobjectives

A. To recognize any evidence of tissue breakdown by criteria of color, sensation, and response to massage (cognitive, comprehension; psychomotor, perception)

B. To reposition the patient at least every 2 hours, so that the body is resting on the same surface only every fourth time (psychomotor, mechanism; cognitive, comprehension)

C. To keep all linen wrinkle free (psychomotor, mechanism; cognitive, knowledge)

D. To massage vigorously, at every turning, the skin that has been receiving pressure from body weight (psychomotor, mechanism)

E. To report to the nurse evidence of incontinence or skin breakdown, within 4 hours after it is observed (cognitive, knowledge)

F. To maintain adequate instructional intake (cognitive, knowledge)

Examples of general nonspecific verbs and the much more useful specific verbs follow[16]:

Nonspecific	Specific
Knows	Defines, describes, identifies, lists, names, selects
Understands	Distinguishes, estimates, explains, gives examples
Applies	Predicts, prepares, solves, uses

TAXONOMIES (CLASSIFICATION SYSTEMS) OF EDUCATIONAL OBJECTIVES

Behaviors are divided into three domains: (1) cognitive, dealing with intellectual abilities, (2) affective, including expression of feelings in the areas of interests, attitudes, values, and appreciations, and (3) psychomotor, dealing with skills commonly known as motor skills. Each domain is ordered in taxonomic form of hierarchy; that is, those complex behaviors at the upper end of the taxonomy (number 5.00 or 6.00) diminish to the simple behaviors at the lower end (numbered 1.00). (The taxonomies appear on pp. 35-38.) The cognitive and psychomotor domains are ordered on the concept of complexity of behavior, whereas the affective domain represents increasing internalization or commitment to a feeling, thus also requiring more complex behavior at higher levels.

Besides establishing definitions that facilitate communication, the taxonomy of educational objectives also clarifies certain teaching decisions. In the cognitive domain, learning at the lowest level—acquiring information—can be achieved by a great variety of learning experiences, including lectures, printed material, and pictures or illustrations. Attainment of the higher categories of the domain requires much more investment of time and energy on the part of the teacher and the learner, with the learner actively working through problems and the teacher helping the learner attain insight into the processes to be learned.

■ TAXONOMY OF COGNITIVE DOMAIN

1.00 Knowledge
Knowledge, as defined here, involves recall or remembering of information.

1.10 Knowledge of specifics
Terminology, specific facts

1.20 Knowledge of ways and means of dealing with specifics
Corrections, trends and sequences
Classification, categories
Criteria, methodology

1.30 Knowledge of the universals and abstractions in a field
Principles and generalizations, theories and structures

2.00 Comprehension
This represents the lowest level of understanding. It refers to a type of understanding. The individual knows what is being communicated and can make use of the material or idea being communicated without necessarily relating it to other material or seeing its fullest implications.

2.10 Translation
Comprehension is evidenced by the care and accuracy with which the communication is paraphrased or rendered from one language or form of communication to another. Translation is judged on the basis of faithfulness and accuracy, that is, on the extent to which the material in the original communication is preserved although the form of the communication has been altered.

2.20 Interpretation
The explanation or summarization of a communication. Whereas translation involves an objective part-for-part rendering of a communication, interpretation involves a reordering, rearrangement, or new view of the material.

From Bloom BS and others: *Taxonomy of educational objectives. Handbook I: Cognitive domain,* New York, 1984, Longman.   *Continued.*

TAXONOMY OF COGNITIVE DOMAIN—cont'd

2.30 Extrapolation

The extension of trends or tendencies beyond the given data to determine implications, consequences, corollaries, effects, and so forth which are in accordance with the conditions described in the original communication.

3.00 Application

The use of abstractions in particular and concrete situations. The abstractions may be in the form of general ideas, rules of procedures, or generalized methods. The abstractions may also be technical principles, ideas, and theories, which must be remembered and applied.

4.00 Analysis

The breakdown of a communication into its constituent elements or parts, that the relative hierarchy of ideas is made clear or the relations between the ideas expressed are made explicit, or both. Such analyses are intended to clarify the communication, to indicate how the communication is organized and the way in which it manages to convey its effects, as well as to indicate its basis and arrangement.

4.10 Analysis of elements

Identification of the elements included in a communication.

4.20 Analysis of relationships

Identification of the connections and interactions between elements and parts of a communication.

4.30 Analysis of organizational principles

Identification of the organization, systematic arrangement, and structure which hold the communication together. This includes the "explicit" as well as "implicit" structure. It includes the bases, necessary arrangement, and mechanics which make the communication a unit.

5.00 Synthesis

The putting together of elements and parts to form a whole. This involves the process of working with pieces, parts, elements, and so forth, and arranging and combining them in such a way as to constitute a pattern or structure not clearly present before.

5.10 Production of a unique communication

The development of a communication in which the writer or speaker attempts to convey ideas, feelings, or experiences or all three to others.

5.20 Production of a plan, or proposed set of operations

The development of a plan of work or the proposal of a plan of operations. The plan should satisfy the requirements of a task that may be given to the student or that he may develop for himself.

5.30 Derivation of a set of abstract relations

The development of a set of abstract relations either to classify or explain particular data or phenomena, or the deduction of propositions and relations from a set of basic propositions or symbolic representations.

6.00 Evaluation

Judgments about the value of material and methods for given purposes: quantitative and qualitative judgments about the extent to which material and methods satisfy criteria; use of standard of appraisal. The criteria may be determined by the student or given to him.

6.10 Judgments in terms of internal evidence

Evaluation of the accuracy of a communication from such evidence as logical accuracy, consistency, and other internal criteria.

6.20 Judgments in terms of external criteria

Evaluation of material with reference to selected or remembered criteria.

■ PSYCHOMOTOR DOMAIN: A TENTATIVE TAXONOMIC SYSTEM

1.00 Perception
Process of becoming aware of objects, qualities, or relations by way of the sense organs.

1.10 Sensory stimulation
Impingement of a stimulus(i) on one or more of the sense organs.

    1.11 Auditory
    1.12 Visual
    1.13 Tactile
    1.14 Taste
    1.15 Smell
    1.16 Kinesthetic

1.20 Cue selection
Identification of the cue or cues, associating them with the task to be performed, and grouping them in terms of past experience and knowledge. Cues relevant to the situation are selected as a guide to action; irrelevant cues are ignored or discarded.

1.30 Translation
The mental process of determining the meaning of the cues received for action; it involves symbolic translation, that is, having an image or being reminded of something, "having an idea," as a result of cues received; insight; sensory translation; and "feedback."

2.00 Set
A preparatory adjustment or readiness for a particular kind of action or experience.

2.10 Mental set
Readiness, in the mental sense, to perform a certain motor act. This involves, as prerequisite, the level of perception already identified. Discrimination, using judgments in making distinctions, is an aspect.

2.20 Physical set
Readiness in the sense of having made the anatomic adjustments necessary for a motor act to be performed, including sensory attending and posturing of the body.

2.30 Emotional set
Readiness in terms of attitudes favorable to the motor act's taking place.

3.00 Guided response
The overt behavioral act of an individual under the guidance of the instructor. Prerequisite to performance of the act is readiness to respond and selection of the appropriate response.

3.10 Imitation
The execution of an act as a direct response to the perception of another person performing the act.

3.20 Trial and error
Trying various responses, usually with some rationale for each response, until an appropriate response is achieved.

4.00 Mechanism
Learned response has become habitual. The learner has achieved a certain confidence and degree of skill. The act is a part of his or her repertoire of possible responses to stimuli and to the demands of situations where the response is an appropriate one. The response may be more complex than at the preceding level; it may involve some patterning of response in carrying out the task.

5.00 Complex overt response
Performance of a motor act that is considered complex because of the movement pattern required. A high degree of skill has been attained, and the act can be carried out with minimum expenditure of time and energy.

5.10 Resolution of uncertainty
Performance of a complex act without hesitation.

5.20 Automatic performance
Performance of finely coordinated motor skill with a great deal of ease and muscle control.

6.00 Adaptation
Altering motor activities to meet the demands of new problematic situations requiring a physical response.

7.00 Origination
Creating new motor acts or ways of manipulating materials out of understandings, abilities, and skills developed in the psychomotor area.

Modified from Simpson EJ: In *Contributions of behavioral science to instructional technology: the psychomotor domain,* Mt Rainier, Md, 1972, Gryphon Press.

■ TAXONOMY OF AFFECTIVE DOMAIN

1.00 Receiving (attending)
1.10 Awareness
Awareness is almost a cognitive behavior. But unlike knowledge, the lowest level of the cognitive domain, awareness is not so much concerned with a memory of or ability to recall an item or fact as with the phenomenon that, given an appropriate opportunity, the learner will merely be conscious of something—that he or she will take into account a situation, face or event, object, or stage of affairs.

1.20 Willingness to receive
At a minimum level we are describing here the behavior of being willing to tolerate a given stimulus, not to avoid it.

1.30 Controlled or selected attention
There is an element of the learner's controlling the attention here, so that the favored stimulus is selected and attended to despite competing and distracting stimuli.

2.00 Responding
2.10 Acquiescence in responding
The student makes the response but he or she has not fully accepted the necessity for doing so.

2.20 Willingness to respond
There is the implication that the learner is sufficiently committed to exhibiting a behavior so that he or she does so not just because of a fear of punishment, but "on his own" or voluntarily.

2.30 Satisfaction in response
Behavior is accompanied by a feeling of satisfaction, an emotional response, generally of pleasure, zest, or enjoyment.

3.00 Valuing
3.10 Acceptance of a value
The learner is sufficiently consistent that others can identify the value and sufficiently committed that he or she is willing to be so identified, but there is more of a readiness here to reevaluate his or her position than would be present at higher levels of valuing.

3.20 Preference for a value
Behavior at this level implies not just the acceptance of a value to the point of being willing to be identified with it, but more, a seeking it out and wanting it.

3.30 Commitment
Belief at this level involves a high degree of certainty. There is a real motivation to act out the behavior.

4.00 Organization
4.10 Conceptualization of a value
At this level the quality of abstraction or conceptualization is added. It permits patients to understand how the value relates to those that they already hold or to new ones that they are learning to hold.

4.20 Organization of a value system
Objectives properly classified here as those that require the learner to bring together a complex of values, possibly disparate values, and to relate them in an ordered fashion with one another. Ideally, the ordered relationship will be one which is harmonious and internally consistent.

5.00 Characterization by a value or value complex
5.10 Generalized set
A generalized set is a basic orientation that enables individuals to reduce and order the complex world about them and to act consistently and effectively in it. The generalized set may be thought of as closely related to the idea of an attitude cluster.

5.20 Characterization
Here are found those objectives that concern the individual's view of the universe, his or her philosophy of life . . . a value system having as its object the whole of what is known or knowable.

From Krathwohl DR, Bloom BS, Masia BB: *Taxonomy of educational objectives. Handbook II: Affective domain,* New York, 1984, Longman.

The accompanying boxed material has been prepared to give the reader an opportunity to relate the taxonomy to behaviors that are being taught.

INSTRUCTIONAL FORMS

Instruction is designed to ensure conditions that support learning. The following summary highlights the guidelines from motivation and learning introduced in the first two chapters[24]:

- Begin with objectives and keep objectives in focus from planning to evaluation.
- Design instruction according to learner abilities, knowledge structures, and expectations.
- Provide advance organizers to constitute "ideational scaffolding" in learning. These

---

■ EXAMPLES OF HEALTH TEACHING OBJECTIVES ACCORDING TO TAXONOMIES OF EDUCATIONAL OBJECTIVES

Cognitive domain

Knowledge
To describe three main purposes of the cough, turn, deep-breathe regimen following surgery
To state why the mother's diet may affect breast-feeding

Comprehension
To recognize, in changing a surgical dressing, when something has been contaminated
To translate instructions on a medicine bottle into appropriate action

Application
To apply principles of asepsis to washing a wound with pHisoHex
Given a general knowledge of safety, to plan how to rid a house of safety hazards

Analysis
To identify factors that cause bowel upsets
To distinguish how an uninformed argument differs from scientific reasoning

Synthesis
To design an ileostomy bag that suits the patient's needs better than do available commercial ones
To interpret to others the feelings experienced during illness

Evaluation
To assess the health care the patient is receiving in terms of its completeness, the patient's satisfaction with it, and the results obtained

Affective domain

Receiving
To be aware that others are available to help
To tolerate having a retention catheter

Responding
To cooperate with the insertion of a nasogastric tube
To feel some satisfaction in caring for a baby

Valuing
To accept many of the limitations in life imposed by heart disease
To desire good health rather than mere absence of disease

Organization
To relate to others in a manner consistent with rehabilitation goals
To regularly choose those alternatives of action that are consistent with good parenting

Characterization by a value or value complex
To develop a code of behavior consistent with respect for the health of the patient and others

Continued.

■ EXAMPLES OF HEALTH TEACHING OBJECTIVES ACCORDING TO TAXONOMIES
OF EDUCATIONAL OBJECTIVES—cont'd

Psychomotor domain

Perception	To recognize the "feel" of holding a baby with good balance
	To recognize the difference between systolic and diastolic blood pressure sounds
Set	To demonstrate a well-balanced stance with crutches
	To demonstrate correct placement of sphygmomanometer and stethoscope
Guided response	To discover the most efficient method of diapering a baby through trial of various procedures
	To imitate the blood pressure measurement procedure after demonstration
Mechanism	To control the fall of mercury in the sphygmomanometer at 2 to 3 mm Hg per heartbeat
Complex overt response	To pass a tube through the nose into the stomach skillfully with a minimum of discomfort or danger to the patient
	To measure blood pressure in 1 minute, accurate to ±5 mm Hg (mercury), in comparison with an expert
Adaptation	To perform one's own design for turning, moving, and transferring a hemiplegic person, weighing 100 pounds more than oneself, in a home environment
Origination	(Rarely used in patient education)

statements summarize the essence of the lesson and integrate it with previously learned material.

- Divide a complex task into smaller, achievable sequential learning units so that the learner can experience satisfaction and a feeling of self-efficacy.
- Organize complex information in easy-to-remember structures such as graphics or schematics.
- Practice instruction in a variety of ways to match different learning styles. At least one third of learning time should be used for practice, using different senses.
- Provide immediate feedback so that the learner can improve his or her responses.
- Conclude instruction by recapitulating salient points and linking with future learning.

Most instructional forms are familiar to readers of this book. They have three basic components: (1) a delivery system, which is the physical form of the materials and hardware used to present stimuli to the learners, such as handouts, slides, computer-assisted instruction, or a person; (2) a content or message; and (3) a form or condition of abstractness. Figure 3-1 shows an example of the abstract-concrete continuum. Methods are also instructor-centered, interactive, individualized, or experiential (see box, p. 42) and can be matched with domains and levels of learning (Table 3-1).

Patient education also fits within taxonomies of interventions describing the practice of particular professions. One of the several taxonomies for nursing is the Iowa Intervention Project, which describes patient education as one class of intervention within the behavioral domain. The

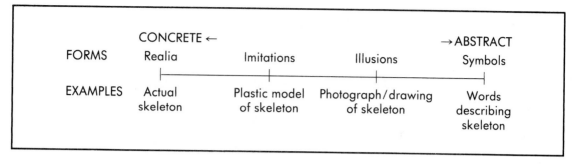

Figure 3-1 Form of instructional materials: the abstract-concrete continuum. (From Weston C, Cranton PA: *J Higher Educ* 57[3]:259-288, 1986.)

Table 3-1 Matching domain and level of learning to appropriate methods

DOMAIN AND LEVEL	METHOD
Cognitive domain	
Knowledge	Lecture, programmed instruction, drill and practice
Comprehension	Lecture, modularized instruction, programmed instruction
Application	Discussion, simulations and games, computer-assisted instruction, modularized instruction, field experience, laboratory
Analysis	Discussion, independent/group projects, simulations, field experience, role-playing, laboratory
Synthesis	Independent/group projects, field experience, role-playing, laboratory
Evaluation	Independent/group projects, field experience, laboratory
Affective domain	
Receiving	Lecture, discussion, modularized instruction, field experience
Responding	Discussion, simulations, modularized instruction, role-playing, field experience
Valuing	Discussion, independent/group projects, simulations, role-playing, field experience
Organization	Discussion, independent/group projects, field experience
Characterization by a value	Independent projects, field experience
Psychomotor domain	
Perception	Demonstration (lecture), drill and practice
Set	Demonstration (lecture), drill and practice
Guided response	Peer teaching, games, role-playing, field experience, drill and practice
Mechanism	Games, role-playing, field experience, drill and practice
Complex overt response	Games, field experience
Adaptation	Independent projects, games, field experience
Origination	Independent projects, games, field experience

From Weston C, Cranton PA: *J Higher Educ* 57(3):259-288, 1986.

■ SUMMARY OF INSTRUCTIONAL METHODS

Instructor-centered	Interactive	Individualized	Experiential
Lecture Students are passive Efficient for lower learning levels and large classes	**Class discussion** Class size must be small May be time-consuming Encourages student involvement	**Programmed instruction** Most effective at lower learning levels Very structured Students work at own pace Students receive extensive feedback	**Field or clinical** Occurs in natural setting during performance Students are actively involved Management and evaluation may be difficult
Questioning Monitors student learning Encourages student involvement May cause anxiety for some	**Discussion groups** Class size should be small Students participate Effective for high cognitive and affective learning levels	**Modularized instruction** Can be time-consuming Very flexible formats Students work at own pace	**Laboratory** Requires careful planning and evaluation Students actively involved in a realistic setting
Demonstration Illustrates an application of a skill or concept Students are passive	**Peer teaching** Requires careful planning and monitoring Utilizes differences in student expertise Encourages student involvement	**Independent projects** Most appropriate at higher learning levels Can be time-consuming Students are actively involved in learning	**Role playing** Effective in affective and psychomotor domains Provides "safe" experiences Active student participation
	Group projects Requires careful planning, including evaluation techniques Useful at higher learning levels Encourages active student participation	**Computerized instruction** May involve considerable instructor time or expense Can be very flexible Students work at own pace Students may be involved in varying activities	**Simulations and games** Provide practice of specific skills Produces anxiety for some students Active student participation
			Drill Most appropriate at lower learning levels Provides active practice May not be motivating for some students

Modified from Weston C, Cranton PA: *J Higher Educ* 57(3):259-288, 1986.

Project describes more than 400 nursing interventions categorized into 27 classes and six domains.[18] This work creates a standardized language for nursing treatments. More specific "Intervention Labels" within the class of patient education include childbirth preparation, learning-readiness enhancement, parent education, preparatory sensory information, teaching: disease process, teaching: group, teaching: individual, teaching: infant care, teaching: preoperative, teaching: prescribed activity/exercise, teaching: prescribed diet, teaching: prescribed medication, teaching: procedure/treatment, teaching: psychomotor skill, teaching: safe sex. The accompanying box shows one of the teaching interventions with its definition and activities. This class of teaching interventions is among those with the highest use among practicing nurses.[6]

Yet another taxonomy describes pediatric primary care nursing interventions. A major focus here is on self-care and patient education, which Kilmon[20] describes as:

an effort to assist parents with self-management of identified health problems. Anticipatory guidance entails education for healthy families with the goal of promoting healthy child and family development while avoiding injuries and other preventable health problems. The category of health problem supportive services includes teaching parents of a child with a significant health problem how to effectively utilize health care resources.

The seven major elements of Kilmon's taxonomy are anticipatory guidance, health problem supportive services, counseling, dietary modifications, immunizations, procedures, and medications. A number of other taxonomies also describe practice, all of which include patient education as a major intervention.

Interpersonal teaching forms

Groups provide an economical way to teach, and the experience of having the support of a group and modeling the behavior of other individuals may be the best way for patients to meet their objectives.

■ TEACHING: PRESCRIBED DIET

Definition: Preparing a patient to correctly follow a prescribed diet

Activities

Appraise the patient's current level of knowledge relating to prescribed diet

Determine the patient's/significant other's feelings/attitude toward prescribed diet and expected degree of dietary compliance

Instruct the patient on the proper name of the prescribed diet

Explain the purpose of the diet

Inform the patient how long the diet should be followed

Instruct the patient how to keep a food diary as appropriate

Instruct the patient on allowed and prohibited foods

Inform the patient of possible drug/food interactions as appropriate

Assist the patient to accommodate his/her food preferences into the prescribed diet

Assist the patient in substituting ingredients to conform his/her favorite recipes to the prescribed diet

Instruct the patient how to read labels and select appropriate foods

Observe the patient's selection of foods appropriate to prescribed diet

Instruct the patient how to plan appropriate meals

Provide written meal plans as appropriate

Recommend a cookbook that includes recipes consistent with the diet as appropriate

Reinforce information provided by other health care team members as appropriate

Refer patient to dietician/nutritionist as appropriate

Include the family/significant others as appropriate

From McCloskey JC, Bulechek GM, editors: *Nursing interventions classifications (NIC),* St Louis, 1992, Mosby.

For example, caregivers of persons with Alzheimer's disease and related disorders need groups that focus on education and support. Such help is necessary because of the patient's progressive deterioration over a 7- to 10-year period. The family experiences role reversals, little family or peer support, absent or misinterpreted feedback from the patient, and withdrawal from social networks. These unpleasant changes can result in progressive deterioration of the family system and depression of caregivers. Caregivers can learn specific skills, such as how to respond to the patient's behavior and cognitive impairments, how to modify his or her environment, and how to deal with legal and financial problems, sadness, frustration, and anger. It is less expensive for the family to attend effective educational and support groups than it is to institutionalize the patient if the caregiver fails to cope. One study of caregivers for frail elderly persons in the community found the institutionalization rate reduced from 17% to 5%. The educational program focused on assisting caregivers in dealing constructively with negative feelings, as well as how to lift, to move, to bathe, and to administer medication. Social skills in dealing with the patient and other family members and relaxation training were also taught. The availability of a secondary caregiver was important.[15]

Annually, 6.4 million individuals participate in member-governed, problem-specific, low-fee self-help groups. Health professionals are involved with these groups in various ways but usually are not central to them. Some groups are small and local; others are nationally networked assemblies. Members are psychologically bonded by the compelling similarity of their concerns. They rely primarily on the collective experiential knowledge possessed by the membership. Acceptance by the group seems to be a vital step toward making cognitive, emotional, and behavioral changes necessary for more effective functioning and an improved quality of life. One data base in California found 188 distinct problem categories around which groups were formed. The support groups address such problems as alcoholism, anorexia, arthritis, parental bereavement, coping with various cancers, caretaking of patients with Alzheimer's disease, diabetes, burn victims, drug abuse, impact of incest, and parental coping with handicapped children, as well as many others.[19]

Some groups form spontaneously. For example, informal support groups were evolving as patients with ventricular tachycardia in the hospital for electrophysiologic studies and treatment socialized in their rooms and the lounge. The disadvantage of this development was that misinformation could easily be perpetuated. Because the disease was life threatening and the treatment invasive, the disruption from misinformation could be serious. A formal program was therefore developed with a teaching component that included information on normal electrical conduction in the heart and pathology of ventricular tachycardia, electrophysiologic studies, telemetry monitoring, medications, and preparation for discharge. Cardiopulmonary resuscitation certifications for family members and friends were also offered. Patients exhibiting severe anxiety, frank denial, or overt hostility were screened out of the group and taught individually.[10]

In another example, Kulik and Mahler described groups that formed even when not intended.[22] Patients who had a postoperative roommate before their own operations were less anxious preoperatively, they were more ambulatory postoperatively, and they were released 1.4 days more quickly than were patients whose preoperative roommates were also preoperative. Social comparison theory predicts that evaluative needs of individuals in unusual and stressful situations are best served by comparison with others who are in similar situations. Roommates' experiences may also provide patients with information preoperatively that will enable them to interpret postoperative sensations and events in a more accurate and less personally threatening manner. With today's brief preoperative stays, such opportunities may no longer exist.

Sometimes it is important to form separate groups for patients and for families. It is also useful to prescreen individuals entering a group to assess whether their learning needs are generally the same or whether one individual would be disruptive to the group.

Role playing

Role playing is an excellent technique for diagnosis of motivation and readiness to learn, as well as for teaching ideas and attitudes. People are assigned to play themselves or someone else. A related technique is for the teacher to enact a role that the learner can model. For example, the teacher could enact a positive or desirable parental role in relation to a child's specific behavior and then discuss and label the behavior that has been portrayed.

Through role playing, a desired behavior is rehearsed. Thus a person is taught the skills required and gains the confidence needed to carry them out. Reversal of the roles is a technique useful for sensitizing one person to the other's situation. Role playing provides a kind of behavioral and mental rehearsal that is a form of practice. It is also a means of increasing retention in learning.

Role-playing techniques have been cited as useful in teaching persons from disadvantaged backgrounds. These techniques are effective in situations that have been described as physical, action-oriented, concrete, and problem-directed rather than those that are introspective. They are most effective when instruction is easy and informally paced. Role playing may also reduce the role distance between client and professional. The technique has considerable potential for reducing overintellectualization and for uniting understanding and feeling.

For all these reasons, school-aged children are taught how to deal with their asthma by using puppets to role-play. At this stage of child development, the chief learning mode is visual and psychomotor (puppets). Teachers focus on helping the children develop an "I can do" attitude (role playing). The accompanying box contains suggested role-playing situations using the puppets. The role play is designed to help children

---

■ SUGGESTED ROLE-PLAY SITUATIONS

Lesson 1
Wheezing Willie is very allergic to grass. If he is near it, he will wheeze and may even have an asthma attack. He is at his friend's house for a birthday party and the children decide to do somersaults and cartwheels on the freshly cut grass. What should Wheezing Willie do?

Lesson 2
Healthy Heather has been given the assignment to tell the class what happens to the human body when it has an asthma attack.

Lesson 3
Wheezing Wendy and her family have just moved to a new neighborhood and she is going to a new school. In the morning of her first day, she begins to wheeze. The person sitting next to her hears her wheezing and starts to call her names. What should Wheezing Wendy do?

Lesson 4
Wheezing Willie has to take a breathing treatment and other medication every day at school during the lunch period. Because he has to take a treatment, he misses half of recess. Lately, Willie has been feeling well and has stopped going to the office to take his breathing treatment and medication. Do you think Wheezing Willie is doing the right thing? What should he do?

Lesson 5
Wheezing Wendy is at her friend Healthy Heather's house. She is having fun playing with Barbie dolls when she begins to have a headache and her throat starts to feel scratchy. These are two of Wheezing Wendy's early warning signs. Wheezing Wendy's mother is at work and won't be home for 2 more hours. What should she do?

From Ramsey AM, Siroky AS: *Pediatr Nurs* 14:187-190, 1988.

---

manage an asthma attack, take their medications correctly, and cope with teasing from peers.

Role playing is often incorporated as one technique in a program. For example, one educationally oriented support group for teenagers with diabetes began with a weekend camping experience to bond the group. The group wore identical T-shirts with a logo to aid in group identity. The members quickly discovered that the group was a place to meet with friends. Role playing on how to relate to parents and other family members was a critical element of the program. Snacks were cooked, and awards were given for each teenager's special trait. Blood glucose was tested before and after exercise. The teenagers gained experience in solving actual problems, and they signed contracts agreeing to certain future behaviors.[8]

Verbal teaching

Inasmuch as teaching is communicating, which is accomplished in large part by language, the teacher must be skilled in the use of language. Clinicians need special knowledge of language because of two conditions inherent in health teaching: medical terminology is foreign to much of the public, and individuals with considerable health needs often have poorly developed language skills that result in low levels of understanding.

The use of written information no doubt improves patients' retention of information. The use of another device, called "advanced organizers," produced significant increases in recall in a study by Ley and others.[23] The advanced organizers were category names to organize the material, which consisted of the following statements:

1. You have a chest infection.
2. And your larynx is slightly inflamed.
3. But I think your heart is all right.
4. We will do some heart tests to make sure.
5. We will need to take a blood sample.
6. And you will have to have your chest x-rayed.
7. Your cough will disappear in the next two days.
8. You will feel better in a week or so.
9. And you will recover completely.
10. We will give you an injection of penicillin.
11. And some tablets to take.
12. I'll give you an inhaler to use.

13. You must avoid cold draughts.
14. You must stay indoors in fog.
15. And you must take two hours' rest each afternoon.

The advanced organizers were used as follows[23]:

> I am going to tell you:
>   what is wrong with you;
>   what tests we are going to carry out;
>   what I think will happen to you;
>   what treatment you will need; and
>   what you must do to help yourself.
>   First, what is wrong with you . . . (statements 1-3)
>   Secondly, what tests we are going to carry out . . . (statements 4-6)
>   Thirdly, what I think will happen to you . . . (statements 7-9)
>   Fourthly, what the treatments will be . . . (statements 10-12)
>   Finally, what you must do to help yourself . . . (statements 13-15)

Notice that the category names are not medical terms; rather, they are categories meaningful to patients.

Because of their backgrounds, health professionals may tend to overuse verbal instruction. They often value independence and symbolic learning. They may therefore choose a verbal means of instruction to motivate a person, when joining the patient in the health action would be more effective. Expressing the idea in words can serve to maintain a professional distance from patients and at the same time create a student-teacher role hierarchy and a status gap between helper and patient. It may fail as a teaching technique, especially if used exclusively.

Demonstration and practice

Demonstration is a performance of procedures or psychomotor skills, which, combined with practice, is the method most suited to attaining skills. The purpose of the demonstration is to give the learner a clear mental image of how the skill is performed. Presentations of a prime view by television or motion picture may be necessary if the groups are large. In some instances an over-the-shoulder view of the demonstrator provides the learner with a clear idea of the way he or she must perform the action. When the demonstrator is removing fluids from a vial and giving an injection, the mirror image that the viewer receives by *facing* the demonstrator is not entirely realistic.

Learners need practice to develop motor skills; therefore the teaching plan must incorporate a time for patients to practice. When equipment is sufficient and the group is small enough, practice may begin with the learner's redemonstrating the skill immediately after the teacher finishes. Additional practice should take place in a setting similar to that in which the skill will be performed. The teacher must supervise enough to provide feedback for a correct performance and to stimulate motivation if necessary.

Teaching Tools

Much teaching is accomplished by means of tools, both written and audiovisual, used within the context of an instructional plan. If these tools are well-designed and have been shown to be effective in creating learning, and if they are well-matched to the goals of instruction and to the learner's capabilities, they can be almost self-instructional.

Written materials are by far the most frequently used in patient education, despite persistent evidence that they are mismatched to the needs of many patients, particularly in their reading level. Printed teaching material can be described as a frozen language that is selective in its description of reality (which is both a strength and a weakness). It encourages limited feedback but is constantly available. Print partially relaxes time requirements and is more efficient than oral language (except for those who have not learned to read efficiently) because readers can control the speed at which they read and comprehend. Certain kinds of thinking seem to demand written expression. For example, a complex sequence of thoughts that incorporates definitions, qualifications, and logical constraints is expressed best

in writing. Most people who have learned to read well generally prefer to acquire information by reading. Reading is ideal for understanding complex concepts and relationships. If the learning objective primarily requires skill in dealing with persons or things, then demonstrations, concrete experience with the activity, and oral coaching and guidance would be more effective than print media.

The various media that can be used for learning possess cognitively relevant characteristics in their technologies, symbol systems, and processing capabilities. Computers are distinguished by their extensive processing capabilities rather than by their access to a particularly unique set of symbol systems (they use words and pictures). In television the symbols can depict action; however, the symbols are transient.[21]

Although some students can learn a particular task regardless of the medium, others need the advantage of a particular medium's characteristics. For example, experts who learn from text, can skim rapidly, using trigger words to read selectively and nonsequentially. When memory limits are reached, they stop and summarize the material they have learned. Such processing strategies cannot be used with audiotapes or lectures. Novices take advantage of the text's stability to slow the rate of information processing; as a result they are able to review the material. Pictures that illustrate information central to the text help the reader. If, however, the material is too difficult for the reader, he or she must expend a great deal of effort trying to decode the text and possibly increasing the risk of learning failure.[21]

Written materials

Although learning by reading is economical in use of teacher time, some people cannot read well enough to use any printed material. For many others the materials available are written at a higher level than they can comprehend. The reading levels of many individuals may be up to five grades below the grade they report they completed.

Of the plethora of studies on readability, most come to the conclusion that many persons who must use written patient education materials have limited ability to understand those that are available.

- A U.S. government publication, *Dietary Guidelines,* varied in reading difficulty levels from sixth grade to college level; 75% of studied individuals in the Special Supplemental Food Program for Women, Infants and Children (WIC) program would be frustrated or need instructional assistance to understand this publication.[7]
- Analysis of 63 patient package inserts accompanying drugs revealed on average a tenth-grade reading level, with only 11% written at the fifth- to seventh-grade level recommended for documents used by the general public. Half had small type or poor-quality print.[3]
- The reading ability of parents of pediatric outpatients in a large public teaching hospital was at the seventh- to eighth-grade level, although the average last grade reported was 11.5 years. Eighty percent of 129 materials from the American Academy of Pediatrics, the Centers for Disease Control and Prevention (CDC), the March of Dimes, pharmaceutical companies, and commercially available books on baby care required at least tenth-grade reading level, with only 2% written at less than a seventh-grade level. The reading levels of these publications are cited in an article by Davis and others.[9] A federal act that mandates that vaccine information pamphlets be given to parents also mandates that the materials be understandable; yet all three of the CDC vaccine pamphlets analyzed were written at a level well above the reading ability of two thirds of the parents tested in this study.
- Readability of consent forms is especially problematic because they have consistently been estimated to be at a scientific or college level. Analysis of consent forms for studies at the National Cancer Institute

found them to range from grades 12 to 17.5, with a mean grade level of 14.3.[25]

It is important to note that readability formulas indicate reading ease, not comprehension, although when the reading level is beyond the skill of the learner, comprehension is known to be decreased and recall sketchy and inaccurate. In contrast to the amount of attention to measuring readability of materials, little attention has been paid to measuring patient comprehension of or learning from educational literature. In addition, although not commonly used in everyday practice, several brief tests are available to estimate a patient's reading level.[28] Other characteristics not captured in readability formulas are also important in written as in other instructional materials. These include organization, including use of headings and outlines, appropriate sequencing of material, and clarity. Examples of materials written at high levels and revised to read at much lower levels can be found in the boxes on pp. 49-51.

Various readability formulas may be useful for different kinds of text. For example, the Fry readability formula, shown on p. 52 and in Figure 3-2, determines the level of materials from grades 1 through college; however, this formula is not useful with passages of fewer than 300 words. The FOG formula, shown on p. 52, uses the number of sentences and the number of polysyllabic words and is useful for grade 4 through college. The Flesch formula, shown in the box on p. 54, uses average sentence length and word length and is useful for grades 5 through college. The SMOG formula, shown on p. 55 (see rules for testing on p. 56), counts the number of sentences and the number of words with three or more syllables and is useful for grades 5 through college. Meade and Smith have compared readability formulas based on the same health education materials and have found that the Flesch, FOG, and Fry formulas correlate highly with each other.[26]

Of the more than 30 formulas assessing readability,[12] Fry has developed a new one that can assess passages of 40 to 300 words.[13] Fry's formulas use a dictionary that gives grade levels for

EXAMPLES OF READING MATERIALS FOR PATIENTS: ORIGINAL AND REVISED VERSIONS

Example 1: Consent to operation

Original (25th grade level)

I consent to the performance of operations and procedures in addition to or different from those now contemplated, whether or not arising from presently unforeseen conditions, which the above-named doctor or his associates or assistants may consider necessary or advisable in the course of the operation.

Revised (6th grade level)

I agree to other operations or treatments. My doctors may learn more in surgery. They may think I need other treatments. My doctors will decide in surgery. I agree to let them do the things they think are needed.

Example 2: Patient education material

Original (16th grade level)

Angina pectoris is a symptom and not actually a disease. The term refers to a pain in the chest, usually under the sternum (breastbone), which is brought on chiefly by exercise or emotional upsets in a person who has a heart problem. The pain is usually relieved by rest alone, but goes away more quickly with the use of a medicine which helps to bring more blood to the heart muscle.

Revised (7th grade level)

Angina is a feeling. It is not really a disease. The word means a pain in the chest. The pain is felt under the breastbone. A person who has heart trouble may feel this. Exercise or getting upset can cause the pain. The pain usually goes away with rest. It goes away faster if you take medicine. The medicine helps to bring more blood to the heart.

From Davis TC and others: *J Fam Pract* 31:533-538, 1990.

SAMPLE PATIENT INFORMATION HANDOUTS

Sample A

The sample below is a typical patient information handout, written at the reading level of a high school graduate or higher, that would be given to patients whose reading ability appears to be at that level. Sample B [see p. 50] is the same handout, rewritten at a fifth grade level of reading ability, and more appropriate for those patients with less developed reading skills.

Strep throat

The physician will treat your strep throat by first ordering a throat culture to make sure you have the streptococcus organism and, if you do, then prescribing medicine. You could receive either a penicillin injection or have to take oral antibiotic medicine for a prescribed length of time. It is essential that you take all the medicine your physician has ordered because if you don't, the infection could continue. When you have finished the oral antibiotic, you may have to come back and see the doctor and have another throat culture. Ask your doctor if you need to return and then call a week in advance for an appointment.

Here are some things you can do. It is important to rest and get sufficient sleep; naps are recommended. Try to drink plenty of water and juice. For example, drink at least five glasses of water and two glasses of juice every day; more if possible. If your throat is painful or you develop a fever, take one or two Tylenol not any more frequently than every four hours. A simple solution of salt water may help the soreness in your throat. Put ¼ teaspoon of salt in one cup of warm water and gargle gently with this as often as needed.

From Dixon E, Park R: *Nurs Outlook* 38:278-281, 1990.

Continued.

■ SAMPLE PATIENT INFORMATION HANDOUTS—cont'd

Do not return to work or school until your fever is gone and you have improved. In any case, you must wait at least 24 hours after you have had your shot to return to work or school and, if you are taking oral medication, you must wait at least 48 hours after beginning your pills to go back. This is so you will no longer be contagious when you return.

Follow these instructions and you should be feeling better soon. If you don't improve in a couple of days, however, call the office and ask to speak to the nurse.

Sample B

The sample patient handout below contains the same information as Sample A above but is written at a fifth grade level of reading ability for those patients with weaker reading skills. Note the simpler vocabulary and sentence structure, the use of questions to focus reader attention on specific points, and the use of bold type to highlight important information.

Sore throat caused by streptococcus

How will the doctor take care of my strep throat?

1. The doctor will order medicine for me. I may have to get a shot (penicillin). I may have to take __ pills (antibiotic) every day, for __ days.
2. It is very important that I take all my pills. Even when my sore throat goes away, I must finish taking my pills. If I do not take all my pills, I could get sick again.
3. I may have to come back to see the doctor again. When all my pills are gone, I might need a test (throat culture). If so, I will come back on _____.

How can I help myself get better?

1. I need to sleep more. Naps are important to get more sleep.
2. I need to drink lots of water and juice. Try to drink 5 glasses of water and 2 glasses of juice a day.
3. TYLENOL medicine can be taken, if I feel hot or have a sore throat. Only take one or two pills of TYLENOL at one time. Do not take TYLENOL any more often than every four hours.
4. I can gargle with warm salt water to help my sore throat. Put a small amount of salt in a spoon and add to a cup of warm water. Gargle gently with the warm salt water as often as it helps.
5. I will not go back to work or school until _____. If I feel hot or sick, I will stay home and rest. If my sore throat does not go away in __ days, I will call the nurse at __ (telephone number).

When I have a bad sore throat, if I see a doctor and take all my pills and rest and drink lots of water, then I will soon feel better.

■ SAMPLE MATERIAL

Written at the thirteenth grade level

The heart usually receives electrical signals from the sinoatrial node, an area in the top right chamber. In ventricular tachycardia the signals that orchestrate the rhythm originate in the ventricle, located below the atrium. This area of origin results in an erratic beat or rhythm. The erratic beat disables the ventricles from contracting, thus blood is unable to be pumped out adequately. Inadequate blood supply affects all body parts since oxygen and nutrients are located in the blood. When the brain does not receive adequate blood supply, symptoms that include fainting, dizziness, and unconsciousness can occur. Stroke and death are also potential results.

With the knowledge that ventricular tachycardia is an erratic and potentially fatal rhythm that can occur at unpredictable times, physicians usually prescribe medications to control or prevent that rhythm. When medications are unable to keep the erratic beat dormant, the heart may require defibrillation. Defibrillation resets the electrical circuit, allowing the sinoatrial node to once again dominate.

Rewritten on the sixth grade level

Electrical signals from the heart's pacemaker keep the heart beating in a normal way. The pacemaker is called the S-A node and is found in the top part of the heart. Signals can also come from the bottom part of the heart. If they come from the bottom part, an irregular or rapid beat results. Several rapid and irregular beats are called V Tach. V Tach means the heart is not able to pump blood. When this happens, the body is not able to get the blood it needs. Blood carries oxygen and food to the body. One of the body parts that needs blood most is the brain. When the brain does not get blood, it can make a person feel faint or dizzy. It can also cause a stroke or death.

Doctors order medicines to try to control or stop this irregular or rapid beat. The medicines usually control this type of beat. Sometimes they do not work. The heart may then need to be shocked. The shock is given by a machine called a defibrillator. The shock usually helps the heart to reset its signals. It then beats in a regular way. All parts of the body can then get the supply of blood they need.

From Evanoski CAM: *J Cardiovasc Nurs* 4(2):1-6, 1990.

43,000 words. Also, several software packages can calculate readability formulas. The user selects several random samples (representative of the text) of 100 words, types the text into the computer, and receives the calculated readability score.[27]

A sample of a pamphlet for use by the lay public is shown in Figure 3-3 (see pp. 57-58). Consider the objectives that this pamphlet meets. Its statements seem to be correct. Some pictures are used to create interest or explain content. The organization of the pamphlet is clearly outlined and reinforced with visual cues throughout the body of the pamphlet. The final messages left with the reader are important ones about prevention and taking action if one has symptoms of pneumonia. Check the readability level.

Many health agencies prepare some teaching aids of their own, often incorporating schedules or procedures specific to that agency. These written materials must also be considered in light of the objectives they must meet, the validity of the material, and the likelihood of patient comprehension.

Text continued on p. 59.

■ DIRECTIONS FOR USING THE READABILITY GRAPH

1. Select three one-hundred-word passages from near the beginning, middle, and end of the book. Skip all proper nouns.
2. Count the total number of sentences in each hundred-word passage (estimating to nearest tenth of a sentence). Average these three numbers.
3. Count the total number of syllables in each hundred-word sample. There is a syllable for each vowel sound; for example: cat (1), blackbird (2), continental (4). Don't be fooled by word size; for example: polio (3),

through (1). Endings such as -y, -ed, -el, or -le usually make a syllable, for example: ready (2), bottle (2). I find it convenient to count every syllable over one in each word and add 100. Average the total number of syllables for the three samples.
4. Plot on the graph the average number of sentences per hundred words and the average number of syllables per hundred words. Most plot points fall near the heavy curved line. Perpendicular lines mark off approximate grade level areas.

Example

	Sentences per 100 words	Syllables per 100 words
100-word sample page 5	9.1	122
100-word sample page 89	8.5	140
100-word sample page 160	7.0	129
	3)24.6	3)391
Average	8.2	130

Plotting these averages on the graph, we find they fall in the 5th grade area; hence the book is about 5th grade difficulty level. If great variability is encountered either in sentence length or in the syllable count for the three selections, then randomly select several more passages and average them in before plotting.

From Fry E: *J Reading* 11:514, 1968.

■ GUNNING FOG INDEX^{sm} SCALE

1. Select a sample of writing 100 to 125 words long. If the piece is long, take several samples and average the results.
2. Calculate the average number of words per sentence. Treat independent clauses as separate sentences. "In school we studied; we learned; we improved" counts as three sentences.
3. Count the number of words of three syllables or more. In your count, omit capitalized words; combinations of short words like *bookkeeper* or *manpower;* or verbs made into

three syllables by adding *"-es"* or *"-ed."* Divide the count of long words by the passage length to get the percentage.
4. Add 2 (average sentence length) and 3 (percentage of long words). Multiply the sum by the factor 0.4, and ignore the digits following the decimal point.

The result is the years of schooling needed to read the passage with ease. Few readers have over 17 years of schooling, so any passage over 17 gets a FOG Index of "17-plus."

From Gunning R, Kallan R: *How to Take the Fog Out of Business Writing,* Chicago, 1994, Dartnell. The Fog Index^{sm} Scale is a service mark licensed exclusively to RK Communication Consultants by D. and M. Mueller.

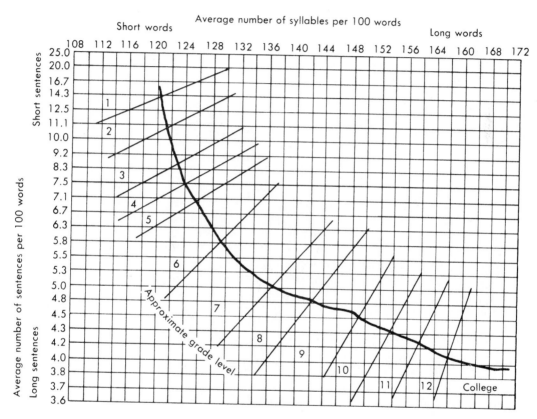

Figure 3-2   Graph for estimating readability. *Directions:* Randomly select three 100-word passages from a book or an article. Plot average number of syllables and average number of words per sentence on graph to determine area of readability level. Choose more passages per book if great variability is observed. (From Fry E: *J Reading* 11:514, 1968.)

■ FLESCH FORMULA

1. For short pieces, test the entire selection. For longer pieces, test at least three randomly selected samples of 100 words each. Do not use introductory paragraphs as part of the sample. Start each sample at the beginning of a paragraph.

2. Determine the average sentence length *(SL)* by counting the number of words in the sample and dividing by the number of sentences. Count as a sentence each independent unit of thought that is grammatically independent, that is, if its end is punctuated by a period, question mark, exclamation point, semicolon, or colon. In dialog, count speech tags (e.g., "he said") as part of the quoted sentence.

3. Determine the word length *(WL)* by counting all the syllables in the sample as if reading the words aloud. Divide the syllables by the number of words in the sample and multiply by 100.

4. These indices are then applied to the formula to compute the reading ease,

$$RE = 206.835 - 1.015\ SL - 0.846\ WL$$

where *RE* is the reading ease score, *SL* is the average sentence length in words, and *WL* is the average word length measured as syllables per 100 words.

Interpretation of Flesch reading ease score

Reading ease	Grade	Description of style	No. syllables/ 100 words	Average sentence length
90-100	5	Very easy	123	8
80-90	6	Easy	131	11
70-80	7	Fairly easy	139	14
60-70	8-9	Standard	147	17
50-60	10-12	Fairly difficult	155	21
30-50	College	Difficult	167	25
0-30	College graduate	Very difficult	192	29

From Flesch R: *The art of readable writing,* New York, 1974, Harper & Row, pp 184-186, 247-251.

■ SMOG TESTING

The SMOG formula was originally developed by G. Harry McLaughlin in 1969. It will predict the grade-level difficulty of a passage within 1.5 grades in 68% of the passages tested. That may be close enough for your purposes. It is simple to use and faster than most other measures. The procedure is presented below.

Instructions

1. You will need 30 sentences. Count out 10 consecutive sentences near the beginning, 10 consecutive from the middle, and 10 from the end. For this purpose, a sentence is any string of words punctuated by a period (.), an exclamation point (!), or a question mark (?).
2. From the entire 30 sentences, count the words containing **three or more syllables,** including repetitions.
3. Obtain the grade level from the table below, or you may calculate the grade level as follows: Determine the nearest perfect square root of the total number of words of three or more syllables and then add a constant of 3 to the square root to obtain the grade level.

Example

Total number of multisyllabic (3 or more syllables) words	67
Nearest perfect square	64
Square root	8
Add constant of 3	11 This is the grade level

TABLE A. SMOG CONVERSION TABLE

Word count	Grade level
0-2	4
3-6	5
7-12	6
13-20	7
21-30	8
31-42	9
43-56	10
57-72	11
73-90	12
91-110	13
111-132	14
133-156	15
157-182	16
183-210	17

Developed by Harold C. McGraw, Office of Educational Research, Baltimore County Public Schools, Towson, Maryland.

From McLaughlin GH: *J Reading* 12:639-646, 1969; Doak CC, Doak LG, Root JH: *Teaching patients with low literacy skills,* Philadelphia, 1985, JB Lippincott.

SPECIAL RULES FOR SMOG TESTING

Hyphenated words are **one** word.

For numerals, pronounce them aloud and count the syllables pronounced for each numeral (e.g., for the number 573, five = 1, hundred = 2, seventy = 3, and three = 1, or 7 syllables).

Proper nouns should be counted.

If a long sentence has a colon, consider each part of it as a separate sentence. However, if possible, avoid selecting that segment of the passage.

The words for which the abbreviations stand should be read aloud to determine their syllable count (e.g., Oct. = October = 3 syllables).

SMOG on shorter passages

Sometimes it may be necessary to assess the readability of a passage of less than 30 sentences. You can still use the SMOG formula to obtain an approximate grade level by using a conversion number from Table B and then using Table A [see box, p. 55] to find the grade level.

First count the number of sentences in your material and the number of words with three or more syllables. In Table B, in the left-hand column, locate the number of sentences, and locate the conversion number in the column opposite. Multiply the word count found earlier by the conversion number. Use this number in Table B to obtain the corresponding grade level.

For example, suppose your material consisted of 15 sentences and you counted 12 words of three or more syllables in this material. Proceed as follows:

1. In Table B, left-hand column, locate the number of sentences in your material. For your material, the number is 15.
2. Opposite 15 in the adjacent column, find the conversion number. The conversion number for 15 is 2.0.
3. Multiply your word count, 12, by 2 to get 24.
4. Now look at Table A to find the grade level. For a word count of 24, the grade level is 8.

TABLE B. SMOG conversion for samples with fewer than 30 sentences	
Number of sentences in sample material	Conversion number
29	1.03
28	1.07
27	1.1
26	1.15
25	1.2
24	1.25
23	1.3
22	1.36
21	1.43
20	1.5
19	1.58
18	1.67
17	1.76
16	1.87
15	2.0
14	2.14
13	2.3
12	2.5
11	2.7
10	3

From McLaughlin GH: *J Reading* 12:639-646, 1969; Doak CC, Doak LG, Root JH: *Teaching patients with low literacy skills,* Philadelphia, 1985, JB Lippincott.

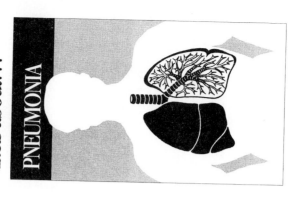

facts about...

PNEUMONIA

AMERICAN LUNG ASSOCIATION®

Continued.

---

medication must be continued according to the doctor's instructions—otherwise the pneumonia may recur. Relapses can be far more serious than the first attack.

Besides antibiotics, patients are given supportive treatment: proper diet and oxygen to increase oxygen in the blood when needed. In some patients, medication to ease chest pain and to provide relief from violent cough may be necessary.

The vigorous young person may lead a normal life within a week of recovery from pneumonia. For the middle-aged, however, weeks may elapse before they regain their accustomed strength, vigor, and feeling of well-being. A person recovering from mycoplasma pneumonia may be weak for an extended period of time. In general, a person should not be discouraged from returning to work or carrying out usual activities but must be warned to expect some difficulties. Adequate rest is important to maintain progress toward full recovery and to avoid relapse. Remember—don't rush recovery!

Prevention is Possible

Because pneumonia is a common complication of influenza (flu), getting a flu shot every fall is good pneumonia prevention.

Vaccine is also available to help fight pneumococcal pneumonia—*one type* of bacterial pneumonia. Your doctor can help you decide if you—or a member of your family—needs the vaccine against pneumococcal pneumonia. It is usually given only to people at high risk of getting the disease and its life-threatening complications.

The greatest risk of pneumococcal pneumonia is usually among people who:

- Have chronic illnesses such as lung disease, heart disease, kidney disorders, sickle cell anemia, or diabetes.
- Are recovering from severe illness.
- Are in nursing homes or other chronic care facilities.
- Are age 65 or older.

If you are at risk, ask your doctor to be vaccinated. The vaccine is generally given only once. Ask your doctor about any revaccination recommendations. The vac-

cine is not recommended for pregnant women or children under age two.

Since pneumonia often follows ordinary respiratory infections, the most important preventive measure is to be alert to any symptoms of respiratory trouble that linger more than a few days. Good health habits—proper diet and hygiene, rest, regular exercise, etc.—increase resistance to all respiratory illnesses. They also help promote fast recovery when illness does occur.

If You Have Symptoms of Pneumonia

1. Call your doctor immediately. Even with the many effective antibiotics, early diagnosis and treatment are important.

2. Follow your doctor's advice. In serious cases, your doctor may advise a hospital stay. Or recovery at home may be possible.

3. Continue to take the medicine your doctor prescribes until you may stop. This will help prevent recurrence of pneumonia and relapse.

4. Remember—even though pneumonia can be treated, it is an extremely serious illness. Don't wait, get treatment early.

To find out more about pneumonia and other types of lung disease, contact your local American Lung Association by dialing 1-800-LUNG-USA (1-800-586-4872).

5

6

Figure 3-3 Sample instructional pamphlet to be used for lay public. (Courtesy American Lung Association.)

What is Pneumonia?

Pneumonia is a serious infection or inflammation of your lungs. The air sacs in the lungs fill with pus and other liquid. Oxygen has trouble reaching your blood. If there is too little oxygen in your blood, your body cells can't work properly—and you may die.

Until 1936, pneumonia was the No. 1 cause of death in the U.S. Then the use of antibiotics brought it under control. Now this deadly enemy is making a comeback, in part because some bacteria can resist antibiotics. Pneumonia and influenza combined have ranked as the sixth leading cause of death since 1979.

Pneumonia affects your lungs in two ways. *Lobar* pneumonia affects a section (lobe) of a lung:

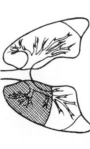

Bronchial pneumonia (or bronchopneumonia) affects patches throughout both lungs:

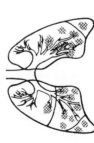

▨ Affected area

Causes of Pneumonia

Pneumonia is not a single disease. It can have over 30 different causes. There are four main causes of pneumonia:

1. Bacteria
2. Viruses
3. Mycoplasmas
4. Other causes, such as pneumocystis

1. Bacterial Pneumonia

Bacterial pneumonia can attack anyone from infants through the very old. Alcoholics, the debilitated, post-operative patients, people with respiratory diseases or viral infections and people who have weakened immune systems are at greater risk.

Pneumonia bacteria are present in some healthy throats. When body defenses are weakened in some way—by illness, old age, malnutrition, general debility or impaired immunity—the bacteria can multiply and cause serious damage. Usually, when a person's resistance is lowered, bacteria work their way into the lungs and inflame the air sacs.

The tissue of part of a lobe of the lung, an entire lobe, or even most of the lung's five lobes becomes completely filled with liquid (this is called "consolidation"). The infection quickly spreads through the bloodstream and the whole body is invaded.

The *pneumococcus* is the most common cause of bacterial pneumonia. It is one form of pneumonia for which a vaccine is available.

Symptoms: The onset of bacterial pneumonia can vary from gradual to sudden. In the most severe cases, the patient may experience shaking chills, chattering teeth, severe chest pain, and a cough that produces rust-colored or greenish mucus. A person's temperature often rises as high as 105 degrees F. The patient sweats profusely, and breathing and pulse rate increase rapidly. Lips and nailbeds may have a bluish color due to lack of oxygen in the blood. A patient's mental state may be confused or delirious.

2. Viral Pneumonia

Half of all pneumonias are believed to be caused by viruses. More and more viruses are being identified as the cause of respiratory infection, and though most attack the upper respiratory tract, some produce pneumonia, especially in children. Most of these pneumonias are not serious and last a short time. *Influenza* virus may be severe and occasionally fatal. The virus invades the lungs and multiplies, but there are almost no physical signs of lung tissue becoming filled with fluid. It finds many of its victims among those who have pre-existing heart or lung disease or are pregnant.

Symptoms: The initial symptoms of viral pneumonia are the same as influenza symptoms: fever, a dry cough, headache, muscle pain, and weakness. Within 12 to 36 hours, there is increasing breathlessness; the cough becomes worse and produces a small amount of mucus. There is a high fever and there may be blueness of the lips. In extreme cases, the patient has a desperate need for air and extreme breathlessness. Other viral pneumonias are complicated by an invasion of bacteria—with all the typical symptoms of *bacterial* pneumonia.

3. Mycoplasma Pneumonia

Because of its somewhat different symptoms and physical signs, and because the course of the illness differed from classic pneumococcal pneumonia, mycoplasma pneumonia was once believed to be caused by one or more undiscovered viruses and was called "primary atypical pneumonia."

Identified during World War II, mycoplasmas are the smallest free-living agents of disease in man, unclassified as to whether bacteria or viruses, but having characteristics of both. They generally cause a mild and widespread pneumonia. They affect all age groups, occurring most frequently in older children and young adults. The death rate is low, even in untreated cases.

Symptoms: The most prominent symptom of mycoplasma pneumonia is a cough that tends to come in violent attacks, but produces only sparse whitish mucus. Chills and fever are early symptoms, and some patients experience nausea or vomiting. The patient's heartbeat is often slow, and in some extreme cases patients may suffer from breathlessness and have a bluish color to lips and nailbeds.

4. Other Kinds of Pneumonia

Pneumocystis carinii pneumonia (PCP) is caused by an organism long thought of as a parasite but now believed to be a fungus. PCP is the first sign of illness in many persons with AIDS, and perhaps 80 percent of AIDS patients (four out of five) will develop it sooner or later. It can be successfully treated in many cases. It may recur a few months later, but treatment can help to prevent or delay its recurrence.

Other less common pneumonias may be quite serious and are occurring more often. Various special pneumonias are caused by the inhalation of food, liquid, gases or dust, and by fungi. Foreign bodies or a bronchial obstruction such as a tumor may promote the occurrence of pneumonia, although they are not causes of pneumonia. Rickettsia (also considered an organism somewhere between viruses and bacteria) cause Rocky Mountain spotted fever, Q fever, typhus, and psittacosis—diseases that may have mild or severe effects on the lungs. Tuberculosis pneumonia is a very serious lung infection and extremely dangerous unless treated early.

Pneumonia Treatment and Recovery

If you develop pneumonia, your chances of a fast recovery are greatest under certain conditions: if you're young, if your pneumonia is caught early, if your defenses against disease are working well, if the infection hasn't spread, and if you're not suffering from other illnesses.

In the young and healthy, early treatment with antibiotics can cure bacterial pneumonia and speed recovery from mycoplasma pneumonia, and a certain percentage of rickettsia cases. There is no effective treatment yet for viral pneumonia, which usually heals on its own.

The drugs used to fight pneumonia are determined by the germ causing the pneumonia and the judgment of the doctor. After a patient's temperature returns to normal,

Figure 3-3, cont'd   For legend, see preceding page.

The "Planning Home Care" guide for care-givers of persons with Alzheimer's disease is presented in the box on p. 60. Its implicit objective is to develop self-efficacy for caregiver coping skills. It is organized around simple suggestions and accompanied with pictures to serve as visual cues to jog memory.

One of five adult Americans is functionally illiterate, reading at or below the fifth grade level. These individuals understand little if any of the written materials provided for them by health professionals. Five percent of the adult population is unable to read. Even the use of audio-taped instructions taxes the language and thinking skills of these persons. Another 33% reads between the sixth and tenth grade levels.[11]

Many individuals who are illiterate have normal or above normal IQs. They will nearly always try to conceal their illiteracy and will use excuses such as not having time or having left their eyeglasses at home. They may be articulate and well dressed. Frequently, they "go along" and react positively even when they do not understand. However, illiterate persons cannot use reference documents or catalogs effectively, cannot follow instruction sheets, or cannot comprehend simple road maps.[15]

The consequences of this problem affect the patient and the caregiver responsible for the patient's well-being; the caregiver also faces the possibility of litigation initiated by a patient acting without knowledge that should have been provided. Thus techniques known to be most effective should be used to teach these individuals.[11]

1. Eliminate everything that is extraneous.
2. Build to complexity when it is necessary; break content into components; and build with review, feedback, and questions.
3. Require patients to demonstrate what they have learned.
4. Those who are insecure in their ability to learn need more rewards than do others to accomplish small tasks.
5. To reduce the reading level and literacy demand, use a conversational style, active voice, short words, and short sentences.
6. Use visuals, especially line drawings, with one idea portrayed by the picture; use captions not longer than ten words.
7. Show only correct behavior.
8. Organize material in the order the patients will use it, and use words that are familiar to them.
9. Pretest all materials.

Computers

Computers are used for instructional purposes: drill and practice in problem solving with feedback until a skill is mastered; games; and as simulators in which one learns how, for example, to adjust insulin level with a program that models the body's blood sugar and responses to insulin, diet, and exercise. Computers can provide highly individualized self-paced learning and can document the learning process. They can be used to elicit information from patients that can help tailor patient education and discharge planning.

ComputerLink is a computer network that has been used to provide information and decision-support functions for caregivers of persons with Alzheimer's disease. A recent study[5] showed that this system enhanced the caregivers' confidence and decreased their sense of isolation, of special importance in that other services are inaccessible because they require leaving home.

A behavioral treatment program for obesity uses an interactive microcomputer small enough to be carried by subjects during their normal daily routines. Learners make self-reports on consumption of food and exercise. If they forget to do so, they are reminded by the computer.

Computer games can help adolescents understand the responsibilities parents face, as well as the costs of childbirth and child rearing. Throughout the game, the teen's readiness for parenting is visually displayed on a thermometer gauge. The program simulates, for example, a 1-year-old with a fever who cries persistently at night or a 2-year-old with temper tantrums. A similar game called "Romance" addresses sex and birth control. It provides simulated outcomes and realistic information. After these games were introduced in clinics, teenage preg-

◼ PLANNING HOME CARE

Dear Caregiver:
Taking care of a patient with Alzheimer's disease requires patience and understanding—and it requires you to look at the patient's environment with new eyes. Then you need to change that environment to help him function as well as possible.

Keeping these points in mind, read over the following tips to help you plan your daily care.

Reduce stress

Too much stress can worsen the patient's symptoms—he can become combative and severely agitated. Try to protect him from the following potential sources of stress:

- A change in routine, caregiver, or environment
- Fatigue
- Excessive demands
- Overwhelming, misleading, or competing stimuli
- Illness and pain
- Over-the-counter medications

Establish a routine

Keep the patient's daily routine stable so he can respond automatically; adapting to change may require more thought than he can handle. Even eating a different food or going to a strange grocery store may overwhelm him.

Also, make a schedule of the patient's daily activities:

- List the activities necessary for his daily care, and include ones that he especially enjoys (such as weeding in the garden). Designate a time frame for each activity.
- Establish bedtime rituals—especially important to promote relaxation and a restful night's sleep for both of you.
- Stick to your schedule as closely as possible (for example, breakfast first, then dressing) so the patient won't be surprised or need to make decisions.
- Keep a copy of the schedule for other caregivers. To help them give better care, include notes and suggestions about techniques that work for you; for instance, "Speak in a quiet voice" or "When helping Mitchell dress or bathe, take things one step at a time, and wait for him to respond."

Practice reality orientation

In your conversations with the patient, orient him to the day and the activity he'll perform. For instance, say "Today is Tuesday and we're going to have breakfast now." Do this every day. The patient will be more aware of his immediate environment, and he'll know what to expect without being challenged to remember events.

Simplify the surroundings

Eventually, the patient won't be able to correctly interpret what he sees and hears. Protect him by trying to decrease the noise level in his environment and by avoiding busy areas, such as shopping malls and restaurants.

Does the patient mistake pictures or images in the mirror for real people? If so, remove the photos and mirrors. Also, avoid rooms with busy patterns on wallpaper and carpets because they can overtax his senses.

To avoid confusion and encourage the patient's independence, provide cues. For example, hang a picture of a toilet on the bathroom door.

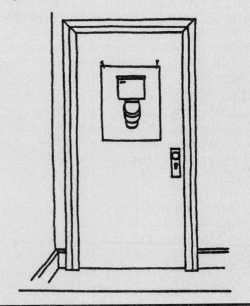

From A Caregiver's Guide, *Nursing 92*, 1992.

■ PLANNING HOME CARE—cont'd

Avoid fatigue

The patient will tire easily, so plan important activities for the morning when he's functioning best; save less demanding ones for later in the day. Remember to schedule breaks. In the early stages of the disease, he'll need about 15 to 30 minutes of listening to music or just relaxing in the morning and in the afternoon. As the disease progresses, schedule longer, more frequent breaks (perhaps 40 to 90 minutes). If the patient naps during the day, have him sleep in a reclining chair rather than in a bed so he won't confuse day and night.

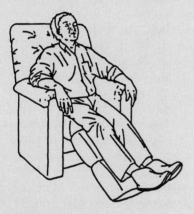

Don't expect too much

Accept the patient's limitations. Don't demand too much from him—this forces him to think about a task and causes frustration. Instead, offer help when needed, and distract him if he's trying too hard. You'll feel less stressed too.

Prepare for illness

If the patient becomes ill, his behavior will deteriorate. He'll have a low tolerance for pain and discomfort.

Never rely on the patient to take his own medicine. He may forget to take it or miscount what he's taken. Always supervise him.

Use the sense of touch

Because the patient's visual and auditory perceptions are distorted, he has an increased need for closeness and touching. Remember to approach him from the front—you don't want to frighten him or provoke belligerent or aggressive behavior.

Respect his need for personal space. Limit physical contact to his hands and arms at first, then move to more central parts of his body, such as his shoulders or head.

Using long or circular motions, lightly stroke the patient to help relieve muscle tension and give him a sense of his physical self. Physical contact also expresses your feelings of intimacy and caring.

Allowing the patient to touch objects in the environment can help relieve stress by providing information. Let him handle, poke, pull, or shake objects—for example, a handbag, a brush, or a comb. Make sure they're unbreakable and can't harm him.

Handle problem behavior

If the patient becomes restless or agitated, divert his attention with appropriate activity. Good choices include walking, rocking in a rocking chair, sanding wood, folding laundry, or hoeing in the garden. These repetitive activities don't require any particular sequence or planning. A warm bath, a drink of warm milk, or a back massage can also be calming.

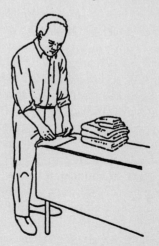

Although problem behavior can be taxing, try to remember that the patient can't help himself. Your understanding and compassion can increase his sense of security.

nancy rates declined by 15%. Computer-assisted instruction uses role modeling and desensitization to raise teens' self-esteem. As teens gain new information, they are empowered with new ways to make decisions.[30]

Computers can generate individualized information leaflets. They incorporate new information easily. On-line, computer-based information systems can educate college students about topics such as AIDS—information that students might not seek at the health centers. Computer information systems can answer questions, offer recent research updates, and display guides to community services. They provide a useful and confidential source of information within a broader AIDS education program.[31]

Despite the versatility of computer-based programs, the results of one study revealed that diabetes educators believed written materials were more useful for patient education than were computers.[1] Respondents indicated that computers have yet to make a major contribution to the teaching and learning process in diabetes education.

Visual materials

When one teaches about actual physical objects, it is often preferable to use the real thing. Nothing but a baby can act like a baby during a bath. However, models are useful when three dimensions must be retained but (1) the real thing is too small, large, complicated, or expensive; (2) the real thing is unavailable; (3) the desired view cannot be exposed; or (4) the object cannot be manipulated. For example, for demonstrating the birth of a baby, a doll may be advanced through an actual-size model of the bony structure of the pelvis. Many times, anatomy and physiology cannot be adequately visualized with the use of a real person because other tissues are in the way or a body part, such as the eye, is too small and complex. A dummy can be useful for showing the position of a tracheostomy and how to remove and reinsert parts of the tube. It can also be used for practicing general movements with the suction tube. The dummy is clearly limited because it lacks functioning muscles and secretions. Some teachers would insist that it would be better to start the learner working with a real tracheostoma. However, if none is available, or if one that is available is difficult to care for, early practice on a model may be helpful. Models in the form of dummies are used to teach resuscitation techniques because someone whose heart or breathing has stopped is not usually available.

Thus models may be used because they can teach better than real objects can or because they are more practical to use. At times they are absolutely essential. However, models frequently are expensive and may not be easily available in many places where patients are being taught.

The research literature on pictorial learning is sparse in comparison with that on verbal learning. Theory about how people learn from pictures is not completely developed. Pictorial learning is superior to verbal for recognition and recall. However, when the subject matter is abstract, it is difficult to communicate with pictures. Media used to convey pictures always distort the various visual dimensions—resolution, color fidelity, and size—to some degree. For example, paintings may eliminate or exaggerate various parts of an object. These distortions may or may not be important to a particular learning task.

Photographs and drawings lack the third dimension but are readily available or can be produced by the teacher. The third dimension is not imperative when the teacher is showing familiar objects or those in which shape and space are not the primary considerations. Examples that fall into these categories and are frequently not available include an infected finger or an abnormal stool in infants. However, the learner must be aware that odor can be important in recognizing abnormal stool. In both of these examples, photographs would be more desirable than diagrams because they more accurately portray the details of the real item.

Drawings are particularly pertinent for removing superfluous detail present in real objects.

During an explanation to a patient about diverticulitis, visualization is obviously desirable. Whereas a photograph shows details of the tissue that the patient does not need to know, a simple line drawing can communicate the concept of a pouch in the intestinal wall. In other instances, drawings in the form of cartoons are used to create interest in a topic.

Pictures may be presented in many ways, depending on the size of the audience and equipment available. For a single individual, visuals on paper 8½ by 11 inches can be used. For small groups, posters can be prepared. Drawings can be made with crayons or felt-tipped pens on flip charts (pads of paper approximately 32 by 26 inches) supported on an easel or chair back. Cutouts can be attached by magnets or flannel to metal or flannel boards. Drawings can be done on the blackboard. Suitable for both large and small groups are 2 × 2 inch slides or filmstrips that can be projected on a screen or wall. Overhead projectors use transparencies (sheets of plastic) prepared with diagrams or drawn at the time of presentation and projected. When teaching is a regular part of the nursing activities, these materials and equipment may be readily available. More commonly, caregivers interact with an individual patient and use an easily obtained visual, such as the pictures in the *Birth Atlas,* sketch the objects needed for a given lesson, or use a prepared teaching aid.

Teaching by television requires many of the same skills as doing an in-person demonstration. Videotapes can be used as "triggers," providing an instructional stimulus that can be followed by discussion groups. In addition, the teacher can use the film of the patient's own cardiac catheterization to teach both the patient and the family about the extent or the absence of cardiac problems. This approach eliminates generic information in other educational tools that may not be immediately useful to a particular patient. The information can be particularly helpful when a decision has to be made. Often, patients need concrete evidence to accept their diagnoses or before they can consider treatment options.[4]

Two reviews have summarized studies of television's power to produce an effect in patient education.[14, 29] Video use is as effective as other presentations. The most suitable educational applications of television are that (1) it presents powerful role models of particular behavior, attitudes, and values; (2) it presents vivid, active illustrative material not otherwise readily available; and (3) it provides direct feedback about a learner's performance of complex interpersonal and psychomotor skills (this assumes the person's performance is videotaped). From a practical point of view, videos are produced cheaply and can be tailor-made for a given patient population. Using video ensures a standard level of teaching. Video presentations can be particularly effective now because of the high rate of functional illiteracy in the United States and because people probably are oriented more to viewing than to reading.

Screening, Preparing, and Testing Teaching Materials

All materials must be viewed and evaluated before they are used for teaching. Previewing is necessary to identify material that the teacher believes is incorrect or is contradictory to other sources being used. It may be necessary to reject an audiovisual aid because it is beyond the level of the learners' understanding or because the aid may be peripheral to the objectives.

Materials must also be culturally relevant. Hall[17] describes designing materials for Mexican-American patients in the California Diabetes Control Program. Nutrition and diabetes educational materials written in Spanish were frequently literal translations of the English-language version. For example, a booklet on diet showed one bread exchange equal to one slice of bread, one half of a bagel, or one half of a cup of cooked cereal. Many Mexican-Americans had never heard of bagels. Tortillas, the starchy food they use daily, were not mentioned. In the new educational package, pictorial exchange lists were modified to reflect Mexican food habits. If possible, the portion sizes on the exchange list were reworked so that one piece of food (banana) represented one exchange. A simplified measuring system was adopted, using only common household measures. For example, three ounces of meat could be estimated by modeling the palm of the hand. Field testing this new material with a target population should determine its effectiveness.

After preview, an instructional material or product should undergo two steps to improve its effectiveness as a teaching tool.

1. *Product verification.* Arrange a tryout of the materials under conditions approximating those in which the finally developed product will be used, using a pretest measure on each instructional objective; record time spent on program components, teacher-learner behavior, and other relevant measures of student use of the material; use a postassessment measure and release the materials for general use if performance is high on all objectives.

2. *Product revision.* Identify the objectives not well met; from data gathered in the verification step, propose revisions; test the revised version.

Learner data are most important in judging learnability. A more complete testing program should be used when there is no precedent for either the content or teaching method; when learning materials are more complex and expensive; when the materials seek to change attitudes rather than increase knowledge; when materials are designed for long-term rather than short-term use; and when the target audience is large. This involves repetitive tryouts with individuals to identify major errors, repetitive tryouts with small groups, and a field test when the materials are well-developed.

Planning and Implementing Instruction

All items necessary for constructing a teaching plan have been introduced. Evaluation, which is also part of the plan, is discussed thoroughly in Chapter 4. Because the purpose of a teaching plan is to force the teacher to examine the relationships among learner receptivity, objectives, content, teaching methods, tools, and evaluation, a plan should be written.

Teaching plans can be written in many formats. The major criterion for judging a format is whether it clearly states the various elements of the teaching process. Are the relationships among assessment-readiness, objectives, teaching actions, and content and evaluation clear? Is the format easy to follow in the urgent state created by teaching in a busy clinical situation? When teaching and learning are a major intervention, it is usual to construct a separate teaching plan, possibly one that can be incorporated into the general nursing care plan. An example appears in Figure 3-4.

Availability of good protocols, teaching tools, and forms for recording teaching are essential to ensure that teaching is actually being delivered to patients.

In purposeful, planned teaching, the caregiver carries out the plan. It cannot work perfectly, but it can be used as a guide unless feedback from the patient indicates clearly that it is inappropriate or ineffective. If this happens, the planning process must be repeated and new data must be added. Experienced teachers can do that on the spot and move ahead. Others will need to break the teaching session and, if possible, to replan and to reimplement.

Staff training is also important to implement programs. Traditional methods of teaching health professionals how to teach often focus only on the theoretical aspects of the teaching-learning process. Frequently, little is offered to help transfer this information into the practice setting. One approach involves apprenticing novice teachers to master teachers, allowing them to observe and participate and gradually do the teaching on their own with feedback from the master teacher. Videotaping teaching interactions provides an opportunity for self-evaluation as well as critique from a master teacher.

SAMPLE STANDARD TEACHING PLAN
Multiple Sclerosis

Patient Learning Objectives	Content	Education Mode	Modifications/Comments	Objective Met (Date/Initials)
Patient will define the remission/exacerbation aspects of the disease process.	Infection, trauma, immunization, delivery after pregnancy, stress, climactic changes How remission/exacerbation is experienced	E D		
Patient will demonstrate how to use various community resources.	Local and national multiple sclerosis society chapters Public health nurse Visiting Nurse Association Community support groups Social workers, therapists Vocational rehabilitation agencies Home health agencies Extended and skilled care facilities Financial counseling	E P V RP		
Patient will specify the safety precautions associated with symptoms.	Decreased sensation ⎤ Visual disturbances ⎬ Safety precautions Motor deficits ⎦	E R P		
Patient will take medications correctly and will recognize expected effects and side effects and interactions with over-the-counter medicines associated with each medication.	Corticosteroids ⎤ Immunomodulators ⎥ How to take— Cholinergics ⎬ recognizing expected Anticholinergics ⎥ effects and Muscle relaxants ⎦ side effects	E R RP		
Patient will perform exercises to promote muscle strength and mobility.	Measures for preventing contractures and skin breakdown Transfer techniques and proper body mechanics Use of assistive devices and other measures to minimize neurological deficits	E R V M		
Patient will diagnosis and self-manage constipation, urinary retention, or urinary tract infection (UTI), including proper self-catheterization technique or care of indwelling urinary catheters.	Constipation ⎤ Urinary retention ⎬ How to diagnosis and UTI ⎦ self-manage	E R		

Figure 3-4 Sample standard teaching plan.

Continued.

Patient Learning Objectives	Content	Education Mode	Modifications/Comments	Objective Met (Date/Initials)
Patient will identify indications of upper respiratory infection and implementation of measures that help prevent regurgitation, aspiration, and respiratory infection.	Cough, increased nasal and respiratory secretions, inability to tolerate breathing of cold air, temperature 100.4° F (38° C), dysphagia How to manage these effects	E V		
Patient will alter diet as necessary.	A nutritious, well-balanced diet Soft food for patients with chewing difficulties High-fiber diet for patients experiencing constipation	E V P M		
Patient will relate the importance of follow-up care to achieve desired outcomes.	Visits to physician Visits to physical therapist Visits to occupational therapists Speech, sexual, or psychological counseling	E P V		

Resource Box (list available patient resources here):

Education Mode Key	Signature	Initials

P = Pamphlet
B = Book
R = Reciprocal demonstration
D = Dialogue
E = Explication
V = Video
RP = Role playing
M = Modeling

Figure 3-4, cont'd   For legend, see preceding page.

SUMMARY

Educational objectives are based on assessment of the patient's readiness and need to learn; they are the framework for the instructional plan. Instructional forms and teaching materials are identified or constructed to provide the learning conditions necessary for meeting the objectives. Teaching plans put these elements together and guide implementation.

? STUDY QUESTIONS

1. A study of patients with lacerations who were treated in an emergency department found that those whose discharge instructional materials contained illustrations were 1.5 times more likely to choose correct responses than those whose instructions did not contain illustrations.[2] Would this finding surprise you?
2. A mother comments to you, "My baby has clumsy fingers." You determine that the child's growth and development are normal for his or her age but that he or she could profit from environmental stimulation to develop his or her eye-hand coordination and prehension. What kinds of general teaching approaches might be used?

REFERENCES

1. Anderson RM, Donnelly MB, Hess GE: An assessment of computer use, knowledge, and attitudes of diabetes educators, *Diabetes Educator* 18:40-46, 1992.
2. Austin PE and others: Discharge instructions: do illustrations help our patients understand them? *Ann Emerg Med* 25:317-320, 1995.
3. Basara LR, Juergens JP: Patient package insert readability and design, *Am Pharmacy* NS34(8):48-53, 1994.
4. Billiard SJ, Beattie S: A nontraditional approach to cardiac education: the use of cardiac catheterization films, *Prog Cardiovasc Nurs* 5:21-25, 1990.
5. Brennan PF, Moore SM, Smyth KA: The effects of a special computer network on caregivers of persons with Alzheimer's disease, *Nurs Res* 44:166-172, 1995.
6. Bulechek GM and others: Nursing interventions used in practice, *Am J Nurs* 94(10):59-64, 1994.
7. Busselman KM, Holcomb CA: Reading skill and comprehension of the Dietary Guidelines by WIC participants, *J Am Diet Assoc* 94:622-625, 1994.
8. Crowe L, Billingsley JI: The rowdy reactors: maintaining a support group for teenagers with diabetes, *Diabetes Educ* 16:39-43, 1990.
9. Davis TC and others: Reading ability of parents compared with reading level of pediatric patient education materials, *Pediatrics* 93:460-468, 1994.
10. DeBasio N, Rodenhausen N: The group experience: meeting the psychological needs of patients with ventricular tachycardia, *Heart Lung* 13:597-602, 1984.
11. Doak LG, Doak CC: Lowering the silent barriers to compliance for patients with low literacy skills, *Promoting Health* 8(4):6-8, 1987.
12. Fry E: A readability formula that saves time, *J Reading* 11:513-516, 1968.
13. Fry E: A readability formula for short passages, *J Reading* 33:594-597, 1990.
14. Gagliano ME: A literature review on the efficacy of video in patient education, *J Med Educ* 63:785-792, 1988.
15. Greene VL, Monahan DJ: The effect of a professional guided caregiver support and education group on institutionalization of care receivers, *Gerontologist* 27:716-721, 1987.
16. Gronlund NE: *How to write and use instructional objectives,* ed 5, Englewood Cliffs, NJ, 1995, Prentice-Hall.
17. Hall TA: Designing culturally relevant educational materials for Mexican-American clients, *Diabetes Educ* 13:281-285, 1987.
18. Iowa Intervention Project: Validation and coding of the NIC taxonomy structure, *Image* 27:43-49, 1995.
19. Jacobs MK, Goodman G: Psychology and self-help groups, *Am Psychol* 44:536-545, 1989.
20. Kilmon C: A taxonomy of pediatric primary care nursing interventions, *Nurs Health Care* 15:150-156, 1994.
21. Kozma RB: Learning with media, *Rev Educ Res* 61:179-211, 1991.
22. Kulik JA, Mahler HIM: Effects of preoperative roommate assignments on preoperative anxiety and recovery from coronary bypass surgery, *Health Psychol* 6:525-543, 1987.
23. Ley P and others: A method of increasing patients' recall of information presented by doctors, *Psychol Med* 3:217-220, 1973.
24. Madhumitan, Kumar KL: Twenty-one guidelines for effective instructional design, *Educ Technol* 35(3):58-61, 1995.
25. Meade CD, Howser DM: Consent forms: how to determine and improve their readability, *Oncol Nurs Forum* 19:1523-1528, 1992.
26. Meade CD, Smith CF: Readability formulas: cautions and criteria, *Patient Educ Couns* 17:153-158, 1991.
27. Meade CD, Wittbrot R: Computerized readability analysis of written materials, *Comput Nurs* 6:30-36, 1988.

28. Murphy PW and others: Rapid Estimate of Adult Literacy in Medicine (REALM): a quick reading test for patients, *J Reading* 37:124-130, 1993.

29. Nielsen E, Sheppard MA: Television as a patient education tool: a review of its effectiveness, *Patient Educ Couns* 11:3-16, 1988.

30. Starn J, Paperny DM: Computer games to enhance adolescent sex education, *MCN* 15:250-253, 1990.

31. Wolitski RJ, Rhodes F: AIDS info on-line: a computer-based information system for college campuses, *J Am Coll Health* 39:90-93, 1990.

4 Evaluation and Research in Patient Education

Evaluation determines the worth of something by judging it against a standard, usually as stated in the learning objective. Evaluation can serve several purposes. It can direct and motivate learning because it provides evidence about patients' accomplishments or skills they need to develop. Evaluation can also be used to judge whether someone ought to be selected or certified for having met a particular level of expertise. Patient education generally has not been used to provide a formal certification; however, evaluative judgments about learning commonly provide the basis for allowing a patient to progress to another setting, such as home. Evaluation also reinforces correct behavior on the part of the learner and helps teachers determine the adequacy of their teaching. In each situation it is important to think through the purpose of the evaluation first.

Once the standard is clear, the next step is to assign learners evaluative tasks. Ambiguous tasks produce faulty evidence and lead to faulty conclusions concerning how much the patient has learned. As a result the learner is confused. Evidence is compared with criteria or standards of adequate performance, and a judgment of adequacy or inadequacy is made. The teaching that follows a judgment of inadequate learning can correct errors in the patient's performance, present correct behavior, and explain the errors and correct behavior, as well as improve teaching.

Evaluation of programs of patient education is also necessary for teaching groups of patients over a period of time. Program evaluation provides direction for improvement of learning in individual patients and leads to judgments about how to improve the program.

Research in patient education is very important to evaluation because it establishes the kind of learning goal that can be attained and what is known about how best to attain it. The research base for patient education is now large, with some of it summarized through review articles or meta-analyses (a statistical approach to summarizing the results from multiple studies on the same question). A summary of the reviews and meta-analyses on patient education is presented in Appendix C.

OBTAINING MEASURES OF BEHAVIOR

All measurement involves observation of behavior. Such observation is more or less direct. Observations are more direct if the method of measurement involves viewing actual behavior as it occurs in natural settings and having access to its intended meaning. They are less direct if the method of measurement involves the subject's response to substitute situations that may be largely verbal and requires much inference of intended meaning. Each method contains certain weaknesses that can produce error in measurement.

Because one of the major purposes of measurement and evaluation activities is to predict how the individual will behave in the future, it is best to base this prediction on observation of actual behavior (direct measurement).

What people say they will do and what they actually do may be different. People often respond in ways that are socially acceptable. Behavior in the affective domain is perhaps the most difficult to measure because the individual can easily control the expression of feelings. Direct observation of behavior when the individual is unaware of being observed is the best opportunity for accurate assessment.

Although indirect measurements are risky, they also possess advantages that can contribute greatly to accurate assessment. Natural behavior is often inaccessible because it occurs in private: in family interactions. Natural behavior might occur infrequently and in various places. For example, it might surface in response to emergencies that require resuscitation measures, such as insulin shock, diabetic coma, or ingestion of poisons by a child.

Natural behavior might also occur infrequently, that is, at times when the observer may not be present. The strategy behind most tests used in indirect measurement is to present the situation in such a way that the provider can elicit the desired behavior in a written, oral, or performance response to a mock situation. Test results for complex behaviors are more accurate if the learner responds to situations on videotape rather than responding to written test situations.

Thus far in this chapter several major sources of error in measurement have been identified. One source of error is the constant possibility that indirect measures may present a false picture of the individual's behavior. A second source of error lies in the complexity of behavior. An observer may be unable to identify the causes of a particular behavior or be unable to measure thought patterns and attitudes even by direct observation. A third source is the bias of human observers. Observers cannot attend to or record all stimuli. They tend to assign meanings according to their own views. A fourth source of error is sampling. It is often not feasible in terms of time and effort expended to observe an individual's or a group's behavior repeatedly to account for the variation in performance from day to day and from situation to situation. It is not possible to inventory all aspects of an individual's knowledge about a particular subject. Obtaining samples over a period of time and in general areas of subject matter decreases error to an acceptable level.

The degree of error allowable depends on the predictions and decisions made and on the precision of the best measuring tool available. The provider should be more concerned with the person who needs to know how to care for a child's tracheostomy at home than with the person who needs to know how to do prenatal exercises. In both cases observing the learner engaged in the behavior would provide appropriate data for evaluation. However, for tracheostomy care the teacher should observe many times, measuring the learner's behavior against objective criteria agreed on by experts. To evaluate the learner's understanding, the caregiver can supplement the observation with oral or written questions asking what to do if the tube becomes dislodged or why suctioning is done a particular way. All methods of measurement are prone to particular errors. To arrive at a decision, the best information often can be gained by using a combination of methods.

Measurement involves obtaining a record of pertinent behavior. Not only is it difficult to record all that occurs, but this mass of information is not useful. The guideline for the pertinence of recording behavior is the objective. If this statement has met all the specifications for preciseness and clarity outlined in Chapter 3, it is much easier to decide which information is useful to record. Envision the difference in trying to evaluate these two patient objectives: (1) to know injection sites and (2) to draw on his or her own skin five areas suitable for injection of insulin. It is difficult to identify and measure the content and behavior of objective number one. Note that no time is stipulated in this objective. Tests limiting time are appropriate only if the learned behavior requires speed.

Rating Scales and Checklists

The most complete recording of behavior is obtained from videotape. This method offers the added advantage that it can be reviewed with the learner to offer feedback on performance. A videotape, however, does not provide access to the learner's thinking, unless he or she verbalizes it while recording. By itself it does not summarize the kind of behavior seen or identify its meaning in relation to objectives. To fill this need, a rating scale that describes pertinent behavior in words (anchored) can be constructed.

To reduce error in measurement, the words must be precise so that misinterpretation is avoided. For example, the rating scale (see accompanying box) can be refined so that several teachers who are observing a learner's behavior can independently classify it at one of the three points with little variation. If the raters cannot agree, the wording probably needs to be clarified. After the scale is refined, individual caregivers can use it by themselves.

Of course, it is possible for an individual to be displaying behavior from two different levels of functioning (see descriptions of behavior in sample rating scale in the accompanying box). For example, the patient may contaminate the syringe and needle fairly often (lowest level) but be quite skilled at removing bubbles from the syringe and measuring accurately (highest level). Usually, the behaviors are at adjacent levels on the rating scale because certain skills involve comparable levels of coordination. The difference may be that the learner is careless about contaminating. Checks can be made beside individual statements at various levels of the description. This will ensure that the teacher does not lose information about the learner's performance by checking just one of the categories on the line.

Another alternative is construction of several scales for this particular subobjective, each dealing with one set of behaviors—maintenance of sterility, obtaining and measuring fluid, or handling errors. Space is usually left below each rating scale for comments. A well-developed scale includes all pertinent points and rarely requires extra written comments. The form is developed to preclude recording behavior by writing it out at great length.

Other factors in the construction of a rating scale besides preciseness of the descriptions contribute to its quality as a measuring instrument. One factor is the number of levels of achievement represented in the behavior descriptions.

■ SAMPLE RATING SCALE

Subobjective: To obtain 1 ml of aqueous fluid for injection from a 2 ml vial with a 2 ml syringe, 22-gauge needle, using sterile technique.

•	•	•
Consistently uses contaminated syringe, needle, or top of vial. Cannot push needle through diaphragm. Is rarely aware of erring and if so usually does not know how to correct the error.	Occasionally contaminates. Can push needle through diaphragm. Has difficulty withdrawing all the fluid and obtaining accurate measurement (within 0.1 ml). Can usually diagnose errors while doing the procedure and correct them.	Rarely contaminates. Can obtain last few drops out of vial without damaging needle. Can measure within 0.1 ml even if bubbles are present. Can change needle or syringe if defective or contaminated. Corrects errors by self.

(Other scales can be developed for other subobjectives of the skill of giving an injection.)

The sample rating scale given here uses three levels of achievement because it is difficult for an observer to discriminate among more than five levels of achievement. Four or five steps could have been used. Note that the kinds of behaviors described in the scale are those that are crucial to the success of the skill as described in the objective: asepsis, accuracy of measurement, and ability to perceive and correct errors. Concerns such as inserting the needle precisely through the center of the rubber stopper or the particular manner in which the syringe is grasped are not considered crucial. The following is an example of a checklist that could be used in lieu of the sample rating scale on p. 71.

❏ Scrubbed top of vial with disinfectant sponge
❏ Punctured rubber vial with needle without contaminating
❏ Withdrew all of fluid from vial
❏ Expelled excess air from syringe without losing fluid
❏ Measured fluid to within 0.1 ml of the correct dose

The accompanying box provides an example of a performance-evaluation tool. Can it elicit critical data? Are the most important steps in this procedure included? Are some steps more crucial than others? If so, should these steps be marked so that patients who cannot do critical steps are identified? Would two health care providers watching a patient perform this procedure give him or her the same number of points? Might it help to include further descriptors of a correct performance for each step?

Oral Questioning

Oral questioning is a flexible form of measurement often used in combination with techniques such as observation. It attempts to reach those behaviors that cannot be easily observed. For example, the caregiver may ask patients questions to determine if they understand the basis for their actions in performing a psychomotor skill. Oral questioning also allows construction of hy-

---

■ VANCERIL INHALER PERFORMANCE EVALUATION

Directions: Give one point if step is done correctly, no point if done incorrectly.

1. Puts inhaler together correctly.   _____
2. Shakes inhaler.   _____
3. Holds inhaler correctly.   _____
4. Gives full expiration with pursed   _____
   lips through mouth.
5. Places mouthpiece in mouth   _____
   correctly.
6. Breathes in deeply through   _____
   mouth.
7. Activates aerosol while breathing   _____
   deeply.
8. Holds breath after activating   _____
   aerosol.
9. Waits between puffs.   _____
10. Shakes inhaler again.   _____
11. Replaces cap when finished with   _____
    entire procedure.

From Heringa P, Lawson L, Reda D: *Health Educ Q* 14:309-317, 1987.

---

pothetic situations that are not present in the actual teaching environment. Examples of these practices include asking a man learning to irrigate his colostomy why he is preparing the equipment as he is or asking a mother what she would do if her baby turned blue, which may include a demonstration of resuscitation techniques.

The method of oral questioning can be expensive in time, particularly if done in a one-to-one teacher-learner relationship. The strength of oral questioning over written testing is that the teacher knows immediately whether the learner understands the question and the teacher can let the learner know immediately whether the answer is right. In a group-teaching situation this kind of direct interchange is limited—although the reaction of one learner responding to another learner's answer can be very educational. In large groups the advantages of oral questioning are somewhat lost because every individual cannot respond to an oral question unless that response is in writing.

The verbal nature of both oral and written questioning may handicap individuals who have difficulty expressing themselves. Individuals probably find it easier to express themselves orally than in writing. In addition, those who are verbally fluent may *seem* to know more. For these reasons combinations of methods, such as observation of behavior and oral questioning, can often provide a truer picture than a single method can.

It is a common misconception that oral questioning does not require much preparation on the part of the teacher. Questions must be very carefully phrased so that (1) the learner can understand them and (2) they test the objective. With knowledge of the individual's previous exposure to an idea, questions can be phrased to stimulate thinking at any level of the cognitive domain. The box on p. 74 shows sample objectives and questions that should test various levels of thinking. Questions need to be carefully phrased to avoid leading the patient to the socially desirable answer or to "the answer" the provider wants, which may be an inappropriate reiteration of the information just presented by the provider. Such a circumstance may indicate that the patient has not comprehended the material well enough to express the idea in alternative ways.

Written Measurement

Written measurement is indirect and demands at least some reading skill and knowledge of test taking on the part of the learner. Well-constructed tests offer an excellent opportunity to measure learning at all levels of the cognitive domain, with considerable efficiency of teacher time.

Tests are prepared by individuals or groups of teachers in a particular institution and are used within that institution. They may be adapted to and published by other institutions, or they may be developed by test experts and sold. Tests sold commercially should provide a manual with in-

formation that explains the purposes of the test. Also, the manual should give evidence that it accurately measures the goals it claims to measure. Evidence should include information that describes how well the test covers the subject matter. If, for example, the test is meant to evaluate knowledge of nutrition, it should include items on all the major concepts in nutrition today. This quality of a test is called *content validity*. Additional information should describe how closely the test score is related to actual patient behavior in the present (*concurrent validity*) or the future (*predictive validity*). For example, if a patient with diabetes scores high on the test, is he or she giving good self-care now? Will he or she be giving good self-care in the future? A similar kind of statement about future self-care would be needed for those doing less well on the test. If a test contains a high degree of validity, its value for decision making is greater than that of a test with a low degree of validity.

Only rarely are locally developed tests studied this carefully. The teachers who use their own tests and have continuing contact with the same patients gain a feeling for how closely the test relates to their patients' actual behavior. However, these teachers rarely perform studies that provide them with accurate test-validity information. Measurement characteristics of certain knowledge tests in the patient education field have been carefully studied. Garrard and others[6] have reported on psychometric study of the Diabetes Information Test, and Devins and others[4] have reported on the initial development of a psychometrically sound instrument for measuring understanding of end-stage renal disease (ESRD). The ESRD test accurately discriminates between groups that differ in relevant knowledge of kidney disease. The test's reading level is grade 9. Consultation with nephrology nurses and physicians determined the content validity. One question arises: "Why was content validity not determined in consultation with patients who have ESRD?" This test comes in parallel forms (see box on p. 75); that is, patients can be retested for the same content without using the same

---

■ SAMPLE OBJECTIVES AND ORAL QUESTIONS FOR EVALUATION

Objectives	Questions
To state what effect worry in the mother may have on her breast milk (level of knowledge)	"What effect can worry have on a mother's breast milk?" (This question presumes that the learner has read or been told of this relationship.)
To translate instructions for time and route on a medicine bottle into appropriate action (level of comprehension)	Present to learners several medicine bottles with directions for time and route different from those on their own bottles. "How and when should these be taken?"
Given general knowledge of safety, to plan how to rid a house of safety hazards (level of application)	"How would you make your kitchen safer?" Repeat the question for bathroom and other rooms, being certain that areas covered include fire safety, electrical hazards, safety from poisons, safety from falling.
To distinguish how an uninformed opinion differs from scientific reasoning (level of analysis)	This can be analysis only if the individual has not been told or has not discussed the difference. Otherwise, he or she will repeat thoughts that are not original thoughts and will be at the level of knowledge or comprehension. Several examples of quack and scientific reasoning may be presented and the learner asked to state differences based on those samples.
To design an ileostomy bag that suits one's needs better than do available commercial ones (level of synthesis)	"For what reasons did you design the bag this way?" This would be combined with observation of the bag.
To assess the health care one is receiving in terms of its completeness, one's satisfaction with it, and the results obtained (level of evaluation)	"What quality of care would you say you have received? Consider its completeness, your satisfaction with it, and the results that have occurred."

---

items. Such tests would need regular updating because knowledge about kidney disease and its treatment changes.

Commercially produced, standardized tests with norms indicating the scores of large numbers of students are widely used in school settings. No such market exists in patient education. Measures of patient education outcomes have been seriously flawed, even in research literature. In reviewing studies on diabetes patient education between 1954 and 1986, Brown concluded that authors often developed new instruments of their own but usually did not address reliability and validity issues.[2]

Nationally distributed tests can have a beneficial effect in widening the staff's view. It is easier to teach patients how something is done in the institution where they receive care than it is to teach them by broad principles that might help them to transfer knowledge to other institutions and situations. Examining the content of a national test can help staff members recognize limitations in their own objectives by reviewing the objectives that others set for their learners.

Evaluation of patients' learning should be tailored to address the material that has been taught. Published tests may not reflect this material. Teachers may want to use a test item bank

KIDNEY DISEASE QUESTIONNAIRE: A TEST FOR MEASURING PATIENT KNOWLEDGE ABOUT END-STAGE RENAL DISEASE

Form A *

1. (1) People normally have two kidneys in the body.
   (a) True
   (b) False
   (c) Don't know

2. (5) When a person has kidney disease, his kidneys must be removed from his body before he can get treatment with a dialysis machine.
   (a) True
   (b) False
   (c) Don't know

3. (3) Kidneys do many important things in the body, but they function only at night while the person is sleeping.
   (a) True
   (b) False
   (c) Don't know

4. (25) What is the term used to describe the vibration or buzzing sensation that can be felt over the vein of a shunt or fistula?
   (a) Hypoplasia
   (b) Lobulation
   (c) Envervation
   (d) Thrill or bruit
   (e) Don't know

5. (11) In CAPD, waste substances pass from the blood, across the peritoneal membrane and into the dialysate fluid by a process called:
   (a) Diffusion
   (b) Transport
   (c) Excretion
   (d) Chemical breakdown
   (e) Don't know

6. (17) In addition to removing wastes from the blood, the artificial kidney also functions to remove excess water from the blood. This water-removal process is called:
   (a) Ultra-filtration
   (b) Ultra-refraction
   (c) Osmosis
   (d) Catharsis
   (e) Don't know

7. (9) A patient with kidney disease can experience high blood pressure, swelling, and rapid weight gain when his body becomes overloaded with:
   (a) Protein
   (b) Urea
   (c) Water
   (d) Don't know

8. (7) Which one of these foods has a lot of potassium?
   (a) Rice
   (b) Ice cream
   (c) Bananas
   (d) Don't know

9. (15) Approximately how many times a week do hemodialysis patients usually have their sessions on the kidney dialysis machine?
   (a) 1
   (b) 3
   (c) 6
   (d) Don't know

10. (14) A patient with chronic kidney diseases may have a living relative who wants to donate a kidney to the patient for transplantation. Which one of the following items about the donor is *FALSE?*
   (a) The donor will have to undergo a series of medical tests before the transplant operation.
   (b) The donor runs very little risk to his own health when he donates one kidney.
   (c) The donor will need to take immunosuppressive drugs for life.
   (d) After the transplant operation the donor's remaining kidney will enlarge in size.
   (e) Don't know.

From Devins GM and others: *J Clin Epidemiol* 43:297-307, 1990.
CAPD, Continuous ambulatory peritoneal dialysis.

Continued.

*Correct responses for Form A of the KDQ are as follows: item 1 (alternative a), 2 (b), 3 (b), 4 (d), 5 (a), 6 (a), 7 (c), 8 (c), 9 (b), 10 (c), 11 (d), 12 (a), 13 (d). Individual item scores (i.e., 0 vs. 1) are summed to generate a total score that can, thus, range between 0 and 13.

■ KIDNEY DISEASE QUESTIONNAIRE: A TEST FOR MEASURING PATIENT KNOWLEDGE ABOUT END-STAGE RENAL DISEASE—cont'd

11. (18) Which one of the following items about kidney transplantation is *FALSE*?
   (a) Sometimes a transplanted kidney will begin to function as soon as the blood vessels are connected on the operating table.
   (b) Kidney transplants are placed in the patient's pelvis rather than in the usual kidney location.
   (c) A person who has recovered from transplant surgery and has a new well-functioning kidney will no longer need dialysis treatment.
   (d) A patient can receive a kidney from a living relative but the donor's kidney must be removed one week before the transplant for close observation.
   (e) Don't know.

12. (20) CAPD is a form of dialysis treatment which is used as an alternative to hemodialysis. One *advantage* of CAPD is that:
   (a) It allows the patient to walk about freely during the course of treatment.
   (b) It only needs to be performed once a week.
   (c) It does not involve any preparatory surgical procedure.
   (d) It makes it easier for the patient to bathe and swim.
   (e) Don't know.

13. (23) Patients with chronic kidney disease are advised to eat limited quantities of potassium-rich foods. Elevated potassium level in the blood is dangerous because:
   (a) It can cause fluid overload.
   (b) It can raise the patient's hematocrit.
   (c) It can decrease the production of white blood cells.
   (d) It can cause the heart to beat irregularly and even stop.
   (e) Don't know.

*Form B**

1. (2) Kidney disease is a problem that comes with old age—young people do not get this disease.
   (a) True
   (b) False
   (c) Don't know

2. (4) Most types of kidney disease last about 5 years. After this the kidneys start to work normally again.
   (a) True
   (b) False
   (c) Don't know

3. (6) Peritonitis, an infection of the abdominal cavity, is one of the major problems for patients on CAPD.
   (a) True
   (b) False
   (c) Don't know

4. Kidney transplantation is the best form of treatment for patients with kidney disease because after the transplant the patients are less likely to get infections from bacteria or virus.
   (a) True
   (b) False
   (c) Don't know

5. (24) There are about one million tiny filters in the human kidney. They are called:
   (a) Ribosomes
   (b) Ureters
   (c) Glomeruli
   (d) Organelles
   (e) Don't know

6. (13) In kidney failure, waste products in the blood build up to abnormal levels and this causes a condition called:
   (a) Absorption
   (b) Uremia
   (c) Libido
   (d) Adaptation
   (e) Don't know

*Correct responses for Form B of the KDQ are as follows: item 1 (alternative b), 2 (b), 3 (a), 4 (b), 5 (c), 6 (b), 7 (d), 8 (a), 9 (b), 10 (a), 11 (b), 12 (b), 13 (a). Individual item scores (i.e., 0 vs. 1) are summed to generate a total score that can, thus, range between 0 and 13.

■ **KIDNEY DISEASE QUESTIONNAIRE: A TEST FOR MEASURING PATIENT KNOWLEDGE ABOUT END-STAGE RENAL DISEASE—cont'd**

7. (16) The artificial kidney is also called:
   (a) Henle's loop
   (b) Transferrin
   (c) BUN
   (d) Dialyzer
   (e) Don't know

8. (21) A new type of dialysis for treating kidney disease is called CAPD. Which part of the body makes this type of dialysis possible?
   (a) Peritoneum
   (b) Bladder
   (c) Renal pelvis
   (d) Don't know

9. (8) Patients with kidney disease are told not to eat salty foods because salt has a lot of:
   (a) Potassium
   (b) Sodium
   (c) Calcium
   (d) Don't know

10. (10) Immunosuppressive drugs are given to transplant patients in order to:
   (a) Prevent and treat rejection of the kidney graft.
   (b) Treat blood clotting in the new kidney.
   (c) Prevent infection of the kidney by virus or bacteria.
   (d) Raise the patient's hematocrit.
   (e) Don't know.

11. (19) Bone disease is a medical problem that could result from chronic kidney disease. It can occur because:
   (a) The diseased kidney can no longer rid the body of excess water in a normal fashion.
   (b) The diseased kidney loses its ability to keep calcium and phosphate levels in the proper range in the body.
   (c) The diseased kidney loses its ability to excrete excess potassium from the bloodstream.
   (d) The body is no longer able to use protein foods.
   (e) Don't know.

12. (12) Which medication is sometimes prescribed to control the level of potassium in the patient's body?
   (a) Riopan
   (b) Kayexalate
   (c) Amphojel
   (d) Aldomet
   (e) Don't know

13. (22) In the regular procedure for CAPD, dialysate fluid is introduced into the patient's abdominal cavity through an implanted tube just below the navel. The dialysate fluid is then:
   (a) Left inside the abdominal cavity for several hours and then drained out.
   (b) Left inside the abdominal cavity until it is completely absorbed into the body.
   (c) Transferred into an artificial kidney through another tube.
   (d) Transferred into an artificial kidney through the same tube.
   (e) Don't know.

NOTE: Items that comprise the 25-item version of the KDQ [not described here] are indicated in parentheses.

as an alternative. Banks contain large numbers of questions that have been keyed to lists of instructional objectives. The items are field tested, reviewed for content validity by experts, and judged technically sound. The developer of a new test on the subject matter covered by the item bank need only specify the objectives of a particular instructional program, suggest a desired number of items per objective, and allow a computer to select the items appropriate for the objectives. A test item bank for diabetes education has been described.[7]

Both so-called objective questions—multiple-choice, true-false, and matching items—and essay questions have their place in measuring health learning. Essay writing requires considerable skill in organizing and expressing ideas. It is more appropriately used in an academic setting than with patients. Thus essay questions for patients are usually shortened and made more specific. They are presented in oral or written form. An example is: "What should be done if your child eats poison, and why should it be done?" Note that this question, whether oral or written, requires recall of information. However, the response will elicit a different behavior than does discriminating among answers that are already present in multiple-choice, true-false, and matching items.

The ability to recall is desirable for information used frequently. It is essential for emergency situations, such as child poisoning, diabetic coma, or seizures. The objective is to be able to act on the information. A person must be able to produce the information from memory, not just recognize it among several alternatives. Periodic self-testing of memory for specific information will strengthen retention of infrequently used material. The strength of the recognition item is that it can enable learners to discriminate between ideas—ideas they might not otherwise consider—thus helping them test their depth of understanding.

As in the box on p. 79, items can be written to test all levels of cognitive behavior. The level measured by a particular question depends on the information the learner has received. The true-false item form is used to test knowledge or comprehension. The multiple-choice form is more flexible and can be used at all levels. Synthesis requires independent thought; therefore it is tested by methods that suggest no answers. At all levels visual materials can be incorporated into written questions. For example, the provider can show a mother four photos of umbilical cords and ask her to indicate the one(s) that need(s) to be called to the attention of the nurse midwife and which one(s) will probably drop off soon.

Numerous possible errors in the construction of single test items and groups of items can prevent an accurate assessment of an individual's cognitive skills.

For open-ended questions the provider can develop criteria for correct responses. The following questions were asked of parents: (1) What would you do if you just saw your child drinking a poison? (2) What would you do if your child just drank some toilet bowl cleaner? (3) What would you do if your child just drank some Drano or Liquid Plumr? Criteria for evaluating answers to these questions are described as follows[3]:

Response	Action
Incorrect response	Immediately make child vomit.
	Use ipecac without medical clearance.
	Give home remedy without seeking medical advice.
	Call ambulance.
	Miscellaneous response without therapeutic merit.
	No answer.
Partially correct	Rush child to emergency department or physician's office (for question 1).
	Follow directions on label of product ingested.
	Check a home reference for instructions.
	Neutralize poison, then call physician or poison control center.
Correct	Call physician immediately.

■ TEST ITEMS ON VARIOUS LEVELS OF THE COGNITIVE DOMAIN

Knowledge T F The hospital is required by law to use isolation with certain diagnoses.

Comprehension T F A patient will not be retained in isolation after a diagnosis is made.

Application Isolation is a means of containing the spread of microorganisms. How can these methods be used with a person at home who has a cold?

Analysis The basic principle(s) of our society that relate(s) to the reason isolation is used is (are):
a. Certain institutions have the right to carry out certain functions for the society.
b. An individual has certain rights.
c. The majority rules.
d. *a* and *b*.
e. *a, b, c.*

Synthesis Suggest a set of rules for isolation that will maximize the well-being of staff, visitors, and patients.

Evaluation It seems necessary to isolate persons with communicable disease to varying extents in order to protect others from the disease. Which one of the following policies would best achieve protection of the public and the welfare of the ill individual?
a. After diagnosis allow the individual and family a choice of sites for care.
b. Have a team of health personnel to enforce the proper degree of isolation in a hospital and the reporting of communicable disease.
c. Allow individual physicians and health agencies considerable latitude in establishing such policies.
(NOTE: The answer must not be in terms of opinion but must show evidence of judgment in terms of particular criteria, such as safety and psychological and sociological well-being.)

Correct—cont'd Call poison control center immediately.
Rush to emergency department (for questions 2 and 3 only).

In the box on p. 80 is a list of guidelines for writing multiple-choice test items.

Testing for trivia or for irrelevant material is an error to avoid. Consider the nurse who shows a film in conjunction with infant care classes. The following question is irrelevant to the objectives of most infant care classes:

The name of the movie you saw about your baby's bath was:
a. "Your Baby's Bath"
b. "Bathing Baby"
c. "Morning Adventure"
d. "Mother Loves Baby"

Clues in the language of the item give away the correct answer to someone who is test-wise. The following example, based on the pamphlet explaining isolation care, suffers from one clue—exactly the same terminology as that used in the teaching presentation:

T F Your illness may be transmitted to others.

In such a case the individual learns to recognize the words without necessarily knowing what they mean. Grammatical clues, such as a plural subject used in the stem, can make some choices in a multiple-choice question grammatically incorrect. An example, using a plural subject and a plural verb, follows:

Areas under the scalp where bone has not yet filled are known as:
a. Meconium

GUIDELINES FOR WRITING MULTIPLE-CHOICE TEST ITEMS

1. Make all distractors plausible.
2. Avoid "None of the above" as an option.
3. Make all the options approximately the same length.
4. Avoid negatively stated items, especially double negatives.
5. Randomly vary the position of the correct answer.
6. Avoid grammatical mistakes. Each option should fit grammatically with the stem.
7. Avoid using "All of the above" as an option.
8. Put as much of the item as possible into the stem. Do not repeat words in the options.
9. The stem should present a definition problem and not lead into a series of unrelated true/false statements.
10. There should be only one correct or best answer.
11. Avoid superfluous wording and irrelevant material.
12. Attempt to measure higher order learning by using novelty.
13. Use three to five options, depending on how many can be logically created for each item.
14. Do not give irrelevant clues to the correct answer.
15. Avoid specific determiners, such as always, never, all, none.

From Ellsworth RA, Dunnell P, Duell OK: *J Educ Res* 83:289-293, 1990.

b. An umbilicus
c. Fontanels
d. All of the above

The following matching item illustrates several problems with clues, ambiguity, and vocabulary level:

Directions: Match the body part with the action that best describes how to wash it.

Body part	Washing action
_____ 1. Vulva	a. With a pointed object
_____ 2. Neck	b. With a soft washcloth
_____ 3. Soft spot	c. Vigorously but gently
_____ 4. Ear	d. With a twisted piece of cotton

Mothers may not know the term *vulva* unless it has been specifically introduced to them. Some learners would eliminate choice *a* because they would know that no one washes the body with pointed objects. The fact that choice *a* is so much easier an item than the others makes it less plausible—a clue.

True-false items are notorious for having clues and can also be ambiguous. Statements containing absolute terms such as *all, always, certainly,* and *entirely* are more often false than true. Statements with words that qualify, such as *generally, sometimes, as a rule,* or *may,* are more often true than false. Uncertainty about the correct answer ensues when part of a question is true and part of it is false, as in the following example:

T   F   The umbilical cord may be swabbed with alcohol in order to dry it and sterilize it.

Many times true-false items that are long in text are true.

For all kinds of items, the best distractors (incorrect choices) are misconceptions that are common among learners. It is easy to learn about these misconceptions by listening to patients talk among themselves, with visitors, or with nurses or by watching them perform certain skills. The following is an example:

T   F   The soft spot should not be touched when the baby is being bathed.

Multiple-choice items suffer from high complexity and readability levels. The Kidney Disease Questionnaire on p. 75 is not atypical. The goal in test construction is to produce items that will assess the learner accurately. Clues and implausible distractors help the learner choose the correct answer by guessing. Individuals appear to know more than they do. By contrast, ambiguity makes it difficult for learners to demonstrate the knowledge that they actually have. Testing for trivia may be reliable in providing information, but it is information about unimportant learning. Such errors should be avoided.

Current test theorists suggest generating a number of items representing a domain (an objective) and randomly drawing a sample of items from each domain. For example, a major objective for instruction about bathing infants might be to cleanse the infant safely. First of all, much of the evaluation of learning in this situation should be accomplished by observing the mother's motor skills. For evaluation of cognitive skill a group of written items may be collected that test the objectives. Table 4-1 presents a summary of the advantages and disadvantages of various measures in evaluating patient education.

Earlier chapters placed emphasis on the emerging importance of self-efficacy as an outcome measure of patient education. Two examples of measures of self-efficacy in particular areas and for particular tasks are shown in the boxes on pp. 84 and 85.

EVALUATIVE JUDGMENTS

Measurement is carried out so that the teaching-learning process can be evaluated more accurately than it could be by general impressions. Evaluation must go beyond measurement. It requires a value judgment about learning and teaching. Evaluation must summarize the evidence and determine how well the objectives are being met.

Measurement and evaluation occur continuously during teaching, serving to redirect the activities of the teacher and the learner. Information about learners' progress is gathered by having learners respond to questions or perform periodically, or both. The expressions of boredom, interest, confusion, or enlightenment on learners' faces give clues about their understanding of the material being taught.

Some individuals are able to tell the teacher that they do not understand. Others cannot identify or express their uncertainty. To identify material that is not clear to the learner, the provider can retrace the explanation or the skill demonstration, can ask questions at intervals, or can observe and critique the performance of a skill by the learner. Such technique will point up terms used by the teacher that the learners may not understand, or it may reveal that the learners are overloaded with complex instructions. Trying to reteach without determining the nature of the learning problem may cause the caregiver to make the same error again. It is unwise to teach for a long time (or even one lesson period) without requiring the learner to respond so that teaching and learning errors can be corrected.

Adequacy of learning must eventually be evaluated in terms of meeting the final objectives. Of course, if satisfactory evaluation takes place as the teaching is going on, the degree of attainment of final objectives or the time needed to meet the final objectives can be quite accurately predicted.

Critical paths, which are discussed in more depth in Chapter 5, provide a structure of expected outcomes within particular time frames that guide all care, including patient education.

Crucial decisions regarding patients, such as whether they can live alone, rest on the outcome of learning. The minimum performance necessary for the individual to function must be identified. Certain basic information and skills must be learned because they are essential to the performance of a particular task. Other information and skills may also be crucial, depending on how independently the individual will be functioning. Therefore an adequate level of performance for one individual may not be sufficient for another.

When measuring learning, teachers focus on the element they have identified as crucial. In a test the learner should probably be able to answer or perform nearly 94% of all crucial behaviors. This figure allows for some error in the measurement tool. Patient education must be followed by questioning and the reteaching of crucial items when patients give incorrect responses. In giving a written test, the teacher may easily lose sight of the difference between essen-

Text continued on p. 86.

Table 4-1 Types of measurement

TECHNIQUE	ADVANTAGES	DISADVANTAGES
Direct observation	Performance under real or simulated conditions can be assessed Task is credible to patient Measure has good content validity	Awareness of the observer may affect performance Training, supervising, using observers are costly Number of patients who may be studied and their locale may be restricted because of the high per-patient cost of observing
Observational checklist	Simple, objective task to record observations Observer error low	Checklist may be long if a multi-faceted behavior is measured
Anchored rating scale	Simple, objective task to record observations Observer error low More gradations of judgment allowed than typical of an observational checklist	Difficult to write behavioral descriptions that differ by equal amounts over an ordered scale Descriptions may introduce several dimensions into a single rating
Observational record	Permits routine recording of simple, repetitive behaviors	Inferences depend on sample of time and fineness of recording unit
Anecdotal notes	May provide unique insights, illustrations	May be irrelevant to outcomes of interest
Critical incidents	Characterize adaptive and maladaptive behavior May serve as the basis for more structured measurement	Time-consuming to collect and analyze Focus on behavioral extremes; ignore typical behavior that is not outstandingly adaptive or maladaptive
Physiological measures	Measure is accurate Measure is a good indicator of health status Measure is responsive to compliance with health care regimen	Measure may be multiply determined; not affected by teaching outcomes alone Measure may depend on patient's willingness and ability to perform routine self-testing and recording Measurement may be costly to obtain and analyze Measurement may be invasive
Self-report	Provides data and insights not available from other sources Measures cognitive, affective, and performance outcomes directly	Subject to faking, socially desirable response set Requires skill in construction of instrument
Oral self-report	Little reading and no writing required of patient Contingent questions, probing, and question clarification possible Cheap, group administration of instruments is possible	Recording burden for interviewer Responses may be biased by interviewer Data collection individualized and costly

From McSweeney M: *Diabetes Educ* 7(3):9-15, 1981.

Table 4-1   Types of measurement—cont'd

TECHNIQUE	ADVANTAGES	DISADVANTAGES
Written self-report	Cheap, group administration of instruments is possible	Reading and recording burdens are placed on patient Questions are fixed; probes and clarifications cannot be introduced Possible reduction in response rate or quality resulting from respondent burden
Open-ended questions	Respondent free to shape reply	Extent of reply depends on verbal fluency of respondent Heavy recording burden for respondent or interviewer Inconsistent dimensions of response across patients Responses difficult to code and analyze
Closed, fixed-alternative questions	Easy recording, coding, processing of data Limited dimensions for replies Relative insensitivity to verbal fluency	Construction of instrument is time-consuming Dimensions on which choices will vary must be anticipated Choices may be forced among non-salient options
Single questions per topic	Speed, ease of response	Instability of response
Scales of questions per topic	Stability of response	Increased length of instrument
Self-monitoring	Recording occurs concurrently with behavior Access to all behaviors, covert and overt, is possible	Recording process may be reactive Quality of record is dependent on patient's cooperation Self-monitored data may differ from externally observed data
Records	*Noninvasive*—supply data without added demands on patients *Nonreactive*—relatively insensitive to external manipulation to claim desired outcomes Relatively low cost of collection	May not be organized to permit easy access retrieval Incomplete and/or inconsistent records Indirect measures; may not be directly relevant to teaching outcomes
Patient charts, physician records		May require health care professional to record and interpret relevant data Privacy considerations may restrict access to records or require hierarchy of obtained consents
Agency service records, public records and reports	Data may be collected by relatively unskilled workers	Data come from a variety of sources with varying degrees of accessibility, reporting standards, and variable conceptualization

■ COPD SELF-EFFICACY SCALE

Read each numbered item below, and determine how confident you are that you could manage breathing difficulty or avoid breathing difficulty in that situation. Use the following scale as a basis for your answers:

(a) = Very confident
(b) = Pretty confident
(c) = Somewhat confident
(d) = Not very confident
(e) = Not at all confident

1. When I become too tired.
2. When there is humidity in the air.
3. When I go into cold weather from a warm place.
4. When I experience emotional stress or become upset.
5. When I go up stairs too fast.
6. When I try to deny that I have respiratory difficulties.
7. When I am around cigarette smoke.
8. When I become angry.
9. When I exercise or physically exert myself.
10. When I feel distressed about my life.
11. When I feel sexually inadequate or impotent.
12. When I am frustrated.
13. When I lift heavy objects.
14. When I begin to feel that someone is out to get me.
15. When I yell or scream.
16. When I am lying in bed.
17. During very hot or very cold weather.
18. When I laugh a lot.
19. When I do not follow a proper diet.
20. When I feel helpless.
21. When I drink alcoholic beverages.
22. When I get an infection (throat, sinus, colds, the flu, etc.).
23. When I feel detached from everyone and everything.
24. When I experience anxiety.
25. When I am around pollution.
26. When I overeat.
27. When I feel down or depressed.
28. When I breathe improperly.
29. When I exercise in a room that is poorly ventilated.
30. When I am afraid.
31. When I experience the loss of a valued object or a loved one.
32. When there are problems in the home.
33. When I feel incompetent.
34. When I hurry or rush around.

From Wigal JK, Creer TL, Kotses H: *Chest* 99:1193-1196, 1991.
COPD, Chronic obstructive pulmonary disease.

■ ARTHRITIS SELF-EFFICACY SCALE*

Self-efficacy pain subscale

In the following questions, we'd like to know how your arthritis pain affects you. For each of the following questions, please circle the number which corresponds to your certainty that you can *now* perform the following tasks.

1. How certain are you that you can decrease your pain *quite a bit*?
2. How certain are you that you can continue most of your daily activities?
3. How certain are you that you can keep arthritis pain from interfering with your sleep?
4. How certain are you that you can make a *small-to-moderate* reduction in your arthritis pain by using methods other than taking extra medication?
5. How certain are you that you can make a *large* reduction in your arthritis pain by using methods other than taking extra medication?

Self-efficacy function subscale

We would like to know how confident you are in performing certain daily activities. For each of the following questions, please circle the number which corresponds to your certainty that you can perform the tasks as of *now, without* assistive devices or help from another person. Please consider what you *routinely* can do, not what would require a single extraordinary effort.

AS OF NOW, HOW CERTAIN ARE YOU THAT YOU CAN:

1. Walk 100 feet on flat ground in 20 seconds?
2. Walk 10 steps downstairs in 7 seconds?
3. Get out of an armless chair quickly, without using your hands for support?
4. Button and unbutton 3 medium-size buttons in a row in 12 seconds?
5. Cut 2 bite-size pieces of meat with a knife and fork in 8 seconds?
6. Turn an outdoor faucet all the way on and all the way off?
7. Scratch your upper back with both your right and left hands?

8. Get in and out of the passenger side of a car without assistance from another person and without physical aids?
9. Put on a long-sleeve front-opening shirt or blouse (without buttoning) in 8 seconds?

Self-efficacy other symptoms subscale

In the following questions, we'd like to know how you feel about your ability to control your arthritis. For each of the following questions, please circle the number which corresponds to the certainty that you can *now* perform the following activities or tasks.

1. *How certain* are you that you can control your fatigue?
2. *How certain* are you that you can regulate your activity so as to be active without aggravating your arthritis?
3. *How certain* are you that you can do something to help yourself feel better if you are feeling blue?
4. As compared with other people with arthritis like yours, *how certain* are you that you can manage arthritis pain during your daily activities?
5. *How certain* are you that you can manage your arthritis symptoms so that you can do the things you enjoy doing?
6. *How certain* are you that you can deal with the frustration of arthritis?

*Each question is followed by the scale:

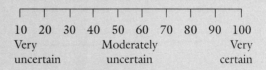

| 10 | 20 | 30 | 40 | 50 | 60 | 70 | 80 | 90 | 100 |

Very
uncertain

Moderately
uncertain

Very
certain

Each subscale is scored separately, by taking the mean of the subscale items. If one-fourth or less of the data is missing, the score is a mean of the completed data. If more than one-fourth of the data is missing, no score is calculated. (The authors invite others to use the scale and would appreciate being informed of study results.)

From Lorig K and others: *Arthritis Rheum* 32:37-44, 1989.

POSSIBLE ERRORS IN TEACHING-LEARNING PROCESS IF GOALS ARE NOT BEING MET

Readiness/motivation goals

1. Did the learner ever accept the goals, or were you teaching only what *you* believed to be important?
2. What evidence do you have that the goals were appropriate?
3. Were the goals clearly written and understood by teacher and learner?
4. Were the goals broken into sufficient intermediate steps to provide guidance?

Teaching-learning

1. Had teaching materials previously been tried with persons of ability similar to your patient and found successful?
2. If previous experience with the materials was not available, in what ways did their characteristics match the patient's readiness?
3. Were evaluative data gathered often during teaching, to give evidence of areas of success and lack of success?
4. Was teaching continued for sufficient time for learning to be thorough?
5. Were the data gathered for evaluation sufficiently valid and reliable to form an adequate basis for the evaluative decision?
6. Were baseline data obtained for measuring change? People rarely start with no knowledge or skill.

ual's ability to transfer knowledge and skills gained in the instructional situation to other situations described or suggested by the objectives. Thorough testing of transfer is necessary because knowledge about ways to produce and verify transfer without careful measurement is insufficient. Initial learning must be established well enough to allow for transfer. Stimulus variation (a variety of situations and tasks) in the initial learning produces transfer and determines how much time instruction and learning difficult tasks should take at various stages in the process of learning.

Suppose that related objectives are as follows:

- To take a diuretic in the prescribed dosage and at the prescribed time
- To recognize the desired and undesired effects of the medication
- To contact the nurse practitioner when undesired effects occur

Instruction for such objectives would no doubt include information about the purpose of the medication, the skills needed to take it, the monitoring of desired and undesired effects, the behavioral reinforcements for adherence, and the practice in problem situations related to taking the medication correctly. It is not feasible to give instruction that represents all possible situations an individual will encounter. If representative situations are used for teaching, most individuals can transfer information to similar situations. To check the amount of transfer the patient actually can make, questions should be constructed to deal with variations or combinations of themes already presented that represent situations the patient might encounter. With a series of questions it is possible to map the areas that the patient does and does not know. The following questions should require transfer (if they have not been used in original instruction):

1. Suppose you have intestinal flu with vomiting and diarrhea for several days. How would this affect the taking of your diuretic?
2. If the belts on your clothes feel tighter over a period of 3 days, what should you do?

tial learning and other items. The score may be added up, and the observer may decide that the learner, who has passed half the items, has learned adequately. The question may never be asked: Exactly what does he or she know? Observers of motor skills are more likely to realize intuitively that the individual who is not placing the crutches in the proper position will have difficulty learning to walk with them.

The person constructing the series of items must be sure that the plan measures an individ-

3. You are visiting friends for a few days, and you find that they do not have any citrus fruit. What should you do?

The interpretation of evaluation by teacher and learner is of utmost importance. Learners will have varying degrees of insight into their progress. Allowing for teacher bias, teachers and learners will agree more or less on the amount of progress that has been made. Learners should assess their progress and should discuss differences and similarities with regard to the teacher's assessment. This kind of interchange will help each party. However, when differences of opinion persist, the caregiver must maintain responsibility.

For example, a home health nurse may be teaching a daughter to give bed care to her older adult mother. After several sessions, the daughter believes that she is performing adequately. However, the nurse observes that the daughter is careless about regular turning and that foot support is not being used—lessons that have been taught. Whatever the daughter's reason, emotional or otherwise, for not giving essential care, the nurse is faced with a choice. One alternative is to find the basis for the lack of learning and reteach the learner, weighing the likelihood that the learner will change against the relative adequacy of the care. The other is to suggest that the learner make other arrangements for care because the nurse is responsible for supervision of care. Sometimes the learner becomes hostile toward the nurse. It is a way of expressing a desire to get out of the situation. Evidence of positive change in the learners is rewarding for the teachers as well as the learners.

The relationship between the learner's competence and the teacher's competence is entangled in evaluation. To some extent this relationship depends on which person is regarded as more responsible for learning. Sometimes it is obvious that a teacher cannot communicate or does not understand the subject matter. In this case the teacher needs to be helped to develop teaching skill. Teaching has the potential for being both harmful plus ineffective, and professional incompetence exists in this area of nursing or medicine,

as well as in any other. Possible harmful effects include leaving the patient with incapacitating confusion, a loss of self-confidence, or an inability to accomplish necessary reintegration into a family or other social group.

Evaluation of teaching and learning also includes a perspective of the known limitations of teaching today—particularly in the area of motivating individuals. Knowledge of the determinants of behavior at the present time is both limited and fragmented, and a practical means of assessing the relative influence of each factor is virtually nonexistent. Therefore in a particular situation it is difficult to estimate how each factor that is already present is influencing particular behavior and how new factors might affect behavior. In many of the complex situations that require learning, reality factors, such as poverty, health, and family crisis, limit the effect that teaching can have. In such situations small but important effects are characteristic even of the "good" programs.

One solution has been to use several complementary kinds of interventions (teaching may be one) to maximize the effect. Sometimes nothing seems to have an effect, and the individual or family does not recover from illness or achieve high-level wellness. Explanation may be sought through inquiry into the patient's perceptions, motives, values, intelligence, and grasp of relevant knowledge. It has also been suggested that the patient's situation might reflect a condition such as powerlessness, and his or her ability to learn may be only one of the behaviors affected.

Thus evaluation during and at the conclusion of a segment of teaching-learning is a summation and interpretation of the results of measurement. It reinforces successful behaviors of learners and teachers. It also provides a time to analyze progress and to redirect activities.

PROGRAM EVALUATION

Increasingly, patient education services are being organized into programs of common goals: teaching and evaluation approaches for patients with similar conditions and learning needs. The remainder of this book provides many examples of such programs.

Several preconditions must be met to evaluate an educational program. If they are not, proceeding may not be worthwhile. For example, the instructional program must have a reasonable design that can produce observable effects. If the goals are not clearly defined or if the teaching intervention will not yield the goals, the program should be redesigned before an institution spends the resources that a thorough evaluation requires. For example, if (1) the outcome of a program is to ensure patient adherence to a drug regimen, (2) needs assessment shows low adherence in the target group, yet (3) the program's design involves only a pharmacist who hands out drug information sheets when he or she has time, it is unlikely that the program as designed can meet its goals. Effecting adherence requires more than drug information, and a delivery system that is haphazard, diffuse, or unclear will not be effective.

Evaluation is especially important in the initial implementation of a recently designed program, when problem areas have been identified in a refined program, or when the program is introduced at a new site. It is also increasingly necessary to justify offering the program or to support accreditation or reimbursement requests. Unfortunately, regular collection of evaluative data is rare in patient education; instead, judgments are made on impressions, or teaching is assumed to be effective.

Ruzicki[9] outlines a series of steps in conducting an evaluation and illustrates this process with the evaluation of a cardiac rehabilitation program at her hospital as an example. The target audiences for the evaluation were identified as the hospital's patient education committee, the administration, cardiologists, and cardiac surgeons. Six evaluative questions were formulated: Does the program meet stated objectives for patient learning? Does it have an impact on changes in risk-factor behaviors after discharge? As a result of their participation in the program, do patients believe that they can manage their own care after discharge? Which teaching techniques are viewed as most helpful by patients? Are physicians satisfied with the program, and do they notice differences after discharge in patients who have participated? Are teaching staff members satisfied with the program, and do they implement it consistently? It is essential to focus the evaluation through development of questions. Because resources for evaluation in this example were limited, questionnaires were used and sample patients were studied.

Results of the evaluation showed that overall the program was functioning as it should. However, the evaluation revealed that there was a lack of documentation and that the nurses were not familiar with some of the information they were expected to teach or with the closed-circuit television films available. The evaluation clearly served as a management tool for improvement of the program.[9]

Some of Ruzicki's questions relate to evaluation of the outcomes of the program and some to process. Administrators are frequently interested in the cost per infection averted after a patient education program and in whether the program could be more cost efficient. Costs usually include personnel, equipment and depreciation, materials, other operating expenses, and sometimes a portion of overhead costs. The easiest way to get a sense of efficiency is to compare one program with another one that shows the same outcomes and utilization. Administrators also are interested in such statistics as unplanned readmissions that can be traced to inadequate or prematurely terminated care, including incomplete patient learning. Readmission data have been used by many payers to screen for quality of care. Ashton and others[1] have developed readiness-for-discharge criteria covering clinical stability, education of the patient and family, and follow-up medical care among patients with diabetes, heart failure, and obstructive lung disease. Use of these criteria to time discharge appropriately will diminish costly early readmission, a significant financial concern in today's payment climate.

RESEARCH IN PATIENT EDUCATION

Reference to the research base that strengthens patient education practice is made throughout this book. In addition, Appendix C presents 42 meta-analyses or research reviews of bodies of studies in patient education. This work, which began to appear in the literature in 1979, continues to accumulate. Although it covers a wide range of topics, most of the work has focused on diabetes education and preprocedure and postprocedure (including preoperative and postoperative) education. Overall, these research summaries show that patient education or psychoeducational interventions (which implies a strong behavioral focus) studied in this research were effective on a wide variety of patient outcomes and contributed significantly to patient welfare.

This body of work shows limitations in the research base for patient education. Few studies have addressed the costs of patient education and the savings it produces; this is a serious omission. Study designs frequently do not provide evidence about what mechanisms in the educational interventions were effective, and sometimes whole bodies of work do not appear to include educationally relevant elements, such as feedback, in their interventions. In addition, studies of culturally diverse populations tend to be limited, thus providing little guidance for educational interventions for these groups.

Summaries of research, particularly meta-analyses, allow us to determine when enough attention has been paid to particular research questions, so that available resources are used for more relevant questions. In general, simple tests of the efficacy of educational interventions have been well studied; attention should rather be turned to more direct comparisons of different kinds of educational interventions.

An example of process, outcome, and, to a certain extent, efficiency outcome in a public health setting has been reported by Dignan and others.[5] The Forsyth County Cervical Cancer Prevention Project is a community-based health education program designed to encourage African-American women in the target population to obtain Pap smears on a regular basis and to return for follow-up care when necessary. Process monitoring is done to ensure documentation of program activities, such as distribution of printed materials and coverage of the target population. Those monitoring the process discovered that leaflets distributed in grocery stores were not reaching low-income women often enough. Thereafter distribution of the leaflets was timed to coincide with receipt of Social Security payments. Interviewing members of the target population provided perspective about which materials and activities were having the greatest impact in raising awareness of cervical screening. In addition, morbidity and mortality data were used. Evaluation served to redirect and improve the campaign as it went along at a cost of 7% of the project's annual expenditures.

SUMMARY

Although evaluation is the final step in the process of teaching-learning, it is forward-looking because its message redirects activity (box, p. 86). Information necessary for an evaluation of how well objectives have been met is gathered by various measurement techniques. A concerted effort is made to gather reliable information by perfecting measuring tools and by using them in conjunction with one another. This method provides a sounder basis for decisions about the competence of the learner to behave in the manner specified in the objectives.

A large body of research results have accumulated that support the efficacy of the patient education interventions tested in those studies.

❓ STUDY QUESTIONS

1. You observe a nurse who has been teaching a patient how to give himself an injection. The nurse asks the patient the following questions as he goes through the procedure: Is it all right to give the injection with the same sy-

ringe and needle you used yesterday? Review why you are wiping the skin a particular way.

What would you do if the tip of the needle touched the table as you were picking up the syringe?

What would you do if you touched the skin now (after it has been cleansed with the alcohol sponge and before the injection is given)?

State the subobjective that the nurse is evaluating.

2. How is the notion of transfer used in evaluation?

3. You are trying to teach a mentally disabled youngster self-dressing skills, and he is inattentive and rebellious. It is obvious that he is showing lack of motivation to learn. List three possible factors that might be producing this behavior, and indicate the action a caregiver might take in response to each.

4. You are the teacher in a class for patients with diabetes, who make the following comments. What evidence does each question or comment give about the individual's understanding?

   a. "Would blood sugar be the same for man, woman, or child?"

   b. "I don't feel I'm really a diabetic because I don't have to take insulin." (Patient is a 19-year-old girl in whom pregnancy precipitated signs and symptoms of diabetes. The physician has ordered that her diabetes be controlled by diet.)

   c. Father whose 8-year-old son has newly diagnosed diabetes, talking to a college student who has been insulin-dependent for 2 years: "Are you able to hunt?"

5. Read the article by Frances Taira on individualized medication sheets,[10] and study Table 3, Medication Knowledge Tool: Interview and Assessment. Do the test items adequately test the objectives? Would two different providers using this test come to the same conclusion about the patient's knowledge?

6. Read the article by Margaret Reuter on parenting needs of abusing parents.[8] Focus on the evaluation tool reproduced in the appendix to the article. Is this tool a measure of feelings, as indicated in the directions?

REFERENCES

1. Ashton CM and others: The association between the quality of inpatient care and early readmission, *Ann Intern Med* 122:415-421, 1995.
2. Brown SA: Quality of reporting in diabetes patient education research: 1954-1986, *Res Nurs Health* 13:53-62, 1990.
3. Dershewitz RA, Posner MK, Paichel W: The effectiveness of health education on home use of ipecac, *Clin Pediatr* 22:268-270, 1983.
4. Devins GM and others: The Kidney Disease Questionnaire: a test for measuring patient knowledge about end-stage renal disease, *J Clin Epidemiol* 43:297-307, 1990.
5. Dignan MB and others: Use of process evaluation to guide health education in Forsyth County's Project to Prevent Cervical Cancer, *Public Health Rep* 106:73-77, 1991.
6. Garrard J and others: Psychometric study of patient knowledge test, *Diabetes Care* 10:500-509, 1987.
7. Nowacek GA, Pichert JW: An item bank of diabetes related test questions, *Diabetes Educ* 11(3):37-41, 1985.
8. Reuter MM: Parenting needs of abusing parents: development of a tool for evaluation of a parent education class, *Commun Health Nurs* 5:129-140, 1988.
9. Ruzicki DA: Evaluation: it's what you do with what you've got that counts, *Promot Health* 6(4):6-9, 1985.
10. Taira F: Individualized medication sheets, *Nurs Econ* 9:56-58, 1991.

II | THE INFRASTRUCTURE FOR DELIVERY OF PATIENT EDUCATION

Introduction to Part II

DELIVERY OF PATIENT EDUCATION

Patient education is currently defined as an essential part of practice in state nurse practice acts, in various federal and state regulations, and in accreditation criteria (see Appendix D for hospital accreditation criteria). Because patient education has not usually been a reimbursable service and does not bring in revenue, the degree of formalization of a structure for delivery of these services seems to have fluctuated and may now be at a lower ebb than it was during the 1980s.

The health care system in the United States is presently in transition to capitated payment arrangements. This change means that the provider/institution is paid a set amount and needs to manage a panel of patients within that preset amount. This situation creates more positive incentives because education can be used to teach people how to manage their own self-care and avoid expensive use of institutional services. In spite of these changed incentives, it is not clear how many patients who are in need of appropriate patient education actually receive it.

Very limited data are available about patient education services. The American Hospital Association reports that 86% of hospitals in the United States offer patient education services on a formal basis[1]; thus it could be assumed that all professional care would incorporate education as part of the provider-patient interaction. Limited survey data of hospitals in various states revealed the following information:

- Rural hospitals in North Carolina were as likely to offer health promotion programs as were larger urban hospitals. Most commonly available programs were education in car-

diopulmonary resuscitation (CPR) and acquired immunodeficiency syndrome (AIDS) education. The most common method of financing these services was to charge participants a small fee.[4]
- In Iowa 99% of rural hospitals offered an average of 7.5 health promotion programs on a regular basis to community residents. The most common types were blood pressure and cholesterol screening, safety and protection, diet/nutrition, prenatal/maternal health, and breast cancer screening programs.[8]
- In New York State a new hospital-reimbursement law requires that all voluntary, nonprofit hospitals develop community service plans; frequently these plans consist of classes for family caregivers on topics identified through community assessment.[10]

Apparently no data about the availability of patient education services in nonhospital sectors of the health care industry are available. Commonly, both individual providers and institutions offer patient education services, including newsletters, as a form of marketing to draw patients to their practices.

Several kinds of initiatives in which patient education is central can be cited.

- The Cooperative Care Unit at New York University Hospital, first established in 1979, is designed especially for the treatment and education of acutely ill patients who face changes in lifestyle.[6] These patients must have a care partner and must be relatively mobile. The patient may be admitted directly from home for a presurgical procedure (e.g., cardiac catheterization) or for medical treatment (e.g., radiation) or the patient may be admitted by transfer from the main hospital. The cost of this care has been documented to be considerably less than the daily hospital charge. The unit has a homelike atmosphere and provides privacy for patient and partner; however, emergency care is always available by telephone. Patients have schedules of appointments, with the Education Center central to the services. Evaluation of this program found that it has significant educational and management advantages and is enthusiastically accepted by its clients.[3]

- The Planetree model[16] operates on a philosophy of compassion, dignity, shared knowledge, and the freedom of informed choice. The first unit was established in 1981; four units have now been established nationally. The physical space for the unit reflects its philosophy—with a homelike, healing environment and a schedule set by patient needs. Patients are assisted in understanding their illness and therapy; and they are guided toward achieving wellness through resources such as a library of printed and videotaped materials.

- Practice guidelines, which define the standard of practice based on research, are now widely used in health care settings to improve the quality of care and to minimize undue variability in care. They frequently contain information to help patients understand the area of treatment and how to determine the quality of the treatment they are receiving. The Agency for Health Care Policy and Research (AHCPR) has developed multiple research-based guidelines, including those for management of acute pain. One institution attempting implementation of these guidelines found a number of problems; for example, parents had a significant lack of knowledge about the role they could take in assisting with their child's pain control. Relevant information frequently was not included in preoperative teaching. This finding prompted the institution to develop the standard of care statement shown in the accompanying box.[15] Note that these are process-oriented standards of care; one would hope for standards that also require attainment of an established level of patient outcome—in this case, in level of pain control.

ILLUSTRATIVE STANDARD OF CARE FOR PEDIATRIC PAIN MANAGEMENT

Education of the patient and family
- The patient and family will receive written and verbal information about pain management preoperatively in the clinic, or on admission to the hospital.
- The nurse will document the goals and expectations identified by the patient and family.

Assessment of pain
- Assessment of pain on the nursing unit will be done immediately on admission and at least every 4 hours for the first 24 hours postoperatively.
- The same pain scale will be used consistently with the patient and family throughout the hospital stay.
- Patients will be reassessed for pain within 30 to 60 minutes after all pain interventions.

Interventions for pain
- Pain control intervention will be provided around-the-clock (e.g., every 4 hours) for at least the first 24 postoperative hours, unless refused by the patient. Interventions can be moved to an "as-needed" schedule at the discretion of the nurse after 24 hours.
- Intervention will be offered on an "as-needed" basis if the child reports a pain rating of 3 or above on the Wong and Baker faces scale or the numeric scales, or if physiological or behavioral indicators of pain are present.
- Equianalgesic conversion charts will be used when converting a patient from IV medications to oral medications.

From Schmidt K and others: *J Nurs Care Qual* 8(3):68-74, 1994.

- Clinical practice guidelines are commonly translated into critical paths, or pathways, now widely used as multidisciplinary care plans, particularly for expensive hospital services provided to patients with predictable courses of recovery. Examples of critical paths are presented for total hip replacement (Figure 1), vaginal delivery (Figure 2), and open heart surgery (Figure 3). These paths serve as the central organizing tool of clinical action across disciplines and are in place around the clock.[17] They offer the advantages of clearly integrating patient education into the plan of care and ensuring that it contributes to meeting both time-based process standards and outcome standards. Variations from the critical path must always be justified. In addition, critical paths serve as educational tools for patients and family members who follow their expected course of recovery.
- A current public education campaign, the National Eye Health Education Program established by the National Eye Institute, addresses eye disease and vision loss, particularly for persons with diabetes.[14] It educates through public service advertisements in magazines and newspapers that stress the importance of an eye examination at least once a year in which the pupils are dilated and that offer information kits to providers.
- Delivery systems for pharmaceutical care have been significantly affected by regulations for patient education. Although a 1990 federal law requires pharmacists to counsel patients on Medicaid about their prescriptions, many states have recently adopted laws requiring the counseling of all patients.[13] In addition, pharmacy benefit managers (PBMs) now serve as more than purchasing and dispensing agents; they monitor drug use and practice disease state management, focused at keeping the disease under control and saving resources. PBMs usually start with diabetes and asthma, two of the most costly conditions for plan sponsors. If the medical claims and test results data suggest that a patient's diabetes may not be controlled adequately, a letter is sent to the primary care physician, noting that the health maintenance organization (HMO) will provide special educational services and coverage of diabetes-specific tests and monitoring devices. If the data base indicates a person with asthma reorders a bronchodilator too often, chances are that the individual does not know how to use it correctly. The plan will alert and pay a pharmacist to counsel the patient on correct use.[12]
- Patient access to medical information in health science libraries has been slow to develop; 58% of these facilities allow patient access without restrictions, and 20% require physician approval. The trend of developing special collections for patients has been slow to develop, and 10% of hospital libraries provided no patient education forum.[7]
- In workplaces workers are being empowered to adopt healthier lifestyles, including smoking cessation, weight reduction and control, blood pressure and cholesterol monitoring, stress management, and nutrition education, as well as being provided access to a fully equipped gym. Employees are coached about how to be more active participants in their own care, including how to prevent and treat ailments and when to call a provider. Ongoing nurse counseling is provided via a toll-free telephone line. Businesses report that such programs yield significant cost savings in health care and in reduced sick days.[2]
- Because of a changed financial environment, some hospitals have eliminated entire education or health promotion departments or individual education positions. Others have reinstituted patient education coordinators or staff members to manage expansion into ambulatory areas.[5] Limited data are available about what portions of the structures common in the 1980s still exist in hospitals—that is, individual departments and interdisciplinary patient education committees that set institutional policy and approve and coordinate individual patient education programs.
- Patient education councils have been growing across the United States since the middle of

Text continued on p. 105.

TOTAL HIP REPLACEMENT (ELECTIVE) CARE PATH

	Pre-hospital	OR Day Inpatient Day 1	Post-op Day 1 Day 2	Post-op Day 2 Day 3	Post-op Day 3 Day 4	Post-op Day 4 Day 5	Post-op Day 5 Day 6	Post-discharge
Outcomes	Patient/family verbalize understanding of plan of care Patient/family will identify post hospital destination Patient satisfied with process of preparation Abnormal labs are identified/addressed Patients who want short-term rehab have initiated application Anesthesia plan in place Pre-surgical evaluation through patient survey: SF-36, WOMAC	Anesthesia plan consistent with pre-op plan	Patient progressing per PT protocol Adequate pain relief Stable HCT	Patient progressing per PT protocol Adequate pain relief	Patient progressing per PT protocol Patient/family confirm pre-hospital discharge plan Adequate pain relief	Patient discharged home with referral to community agency Patient verbalizes understanding of home education program	Patient discharged to SNF or home	Outcome evaluation through patient survey: SF-36, WOMAC (6 months post-op)
Consults needed	Physical therapy Anesthesia Discharge planning Blood bank	Anesthesia Physical therapy Occupational therapy	PT OT Anesthesia (if epidural)	PT OT Anesthesia (if epidural)	PT OT Anesthesia (if epidural)	PT OT	PT OT	Patient at home or SNF
Diagnostic studies	Blood work Urinalysis EKG Chest x-ray Other studies as needed	X-ray in PACU H&H in PACU	HCT in AM Other labs as needed	HCT in AM Other labs as needed	HCT in AM PLTS in AM Other labs as needed	Other labs as needed	Other labs as needed	Lab work per MD order

Figure 1   Example of critical pathway for total hip replacement. (From John Dempsey Hospital, University of Connecticut, Farmington, Conn. Used with permission.) CSM, Circulatory sensation movement; D/C, discontinue; HCT, hematocrit; IS, incentive spirometer; OOB, out of bed; OT, occupational therapy; PACU, postanesthesia care unit; PAS, type of stocking; PLTS, platelets; PT, physical therapy; SNF, skilled nursing facility; TEDS, anti-embolism stockings; VS, vital signs; WOMAC, instrument for measuring functional status.   *Continued.*

	Pre-hospital	OR Day Inpatient Day 1	Post-op Day 1 Day 2	Post-op Day 2 Day 3	Post-op Day 3 Day 4	Post-op Day 4 Day 5	Post-op Day 5 Day 6	Post-discharge
Treatments (procedures)		Pain assessment per appropriate pain protocol VS & CSM q 4 hr Foley to closed drainage TEDS stockings/ PAS Hemovac to suction IS q hour while awake Monitor primary dressing	Pain assessment per appropriate pain protocol VS & CSM q 4 hr Foley to closed drainage TEDS stockings/ PAS Hemovac D/C IS q hour while awake Monitor primary dressing	Pain assessment per appropriate pain protocol VS & CSM q 8 hr Foley to closed drainage TEDS stockings/ PAS IS q hour while awake Primary dressing changed by MD then dressing/ incision care per MD order	Pain assessment per appropriate pain protocol VS & CSM q 8 hr D/C Foley at 8 AM per nursing protocol TEDS stockings/ PAS IS q hour while awake Dressing/incision care per MD order D/C epidural cath	Pain assessment per appropriate pain protocol VS & CSM q 8 hr TEDS stockings/ PAS Dressing/incision care per MD order	Pain assessment per appropriate pain protocol VS & CSM q 8 hr TEDS stockings/ PAS Dressing/incision care per MD order	Incision care per MD order
Treatments (medications)		IV fluids Antibiotics Tx Stool softeners Pain medications Anticoagulation Tx Routine meds	D/C IV fluids when PO adequate Antibiotic therapy Stool softeners Pain medications Anticoagulation therapy Routine meds	Stool softeners Pain medications Anticoagulation therapy Routine meds	Stool softeners Pain medications Anticoagulation therapy Routine meds	Stool softeners Pain medications Anticoagulation therapy Routine meds	Stool softeners Pain medications Anticoagulation therapy Routine meds	Stool softeners Pain medications Anticoagulation therapy Routine meds
Diet		Clear liquids or diet as ordered	Regular or special diet as needed	Regular or special diet as needed	Regular or special diet as needed	Regular or special diet as needed	Regular or special diet as needed	Regular or special diet as needed
Activities allowed		Bedrest in abduction pillow	Dangle with PT BID Abduction pillow while in bed	Progressive activity per PT protocol: OOB to chair Regular pillow between legs while in bed/chair	Progressive activity per PT protocol Regular pillow between legs while in bed/chair	Progressive activity per PT protocol Regular pillow between legs while in bed/chair	Progressive activity per PT protocol	Partial weight bearing × 6 weeks (cemented) Toe touch weight bearing × 6 weeks (uncemented)
Patient education	Patient education video Patient education booklet	Nursing patient education protocol Patient education booklet	Nursing patient education protocol Patient education booklet	Nursing patient education protocol Patient education booklet	Nursing patient education protocol Patient education booklet	Nursing patient education protocol Patient education booklet	Nursing patient education protocol Patient education booklet	
Discharge planning efforts	Referral to discharge planning Application for short-term rehabilitation initiated if needed	Discharge planning education Social work if referral to SNF	Discharge planning education Social work if referral to SNF	Discharge planning education Social work if referral to SNF	W-10 completed with referral to community agency	Discharge summaries completed: Nurse PT	Social work referral to SNF	

HARTFORD HOSPITAL CRITICAL PATHWAY POST PARTUM UNCOMPLICATED VAGINAL DELIVERY
(DRG373)

PATIENT CARE COORDINATOR: _____
ADMISSION DATE: _____   ADMISSION TIME: _____
DISCHARGE DATE: _____   DISCHARGE TIME: _____

LOS: EXPECTED: _____   ACTUAL: _____
PATIENT STATUS:

PATHWAY NOT CLINICALLY APPLICABLE: _____

TX NEW PATHWAY: NAME: _____
CP030302

0-6 HOURS AFTER ADM. TO UNIT
TIME: _____

Columns: N | A(D E) | V

OUTCOMES*
1. Temp/Vital Signs WNL
2. Post partum assessment WNL
3. Demonstrates appropriate breastfeeding skills as indicated
4. If breastfeeding, nipples WNL
5. Verbalizes adequate level of comfort
6. Voiding qs
7. Tolerating diet
8. Ambulates with assistance initially
9. Verbalizes understanding of hospital/unit routine
10. Verbalizes understanding of restrictions regarding 1st time OOB
11. Demonstrates positive parent/infant/family interaction
12. Demonstrates safe infant care skills
13. Maintains safe maternal environment
14.
15.
16.
17.
18.
19.

6-12 HOURS
TIME: _____

Columns: N | A(D E) | V

OUTCOMES
62. Temp/Vital Signs WNL
63. Post partum assessment WNL
64. Demonstrates appropriate breastfeeding skills as indicated
65. If breastfeeding, nipples WNL
66. Verbalizes adequate level of comfort
67. Voiding qs
68. Tolerating diet
69. Ambulates independently
70.
71.
72. Demonstrates positive parent/infant/family interaction
73. Demonstrates safe infant care skills
74. Maintains safe maternal environment
75. Patient receives prevention for RH sensitization if indicated
76.
77.
78.
79.
80.

12-24 HOURS
TIME: _____

Columns: N | A(D E) | V

OUTCOMES
123. Temp/Vital Signs WNL
124. Post partum assessment WNL
125. Demonstrates appropriate breastfeeding skills as indicated
126. If breastfeeding, nipples WNL
127. Verbalizes adequate level of comfort
128. Voiding qs
129. Tolerating diet
130. Ambulates independently
131.
132.
133. Demonstrates positive parent/infant/family interaction
134. Demonstrates safe infant care skills
135. Maintains safe maternal environment
136.
137. Demonstrates and verbalizes understanding of post partum self care, infant care, safety
138. Verbalizes understanding of discharge instruction sheet for self/infant at discharge
139. Immunized against rubella if indicated at discharge
140. Discharged at 24 hours
141.

* Refer to page ④ for key.
HH7013.doc Rev. A 11/95

①

NAME: _____

0-6 HOURS AFTER ADM. TO UNIT

TIME: _____

	N	D	E	V
CONSULT				
20. Evaluate need for and initiate prn				
21.				
ASSESSMENT				
22. Temp/Vital Signs on admission and at 2 hours				
23. Breasts, fundus, lochia, and episiotomy on admission and at 2 hours				
24. Pain level per scale				
25. Urinary Output				
26. Parent/infant/family interaction				
27. Infant care/feeding skills				
28. Environmental maternal safety q shift				
29. Review prenatal ACOG record				
30. Complete admission data base				
31. Complete initial assessment/problem list				
32.				
TESTS				
33.				
NUTRITION				
34. Diet ordered as tolerated				
35.				
MEDICATIONS				
36. Scheduled medications as ordered				
37. PRN analgesics				
38. Dibucaine prn				
39.				
40.				
41.				
TREATMENT/INTERVENTION				
42. Ice to perineum prn				
43. Tucks prn				
44. Breast pump prn				
45.				
46.				

6-12 HOURS

TIME: _____

	N	D	E	V
CONSULT				
81. Evaluate need for and initiate prn				
82.				
ASSESSMENT				
83. Temp/Vital Signs at 6 hours and 10 hours				
84. Breasts, fundus, lochia, and episiotomy at 6 hours and 10 hours				
85. Pain level per scale				
86. Urinary Output				
87. Parent/infant/family interaction				
88. Infant care/feeding skills				
89. Environmental maternal safety q shift				
90.				
91.				
92.				
93.				
TESTS				
94.				
NUTRITION				
95. Diet ordered as tolerated				
96.				
MEDICATIONS				
97. Scheduled medications as ordered				
98. PRN analgesics				
99. Dibucaine prn				
100. Rhogam given if indicated				
101.				
102.				
TREATMENT/INTERVENTION				
103. Ice to perineum prn				
104. Tucks prn				
105. Breast pump prn				
106. Sitz bath prn				
107.				

MEDICAL RECORD# _____

12-24 HOURS

TIME: _____

	N	D	E	V
CONSULT				
142. Evaluate need for and initiate prn				
143.				
ASSESSMENT				
144. Temp/Vital Signs each shift until discharge				
145. Breasts, fundus, lochia, and episiotomy each shift until discharge				
146. Pain level per scale				
147. Urinary Output				
148. Parent/infant/family interaction				
149. Infant care/feeding skills				
150. Environmental maternal safety q shift until discharge				
151.				
152.				
153.				
154.				
TESTS				
155.				
NUTRITION				
156. Diet ordered as tolerated				
157.				
MEDICATIONS				
158. Scheduled medications as ordered				
159. PRN analgesics				
160. Dibucaine prn				
161.				
162. Rubella given if indicated				
163.				
TREATMENT/INTERVENTION				
164.				
165. Tucks prn				
166. Breast pump prn				
167. Sitz bath prn				
168.				

HH7013.doc Rev.A 11/95

②

Figure 2 Example of critical pathway for vaginal delivery. (Courtesy Hartford Hospital, Hartford, Conn.) *ACOG,* American College of Obstetricians and Gynecologists; *RH,* Rh factor; *WNL,* within normal limits.

Continued.

NAME:

MEDICAL RECORD#

0-6 HOURS AFTER ADM. TO UNIT

	N	A — D	E	V
TIME:				
MOBILITY/ACTIVITIES				
47. Initial OOB with assistance				
48.				
PSYCHOSOCIAL MANAGEMENT				
49. Facilitate parent/infant/family interaction				
50.				
EDUCATION				
51. Orient to room, unit, and electronic infant security system				
52. Initiate post partum education sheet				
53. Give post partum education packet				
54. Instruct on TV education				
55. Instruct on peri care				
56. Instruct on infant feeding/care skills and infant safety				
57. Give parents the opportunity to bathe infant				
58.				
DISCHARGE MANAGEMENT				
59. Determine patients support system and plan for home management				
60.				
61.				

6-12 HOURS

	N	A — D	E	V
TIME:				
MOBILITY/ACTIVITIES				
108. OOB ad lib				
109.				
PSYCHOSOCIAL MANAGEMENT				
110. Facilitate parent/infant/family interaction				
111.				
EDUCATION				
112.				
113. Provide teaching for identified needs from post partum educational needs assessment sheet				
114. Follow-up on post partum education packet				
115. Reinforce TV education				
116. Reinforce self peri care				
117. Reinforce infant feeding/care skills and infant safety				
118. Give parents the opportunity to bathe infant				
119.				
DISCHARGE MANAGEMENT				
120. Referrals to preferred providers for follow-up home care as needed				
121.				
122.				

12-24 HOURS

	N	A — D	E	V
TIME:				
MOBILITY/ACTIVITIES				
169. OOB ad lib				
170.				
PSYCHOSOCIAL MANAGEMENT				
171. Facilitate parent/infant/family interaction				
172.				
EDUCATION				
173.				
174. Complete teaching for identified needs from post partum educational sheet at discharge				
175. Review post partum education packet				
176. Reinforce TV education				
177. Reinforce self peri care				
178. Reinforce infant feeding/care skills and infant safety				
179. Give parents the opportunity to bathe infant				
180.				
DISCHARGE MANAGEMENT				
181. Referrals to preferred providers for follow-up home care as needed				
182. Review discharge instruction sheet with patient/family				
183. Give immunization booklet to mother at discharge				

This critical path was developed through the consensus of a multidisciplinary group and depicts the sequence and timing of those critical events which drive the achievement of progressive patient outcomes during an episode of illness. This is not meant to represent the only acceptable way to design the care for a given patient not would all patients' needs necessarily be met by such a path, therefore the content may be tailored to meet the needs of the individual patient.

CRITICAL PATHWAY APPROVED BY Maria J. Hansen, RN ___ ON 8/5/95

The contents of this document incorporate the "Postpartum Care" standards
Tucker, S. Canobbio, M., Paquette, E., and Wells, M. Patient Care Standards Fifth Edition (1992) Mosby Year Book, St. Louis p.724-728 - Revised 1995
cp_ppuvd.doc
HH7013.doc Rev.A 11/95

(3)

HARTFORD HOSPITAL
OBSTETRICS AND GYNECOLOGY

ASSESSMENT PARAMETERS
UNCOMPLICATED VAGINAL DELIVERY

Documentation on the Critical Path "Accomplished" indicates the following outcomes.

LEGEND:

A = Accomplished: intervention/outcome reached
V = Variance: intervention/outcome not reached
NA = Non-applicable: intervention/outcome deemed not
   clinically applicable
X =Write "X" in accomplished column when variance has been
   addressed and outcome/intervention will not be accomplished

OUTCOMES *	EXPECTED FINDINGS
Temp/Vital Signs WNL	Temp ≤ 101° within first 24 hours or ≤ 100.4° after 24 hours. Resp. unlabored. Rate 16-24/minute B/P not < 90/60 - > 140/90. Heart rate regular not < 60 - >100 beats/minute.
Tolerating diet	No nausea or vomiting.
Postpartum Assessment WNL	Fundus firm, midline; level at umbilicus or below. Lochia rubra 1-3 days, no foul odor, amount: scant- moderate, < 1 pad per hour. Small clots may be present; no evidence of placental tissue present with clots. Perineum intact, slight - moderate edema. Edges of episiotomy/laceration repair well approximated. No evidence of infection or hematoma. Hemorrhoids may be present. Breasts soft, nontender, colostrum present, breastmilk in 2 - 4 days, nipples everted. If breastfeeding, nipples without evidence of blisters, cracking, or bleeding.
Voiding q.s.	Voiding q.s. without difficulty, bladder not palpable, fundus firm and midline.
Verbalizes Adequate Level of Comfort (Pain Control)	Rates Pain on Scale of 0-5 0 - 6 hours = 0-3 level of pain 6 hours - Discharge = 0-2 level of pain 0 = No pain 1 = Mild 2 = Discomforting 3 = Distressing 4 = Horrible 5 = Excruciating Reference: Knoll Pharmaceuticals Incorporated Pain Scale
Environmental Maternal Safety	Siderails up. Bed down. Call light within reach. Bed wheels locked. Patient does not get OOB initially without asking for assistance. Assisted with ADLS, as necessary.
Positive Parent/Infant/Family Interaction	Mother or significant other: 1) Asks about the infant (including location and well-being); 2) Holds or cuddles baby; 3) Makes eye contact/talks to infant; 4) Asks questions about taking care of infant.
Safe Infant Care Skills	1) Does not leave infant unattended in unsafe place or while out of room; 2) Holds infant enface position during feeding; 3) Places infant in proper position in crib; 4) Attentive to baby's safety care needs, i.e. holding, choking, spitting, crying.
Appropriate Breastfeeding Skills	1) Feeds infant based on infant's cues of hunger or breastfeed at least q 3 hours and does not limit length of nursing time; 2) Positions baby correctly for latch on; 3) Breaks suction correctly when removing infant from areola, 4) Alternates breast for each feeding; 5) Air dries nipples after each feeding.
Understanding of Postpartum Self Care	1) Washes hands after going to the bathroom; 2) Does own perineal care, i.e. cleaning and changing pads; 3) Cares for breasts and wears supportive bra; 4) Identifies plan for contraception and asks for necessary information.
Understanding of Infant Care and Safety	Performs or verbalizes comfort with: 1) Holding/positioning infant, 2) Diapering, 3) Feeding, burping, 4) Cord care, 5) Circumcision care, as indicated, 6) Bathing Mother does not remove Identabands, Electronic Security Tag, and does not take infant beyond designated areas.

INITIALS:_____ SIGNATURE:_____ TITLE:_____

INITIALS:_____ SIGNATURE:_____ TITLE:_____

INITIALS:_____ SIGNATURE:_____ TITLE:_____

INITIALS:_____ SIGNATURE:_____ TITLE:_____

INITIALS:_____ SIGNATURE:_____ TITLE:_____

INITIALS:_____ SIGNATURE:_____ TITLE:_____

INITIALS:_____ SIGNATURE:_____ TITLE:_____

INITIALS:_____ SIGNATURE:_____ TITLE:_____

INITIALS:_____ SIGNATURE:_____ TITLE:_____

INITIALS:_____ SIGNATURE:_____ TITLE:_____

INITIALS:_____ SIGNATURE:_____ TITLE:_____

INITIALS:_____ SIGNATURE:_____ TITLE:_____

HH7013.doc Rev.A 11/95   CP_PPUVD.doc

④

Continued.

Figure 2, cont'd For legend see p. 99.

PATIENT FLOW SHEET

INTAKE

DATE	11-7	7-3	3-11	24° Total
ORAL				
IV Infused				
8° TOTAL				

OUTPUT

	11-7	7-3	3-11	24° Total
URINE				
STOOL				
EMESIS				
8° TOTAL				

PAIN FLOW SHEET

DATE	TIME	Location of Pain	Pain Level Before Analgesic	Pain Level After Analgesic

HH7013.doc Rev.A 11/95

⑤

RECORD OF VITAL SIGNS

DATE	TIME	BLOOD PRESSURE	PULSE	RESP	TEMP	REMARKS

HH7013.doc Rev.A 11/95

CP_PPUVD.doc

⑥

Figure 2, cont'd For legend see p. 99.

Patient: _____

Spouse: _____

Surgeon: _____

Cardiologist: _____

ANTICIPATED RECOVERY PATH — OPEN HEART SURGERY

POD #2 ____	POD #3 ____	POD #4 ____	POD #5 ____	POD #6 ____
Sit in chair 3× today Bathroom privileges with help	Sit in chair for all meals Walk 2 minutes × 2 and as desired (with help) ( ) ( ) ( )	Sit in chair for all meals Walk 3-4 minutes × 2 and as desired ( ) ( ) ( )	Sit in chair for all meals Walk 4-5 minutes × 2 and as desired ( ) ( ) ( )	Sit in chair for all meals Walk 5-6 minutes × 2 and as desired ( ) ( )
Use incentive spiro-meter every hour _____ cc's Eat regular diet (family may bring favorite foods)	Use incentive spiro-meter every hour _____ cc's Regular diet	Use incentive spiro-meter every hour _____ cc's Regular diet	Use incentive spiro-meter every hour _____ cc's Regular diet	Use incentive spiro-meter every hour _____ cc's Regular diet
	Prune juice and/or laxative if no bowel movement	Bowel function normal for you (suppository if needed)	Dietitian consultation	Discharge after 1:00 PM, if approved by physician
Cardiac rehabilitation in room	Rest period and pain med prior to Cardiac Rehab (in clinic, AM and PM)	Rest period and pain med prior to Cardiac Rehab (in clinic, AM and PM)	Rest period and pain med prior to Cardiac Rehab (in clinic, AM and PM)	Cardiac Rehab in clinic (only in AM on day of dis-charge)
Begin discharge plan-ning				

LEARNING PROGRAM

Pulmonary care incen-tive spirometer TCH Telemetry Splinting	Pain differentiation TEDS and TEDS care Constipation Progressive rest periods Infection symptoms Incisional care	Lifting restriction Emotional reactions Sexual considerations Support groups Read discharge instructions Pamphlet	Pulse-taking demo Develop plan for risk factor modification View discharge video	Review home meds Read Med-in-form cards Evaluate understand-ing of discharge instructions

Figure 3   Example of critical pathway for open heart surgery. (From Zander K, McGill R: *Nurs Manage* 25(8):34-40, 1994.) *POD*, Postoperative day; *TCH*, turn, cough, hyperventilate; *TEDS*, anti-embolism stockings.

the 1970s, reaching 30 in number by the mid 1980s. Councils encourage networking and formal education for coordinators of patient education.[9]

- The preparation of health care professionals to provide patient education has always been less than outstanding. Recent data from medical schools in the United States show that only 65% offer instruction in patient education.[11]

The infrastructure described in the preceding discussion seems scattered, incoherent, and lacking in data. It is accurate to say that there is no concerted direction for patient education or even an organizational structure under which those committed to its development come together. Rather, patient education services have developed in separate practice areas, associated with disease or health states. Although there are some commonalities in their development, it is best to understand each of them in some detail. The following chapters in Part II describe in depth approximately twelve such areas of practice.

AREAS OF PATIENT EDUCATION PRACTICE

Of the areas in which patient education is practiced, perhaps the oldest are diabetes education and pregnancy and parenting education. The field of diabetes has developed a more formal structure than have most other fields; it includes advanced practice specialists who are certified, accreditation of diabetes education programs, and a considerable research base on which to base practice. Other areas of practice, such as education of patients and families with mental health needs, are much newer in development. Exploration of the educational structure on which to base programs for persons with schizophrenia and depression is ongoing and is yet to be formalized. I believe that the single strongest element that distinguishes those fields that are well developed from those that are not is considerable interest on the part of the associations representing health professionals and consumers in the education of patients and the public.

All the chapters in Part II are organized around a common framework: general approach of the field, educational approaches and research base, community-based education and education of special populations, and national standards and tested programs. Each chapter or section also includes assessment/evaluation and teaching tools and methodologies.

REFERENCES

1. American Hospital Association: *Hospital statistics,* Chicago, 1993/94, The Association.
2. Battagliola M: Making employees better health care consumers, *Business and Health* 10(7):22-28, 1992.
3. Chwalow AJ and others: Effectiveness of a hospital-based cooperative care model on patients' functional status and utilization, *Patient Educ Counsel* 15:17-28, 1990.
4. Dorresteyn-Stevens C: The rural hospital as a provider of health promotion programs, *J Rural Health* 9:63-67, 1993.
5. Giloth BE: Management of patient education in U.S. hospitals: evolution of a concept, *Patient Educ Counsel* 15:101-111, 1990.
6. Greico AJ and others, editors: *Family partnership in hospital care; the cooperative care concept,* New York, 1994, Springer.
7. Hafner AW: Medical libraries and patient information services, *Bull Med Libr Assoc* 82(1):43-66, 1994.
8. Hendryx MS: Rural hospital health promotion: programs, methods, resource limitations, *J Commun Health* 18:241-250, 1993.
9. Johnson LJ, Hawkins S: The Maine state patient education forum: networking system for a rural area, *Patient Educ Counsel* 14:243-246, 1989.
10. Keleher S, Stanton MP: Implementing a community health education program in an acute care hospital, *J Healthcare Educ Training* 6(2):13-16, 1991.
11. Little DR: Health education programs in U.S. medical schools, *Academic Med* 67:596-598, 1992.
12. Mandelker J: The expanding role of PBMs, *Business and Health* Special Report, 1995.
13. Meade V: OBRA '90: how has pharmacy reacted? *Am Pharm* NS35(2):12-16, 1995.
14. NEI launches National Eye Health Education Program, *Pub Health Rep* 107(4):3rd cover, 1992.
15. Schmidt K and others: Implementation of the AHCPR pain guidelines for children, *J Nurs Care Qual* 8(3):68-74, 1994.
16. Weber DO: Planetree transplanted, *Healthcare Forum J* 35(5):30-37, 1992.
17. Zander K, McGill R: Critical and anticipated recovery paths: only the beginning, *Nurs Manage* 25(8):34-40, 1994.

5 Cancer Patient Education

GENERAL APPROACH

Education helps individuals detect their own cancer, and aids in treating and rehabilitating them. Perhaps the greatest effort in cancer education has been placed on teaching self-assessment techniques such as breast self-examination and persuading women to seek other screening techniques such as Papanicolaou (Pap) smears. Because minority women are more likely to seek medical care when breast and cervical cancers are in an advanced stage,[1] special attention is being paid to cultural models for assessing how individuals from these populations understand cancer and how interventions can best be delivered to them. Since cancer is a chronic disease, the needs of families and home caregivers and the use of cancer support groups have also received attention, as has the education necessary to adequately manage pain associated with the disease.

The National Cancer Institute's Cancer Information Service operates a nationwide 800 number to facilitate diffusion of new cancer knowledge to health professionals and to the public. Follow-up interviews of patients with cancer and their relatives who called this service revealed that they had strong informational needs and preferred to participate in their treatment plans. Their most common needs were for exploring all treatment options, including experimental treatments and referral to cancer experts.[12]

EDUCATIONAL APPROACHES AND RESEARCH BASE

The most recent and most rigorous review of the effects of psychosocial interventions on adults with cancer[15] is a meta-analysis of 45 studies of nonpharmacological interventions intended to improve the quality of life of patients diagnosed with one of the neoplastic diseases (see Appendix C). Outcomes of interest included emotional and functional adjustment, symptoms, and medical status. The interventions were broader than what is usually considered to be aspects of patient education and included progressive muscle relaxation, meditation, hypnotherapy, systematic desensitization, biofeedback, behavior modification or reinforcement, psychotherapy, and counseling. Most studies focused on white women in the United States. The summary found relatively small effect sizes: 0.31 for emotional adjustment, 0.32 for functional adjustment, and 0.41 for symptoms, with no difference among the various kinds of interventions (behavioral, counseling and therapy, informational and educational methods, or organized social support).[15] An effect size is the change (in standards deviation units) attributable to the experimental intervention.

In addition, Janz and others[10] summarized more than 33 intervention studies of breast self-examination (BSE), which showed that more than 90% of women were aware of recommendations to practice BSE, yet only 25% to 35% did so on a monthly basis. Although the profusion of BSE information has gained women's attention, it has not encouraged many to practice or to become proficient at BSE. Most women have not been taught to detect lumps in a silicone breast model, which is believed to be a very useful method. BSE education can be augmented if the learner practices the technique on her own breasts while the provider stands ready to monitor and correct. One program supplies a silicone model and a 10-minute videotape that demonstrates the correct technique for the learner to use at home.[5]

Prompts and reminders seem to contribute to frequent long-term use of BSE. Reassessment and retraining (which takes 5 to 8 minutes) are also necessary and must be incorporated into such events as annual physical examinations and mammograms. Although researchers have developed an effective technology for training in these skills (use of silicone breast models for lump detection), the actual maintenance of such skills remains questionable. Evidence suggests that performance deteriorates after only one training session, returning to near pretraining levels after 6 months. From a learning perspective it can be understood that BSE skills are not typically performed often, and there is limited opportunity for corrective feedback and reinforcement.[20]

The cost of teaching BSE has been found to be substantial and includes instructional time, take-home kits of a silicone model for practice of skills, and the increased costs of medical care for evaluation of breast problems in the months following teaching. Other instructional approaches, including group teaching and community/mass media campaigns, should be considered. Although for almost 40 years regular BSE has been advocated as an integral part of breast-cancer screening in the United States, its effectiveness has been questioned, and it is recommended that its cost-effectiveness be further studied.[17]

A related issue is education to persuade women to follow up on abnormal screening results. Stewart and others[24] note that there are clear and consistent findings that women with abnormal Pap smear results are more likely to complete recommended treatment and follow-up and to be less emotionally distressed by fear of cancer if they receive appropriate and reassuring educational materials.

Education to support patients in making decisions about their treatment is also of great importance. For example, women need information to choose among alternative treatments for breast cancer the one most consistent with their own values. It has been documented that for obvious reasons many women have greater difficulty concentrating just before having a breast biopsy.[26] A computer-based system contains information, referrals, and decision and social support programs for women with breast cancer. It allows them to talk anonymously with peers, to question experts, to learn where to obtain help, to read stories about people who have survived similar crises, to read relevant articles, to monitor their health status, to consider difficult decisions, and to plan how to regain control of their lives. This kind of system is especially important for those who live in rural areas where there may be less access to state-of-the-art treatment options, libraries, and social support groups. Because health crises are often protracted, an information and support service must be available when and where people need it, not just at a clinic.[8]

Family support is also necessary. Several longitudinal studies of patients and spouses indicate that the stressful effects of cancer extend as long as 1 to 2 years after the initial diagnosis. For the most part spouses report receiving little information about their partner's illness, and their attempts to request information or to contact the physician by telephone were often unsuccessful. It is believed that families need a framework of expectations about emotional aspects of recovery that can serve as a measure against which they can monitor progress and receive encouragement to view their concerns as a normal part of the recovery process.[16] A study of home caregivers[7] found significant needs that were not satisfied (barrier needs); these are identified in the first box on p. 108. Note how many of these barrier needs are amenable to instruction. Both the importance and the satisfaction of most caregiver needs change over time and should be reassessed.

Part of the self-care that patients and families give at home consists of monitoring for signs and symptoms of progression of the disease or side effects of treatment. For example, in one study[13] patients with lymphoma were taught self-diagnosis and self-referral for on-demand treatment for herpes zoster, which can leave painful long-term effects if not treated. In patients who remembered receiving pamphlets with color photos of typical cutaneous zoster lesions, long-term complications were less prevalent.[13] Another example is teaching patients to detect early signs of spinal cord compression (frequently from vertebral metastases), a treatable oncologic emergency that can lead to permanent neurologic deficits.[18] Unexplained back pain, followed by weakness of the lower extremities, is the usual pattern; such symptoms could easily confuse a patient, who might attribute this pain to other sources.

Educational interventions for pain management are important because pain affects 50% to 80% of cancer patients, with pain poorly controlled in an estimated 80%. The content for a pain education program is shown in the box below. Although it would have been helpful if

---

■ TOP 25 BARRIER NEEDS BY ALL SUBJECTS IN PHASE I (N = 492)

1. Information about the underlying reasons for symptoms
2. Information about what symptoms to expect
3. Information about what to expect in the future
4. Information about treatment of side effects
5. Information about community resources
6. Honest and updated information
7. Ways to reassure my patient
8. Ways to deal with my patient's decreased energy
9. Ways to deal with the unpredictability of the future
10. Information about medications (side effects and scheduling)
11. Ways to encourage my patient
12. Information about my patient's psychological needs
13. Methods to decrease my stress
14. Ways of coping with my patient's diagnosis of cancer
15. Information about the type and extent of my patient's illness
16. Ways to cope with role changes
17. Information about the physical needs of my patient
18. Activities that will make my patient feel purposeful
19. Ways to be more patient and tolerant
20. Ways to deal with my depression
21. Ways to maintain a normal family life
22. Ways to discuss death with my patient
23. Ways to deal with my fears
24. Ways to combat fatigue
25. Ways to provide my patient with adequate nutrition

From Hileman JW, Lackey NR, Hassanein RS: *Oncol Nurs Forum* 19:771-777, 1992.

■ PAIN EDUCATION PROGRAM CONTENT

Part I. General overview of pain
  A. Defining pain
  B. Understanding the causes of pain
  C. Pain assessment and use of pain rating scales to communicate pain
  D. Using a preventive approach to controlling pain
  E. Involvement of the family in pain management
Part II. Pharmacologic management of pain
  A. Overview of drug management of pain
  B. Overcoming fears of addiction
  C. Fear of drug dependence
  D. Understanding drug tolerance
  E. Understanding respiratory depression
  F. Talking to the doctor about pain
  G. Controlling other symptoms, such as nausea and constipation
Part III. Nondrug management of pain
  A. Importance of nondrug interventions
  B. Use of nondrug modalities as an adjunct to medications
  C. Review of previous experiences with nondrug methods
  D. Demonstration of heat, cold, massage, relaxation/distraction, and imagery

From Ferrell BR, Rhiner M, Ferrell BA: *Cancer* (Suppl) 72:3426-3432, 1993.

behavioral objectives had also been included, evaluation of the outcome of the program found it effective in decreasing pain intensity and severity, decreasing perception of addiction, decreasing anxiety, increasing use of pain medications, and helping to improve sleep.[3] Patient and professional education about pain relief is so important that 28 states have established initiatives to deal with cancer pain. Inadequate assessment of pain and fear of addiction are two strong educational needs that must be addressed.[6]

Rimer, Kedziera, and Levy[21] note that few systematically developed and carefully evaluated patient education programs on cancer pain control have been reported. Although cancer pain can be controlled, it frequently is not, and fear of pain is a common concern of persons with cancer and their families. During the educational assessment process, it is important to assess not only knowledge and cultural beliefs but also the meaning of pain—perceptions of what is causing it and how it affects life. Often patients use pain as an indicator of advancing disease or resistance to cancer therapy. To set common goals, patients and their families should be encouraged to verbalize expectations, and providers must help them understand what can reasonably be accomplished. Well-ingrained attitudes and beliefs about addiction must be addressed. Addiction refers to psychological dependence and is rare in the cancer patient population.

Patients must be taught how to communicate their pain to their health care teams, including the use of common pain-rating scales, and to describe pain site, quality, intensity, aggravating factors, and amount of relief current measures give as well as how long the relief lasts. They should also be able to participate in pain management, including use of medications and adjunctive strategies such as self-hypnosis, relaxation, and imagery. Pain control is an active process that requires frequent fine tuning to be successful. Whenever possible, the designated caregiver should be included because this person may eventually need to manage the patient's care and can inadvertently undermine a well-designed

teaching plan. The teaching plan is focused on a more recently accepted view that patients have a right to pain control, allowing them to optimize their quality of life.[21]

Teaching tools are widely available from national voluntary and government agencies for the education of patients with cancer. Estimates of the reading levels of standardized patient education materials may be found in Appendix E. As with other areas of practices, there are very few materials written at lower reading levels. Teaching tools are published regularly in professional journals, such as *Oncology Nursing Forum*, which serve to educate the professional nursing community so that practitioners can fulfill their patient education roles.

Two such tools are reproduced in the boxes on pp. 110 and 112. The first focuses on receiving continuous intravenous infusion recombinant interleukin-2 (rIL-2) therapy.[22] This therapy has been prescribed for patients with a wide variety of malignant conditions. The teaching tool is meant to be used within the context of a teaching plan and is appropriate for patients receiving low-dose rIL-2 therapy as outpatients or intermediate-dose rIL-2 therapy in an inpatient setting. The authors indicate that because of the complexities of the immune system, the therapy itself, and potential side effects, the tool is written at the twelfth-grade reading level and could not be written at the grade school level. Such a teaching tool ensures that consistent information is conveyed to patients but may require several teaching sessions to promote comprehension.[22] It is important to exert extra effort to make such a teaching tool accessible for those with a less developed reading ability.

The second box presents a guide that deals with a common screening method, mammography.[11] Provide a critique of this teaching tool. Is the content correct? Would it motivate? On which theories of motivation is it based? Analyze it on the basis of the health belief model. Does the teaching tool correspond to cognitive models of breast cancer for women from various cultures? Does it contain enough pictures and sto-

Text continued on p. 114.

■ CONTINUOUS INFUSION INTERLEUKIN-2: A PATIENT GUIDE TO THERAPY

Introduction to IL-2 therapy

There are four major treatment methods used against cancer: surgery, radiation therapy, chemotherapy, and biotherapy. As part of your cancer treatment, your physician has prescribed treatment with interleukin-2 (IL-2), a form of biotherapy.

Biotherapy utilizes substances and processes that occur naturally in the human body. This includes the cells and interactions within the immune system. The immune system provides the body with a defense mechanism against foreign invaders and certain diseases. The most important cells in the immune system are the white blood cells and the protein substances they produce to stimulate the immune response. Treatment with biotherapy may assist the immune system in killing cancer cells.

In the human body, IL-2 is a naturally occurring protein that is produced in small amounts by a type of white blood cell called a T lymphocyte. IL-2 has many important functions in the immune system, including stimulating lymphocytes and activating killer cells.

IL-2 was identified by scientists in 1976. Since that time, scientific advances in genetic engineering have enabled the production of the manufactured or recombinant form of IL-2 in large quantities. In the human body, recombinant IL-2 acts similarly to natural IL-2 to stimulate the immune system.

After years of clinical trials, IL-2 was approved by the Food and Drug Administration in May 1992 for the treatment of renal cell carcinoma. Physicians may prescribe IL-2 for different types of cancer using a variety of doses, routes, and schedules of administration. This patient teaching tool will review the administration of IL-2 given by the continuous intravenous infusion route. It will provide information about how IL-2 is given, possible side effects, the treatment of side effects, and your role in IL-2 therapy.

Before you begin IL-2 therapy

Before IL-2 therapy begins, your physician will order tests to evaluate your medical condition.

Baseline tests include history and physical, chest x-ray, electrocardiogram (ECG), lab work, and various x-rays or scans for tumor measurements. Consulting physicians may be asked to evaluate your heart and lungs to identify areas of possible complications. After a thorough evaluation, your physician will determine if IL-2 therapy may be of benefit in the treatment of your cancer.

Continuous infusion of IL-2

IL-2 is a clear, colorless liquid mixed with intravenous fluids in the pharmacy. It will be given around the clock for several days through a vein in your arm or a long-term port or catheter. A pump will be used to regulate the infusion rate. The dosage of IL-2 will be based upon your height, weight, and medical condition. Your physician will decide whether you will receive IL-2 in the hospital or at home.

Side effects of IL-2 therapy

It is very important that you communicate with your medical team during IL-2 therapy. Describe how you are feeling and report any change, even if it isn't worrying you. If you receive IL-2 in the hospital, your "vital signs" (temperature, respirations, pulse, and blood pressure) will be closely monitored. Although everyone experiences side effects with IL-2 therapy, the pattern and intensity of the side effects varies with each person. Long-lasting or permanent side effects are uncommon with IL-2.

Most patients experience a **flu-like syndrome,** including fever, chills, nasal stuffiness, muscle aches, and joint pain. Tylenol (McNeil Consumer Products Company, Raritan, NJ) is helpful to reduce fevers. Medications may be prescribed if you experience severe chills. An anti-inflammatory medication may be given to control fevers and relieve muscle and joint aches. A bedside humidifier may relieve the discomfort associated with nasal stuffiness.

Most patients on IL-2 also experience **fatigue** or **weakness.** Try to continue with your daily activities by pacing yourself and taking frequent rest periods. Although you will begin to regain your

From Sharp E and others: *Oncol Nurs Forum* 21:911-914, 1994. Reprinted with permission from Williamson Medical Center, Franklin, Tenn.

■ CONTINUOUS INFUSION INTERLEUKIN-2: A PATIENT GUIDE TO THERAPY—cont'd

strength at the end of therapy, it may take two or three weeks to fully recover.

Loss of appetite or **taste changes** are temporary side effects that you may experience. Meals, snacks, and liquids that are high in protein and calories are recommended to maintain good nutrition. Some patients experience gastrointestinal upset such as **nausea, vomiting,** or **diarrhea.** Medications are available to help ease these side effects. IL-2 may also cause a **sore mouth.** Gentle brushing, oral rinses, and a bland diet are recommended to reduce mouth irritation. Remember, these side effects are temporary and will resolve when therapy ends.

Many patients have **skin reactions** ranging from dry, red skin to severe itching and flaking. The skin on your hands or feet may even peel. Comfort measures include skin lotions and mild bathing solutions. A medication may be given to reduce the itching.

During IL-2 therapy your **urine output** is likely to decrease. Urine may darken and have an unpleasant odor. You may experience **swelling** and **weight gain** caused by fluid accumulation. If this fluid leaks into the lungs, you may begin to **wheeze** or become **short of breath.** Respiratory treatments or oxygen may improve your breathing. To monitor your condition, a daily weight is required. In the hospital, nurses will weigh you daily, measure your urine output, and ask you to record everything you drink. A medication may be given during therapy to remove some of the excess fluid by urination. Any remaining extra fluid will gradually disappear after therapy.

IL-2 may affect the heart and circulatory system. Your blood pressure may become lower than normal, causing you to feel **dizzy** or **light-headed.** Treatment of **low blood pressure** may include bed rest, administration of intravenous medications, or stopping IL-2 therapy until the blood pressure recovers. You may have a rapid or irregular heartbeat. If you experience **chest pain** or **tightness in your chest,** notify your medical team immediately.

Side effects associated with the central nervous system may occur, including **changes in sleep patterns, anxiety, forgetfulness, loss of concentration, unsteady walk, confusion,** and **mood changes.** Family members or friends may be the first to notice any changes. They should report any changes they notice to your medical team. Medications or a reduction of the IL-2 dose may be required to reduce these side effects.

IL-2 may affect your blood counts, liver and kidney function, and blood chemistry values. Routine blood tests will be ordered to monitor your body's response to IL-2 therapy.

Based on the severity of the side effects you experience, your physician may decide to change the IL-2 dose or stop IL-2 therapy at some point in your treatment. Every effort will be made to continue therapy with minimal side effects. The goal is to provide you with the best possible care.

After IL-2 therapy

After IL-2 therapy has been completed, some side effects may persist for several weeks.

Fatigue is the most persistent side effect. Activity combined with periods of rest is encouraged. You may resume activities based upon your energy level including exercise, returning to work, and sexual activity.

Loss of appetite may persist for a few days. Small, frequent meals are usually more appealing during this time. Concentrate on eating a well-balanced diet. Try to drink at least six to eight glasses of water daily.

Skin reactions may also persist. Continue using lotions and mild bathing solutions. Be aware that your skin may be sensitive to sunlight. Sunscreens, hats, and protective clothing are recommended.

Questions may arise once IL-2 therapy has ended. Concerns that should be reported to your physician include:
- Temperature greater than 101 degrees
- Mental confusion
- Development or increase in shortness of breath
- Chest discomfort or pain
- Swelling of neck, hands, or feet

Continued.

You will be given instructions for follow-up lab work, clinical check ups, or readmission to the hospital.

Feelings of discouragement are not uncommon during the recovery period. With time, these side effects will resolve. Your healthcare team will be available to support and assist you throughout therapy.

Notes

_____

_____

_____

_____

_____

_____

_____

_____

_____

■ MAMMOGRAPHY: AN EASY-TO-USE GUIDE

The American Cancer Society estimates that one out of every nine women will develop breast cancer at some point in her life. **EVERY** woman should consider herself at risk. But there is good news. Advances in methods of early detection of breast cancer, combined with better treatment, enable many women to go on to live full lives.

EVERY woman should know the signs of breast cancer and how to detect it early. The following screening recommendations are for women who have not previously shown signs or symptoms of breast cancer.

Signs of breast cancer
- Lump or thickening in the breast or armpit
- Change in the breast skin color, dimpling, or puckering
- Nipple discharge
- Change in the size or shape of the breast
- Change in the direction the nipple points

Recommended breast screening
- Monthly breast self-examination (BSE)

- Annual examination by a trained health professional
- Mammography:
  Age 35 to 40—one baseline screening mammogram
  Age 40 to 49—mammogram every one to two years
  Age 50 and over—mammogram every year

Those women who are at higher risk of breast cancer or who have breast abnormalities should ask their physician for specific guidelines.

Mammography
A mammogram is a low-dose breast x-ray used to find cancers too small to be felt. It makes pictures of the breast on film. A mammogram also can reveal other breast changes that may signal a very early breast cancer. Women need to have regular mammograms whether they have symptoms or not. The illustration on p. 113 demonstrates the importance of mammography.

From Mahon SM, Casperson D: *Oncol Nurs Forum* 18:1375-1378, 1991.

■ MAMMOGRAPHY: AN EASY-TO-USE GUIDE—cont'd

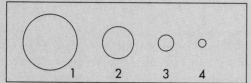

1. Average lump found by a woman practicing occasional breast self-examination
2. Average lump found by a woman practicing regular breast self-examination
3. Average lump found by first mammogram
4. Average lump found by regular mammogram

Safety

It is important to realize that modern mammography equipment uses a very low dose of radiation. The risk of radiation exposure is very small when compared to the benefit of detecting a breast cancer early. Every effort is made to keep exposure to a minimum.

Scheduling a mammogram

Every woman should talk to her personal physician about early detection of breast cancer. In general, it is best to perform breast self-examination, have a professional breast examination, or have a mammogram five to seven days after the menstrual period starts. This is because breasts are least tender and sensitive at this point, and it is easier to detect changes.

What to expect

Mammograms are performed by a trained radiology technologist who works closely with a radiologist (a physician who specializes in working with x-rays). At the time of the examination, you will undress to the waist. The technologist will position the breast on the mammography machine, which flattens the breast. It is important to remember that flattening the breast *does not* cause breast cancer and is very necessary in order to examine as much of the breast tissue as possible. In most cases, two x-rays are taken of each breast—one from above and one from the side. Occasionally, other views are taken. This does not mean that you have breast cancer, but rather that an additional picture was needed to better see more of the breast tissue.

After the mammogram

After the mammogram, the radiologist will examine the films for any sign of breast cancer or breast problems. The results of the mammogram will be given to your physician. Occasionally, women have sore or tender breasts after the test because of the compression necessary for an optimal diagnostic examination.

When regular professional breast examinations are combined with mammography, more than 90% of all breast cancers can be found in their earliest stages. That's when the possibility of a cure is greatest. Women also should learn how to perform breast self-examination and should perform the examination carefully every month. This will allow you to monitor for changes between professional examinations. If you are unsure of how to perform breast self-examination properly, ask your physician or nurse for instructions.

Risk factors

EVERY woman should consider herself at risk of breast cancer, but the risk factors below place a woman at higher than normal risk of breast cancer:

- A family history of breast cancer
- No children, or first birth after age 30
- Beginning menstrual periods early (before age 12)
- Late menopause (after age 50)
- Obesity
- A high-fat diet
- A family history of uterine, ovarian, or colon cancer

Significance of changes

It is important to remember that even if you find a change on self-examination, or if a change is noted during a professional breast examination or mammogram, most changes are not cancerous.

The best defense against breast cancer is to find and treat it during its earliest stages. Regular examinations of the correct type can improve the likelihood of good health in the future.

ries to be attractive to individuals with a variety of levels of formal education? What is its reading level?

Ward and Griffin[26] have developed a test to assess knowledge of treatment options for breast cancer (see box below).

■ **AREA OF KNOWLEDGE TAPPED BY THE ITEMS ON THE BREAST CANCER INFORMATION TEST**

What is removed when one has an MRM
XRT is given after lumpectomy
Percent chance that cancer will recur after lumpectomy
Breast reconstruction
What is removed when one has a lumpectomy
Delay of 1 or 2 weeks between discovery and surgery
Fatigue is a side effect of XRT
Redness and itching are side effects of XRT
Length of time to recuperate after MRM and BC is equal
Definition of metastasis
Frequency and duration of XRT
How common nausea is during chemotherapy and XRT
Lymph nodes are removed with either MRM or BC
Overall life expectancy does not differ for MRM and BC
Not all women have a choice between MRM and BC
For whom hormonal therapy is used
Hair loss is not a common side effect of XRT
MRM does not involve removal of chest wall muscles
Chemotherapy may follow either MRM or BC
Light arm exercise after MRM and BC is a good idea
How XRT is administered
Breast cancer is one of the most curable cancers

From Ward S, Griffin J: *Cancer Nurs* 13:191-196, 1990.
MRM, Modified radical mastectomy; *XRT,* radiotherapy; *BC,* breast conserving surgery.

In addition to instrumental learning, persons with cancer and their families struggle to establish meaning about what is happening to them. In life-threatening illness, meaning affects coping behavior, has an impact of psychosocial well-being, and is important in the struggle to obtain a sense of mastery. Meaning refers to the individual's understanding of the implications an illness has for his or her identity and for the future—the individual's perceptions of the ability to accomplish future goals, to maintain the viability of interpersonal relationships, and to sustain a sense of personal vitality, competence, and power. The constructed meaning scale, shown in the box below, is a measure of such meaning. Each statement allows a response on a scale of 1 to 4: strongly disagree, disagree, agree, strongly agree. The lowest test score, 8, indicates a very negative sense of the meaning the illness holds for one's self and for one's future life. The authors discuss the validity and reliability in the text of their article.[4]

■ **CONSTRUCTED MEANING SCALE**

1. I feel cancer is something I will never recover from.
2. I feel cancer is serious, but I will be able to return to life as it was before my illness.
3. I feel cancer has changed my life permanently so it will never be as good again.
4. I feel I have made a complete recovery from my illness.
5. I feel that I am the same person as I was before my illness.
6. I feel that my relationships with other people have not been negatively affected by my illness.
7. I feel that my experience with cancer has made me a better person.
8. I feel that having cancer has interfered with my achievement of the most important goals I have set for myself.

From Fife BL: *Soc Sci Med* 40:1021-1028, 1995.

Persons with cancer who are undergoing active treatment may have learning difficulties resulting from their therapy in addition to the stress and anxiety caused by their diagnosis and by the obvious effects of cancers of the central nervous system. High-dose chemotherapy may cause transient attentional problems, personality change, and neurological dysfunction such as paralysis and seizures. These effects generally resolve within 72 hours of discontinuing treatment, although more delayed and chronic effects of chemotherapy can occur, particularly when it is combined with radiation therapy. There is also growing evidence that some individuals experience subtle and persistent deficits of cognitive functioning long after treatment with biological modifiers (agents such as interferon and interleukin-2) ceases.[25]

COMMUNITY-BASED EDUCATION AND EDUCATION OF SPECIAL POPULATIONS

Much education for the patient with cancer is community-based, as the preceding examples indicate. Particularly important are programs aimed at the issues of continuing care and remission, with its requirement for self-monitoring. Pillon and Joannides[19] describe a decade-long educational and support group of this type. The "Living With Cancer" program addresses the needs of a family from diagnosis through a disease-free state or until death occurs. In addition to an oncology nurse and a mental health nurse, the program uses volunteers who have been screened regarding their own bereavement and trained as group facilitators. Weekly staff meetings that include volunteers serve to solve the participants' problems and to provide mutual support. Because the needs of cancer patients and their families change quickly, group sessions are scheduled on a weekly basis. A break of several weeks is granted at the conclusion of the series to allow patients to separate from the group. Session topics include chemotherapy and radiation, relaxation techniques, mental imagery and visual-

ization, nutrition, and health insurance. The series of patient education programs is usually marketed through oncologists' offices, hospitals, newspapers, and radio.

The educational needs of a number of special populations with cancer require attention. For example, more than 50% of all cancers occur in the 11% of the population over the age of 65 years; yet very little attention has been paid to the educational needs of this population. Mortality caused by cancer is also higher in minority groups, partially because some ethnic groups are less aware of the signs and symptoms of cancer and may have beliefs that are divergent from the mainstream of the health care system. Each major ethnic population serves as an umbrella for several diverse populations. It is important to look at cancer knowledge, beliefs, and attitudes by socioeconomic status as well as by cultural group. In addition, research has shown that different ethnic groups have different styles of learning. Most efforts to meet the educational and informational needs of different ethnic groups have revolved around translated materials, focus groups conducted to ensure cultural relevance, and community leadership involvement. Past experiences with difficulties in an institutional or a learning environment may make it difficult for any individual to ask questions or seek assistance.[25]

Other special populations include those who are developmentally disabled or who are functionally illiterate, reading at or below the fifth-grade level and able to understand few, if any, of the written materials provided to them by health care professionals. Yet the main intervention in patient education has been the use of written pamphlets. For any of these populations print materials should be culturally specific, clear, and limited to essential information. Visual messages are important in teaching persons with low literacy levels, and complex information must be broken down into individual parts. The National Cancer Institute and the American Cancer Society have developed cancer education materials to teach this population.[25]

A study of low-income African-American women older than 40 years of age in Atlanta, Georgia, found that their cancer models differed significantly from those held by clinicians.[7] The women attending these clinics endured cancer-screening tests that to them seemed to serve only as heralds of a disease that would ultimately kill them and that was outside the realm of physicians' abilities. Many women preferred to remain ignorant of the existence of cancer. Many believed that cancer originates as a bruise or sore that will not heal. Almost 60% believed that surgery just makes the cancer worse by exposing the tumor to air and thereby spreading the disease. Faith in God seemed to be one of the few completely benign and truly powerful treatment alternatives available to an individual with cancer. Given the explanatory models of this group of women, the question to ask is why any women in this group would undergo screening.

Two excellent examples of culturally relevant educational programs appeared recently in *Oncology Nursing Forum*.[2] In an effort to reach African-American adolescents, a video was made setting BSE instruction to rap music. Participants responded to the rap music with laughter, moving their arms in the air and their hands around their breasts in circular motions as directed in the song. A second excellent example gives information about cervical health in a game format called *Loteria*, which is familiar to many adult Hispanic women of Mexican descent.[23] As in the traditional *Loteria* game, pictures are matched with written text that instructs them about the risk factors for cervical cancer, screening guidelines for cervical cancer, and the increased rate for invasive cervical cancer found in adult Hispanic women. Because many members of the target population did not have transportation outside their community, the educational programs were presented in churches, clubs, and clinics, with cosmetic gifts supplied to participants. The importance of staying well by undergoing regular Pap testing was highlighted as allowing the women to continue to perform their roles as mother and wife, important in the Hispanic culture.

A final example of a special population is the mildly handicapped or disabled adolescent girl, instructed in the performance of BSE.[27] Because the population taught was capable of second- to fifth-grade achievement, active participation, im-

Table 5-1   Degree to which "I Can Cope" participants agree that the program met its objectives

OBJECTIVE	N	MEAN*
1. Provided an opportunity to learn about cancer, its causes, diagnosis, treatment, and rehabilitation	905	3.5
2. Learned about medical problems that may arise because of cancer and its treatment	900	3.3
3. Learned ways of dealing with medical problems that arise because of cancer and its treatment	887	3.3
4. Learned about importance of communicating effectively with health care professionals, family, and friends	895	3.5
5. Learned about emotional and social aspects of cancer and how to deal with them	898	3.4
6. Learned to recognize importance of maintaining physical fitness during treatment	888	3.3
7. Learned to identify and use physical and rehabilitative resources in community	864	3.2
8. Learned to identify and use social, psychological, and religious resources in community	872	3.2
9. Learned to identify and use financial and legal resources in community	835	3.1
10. Provided a climate of understanding by sharing common needs and experiences	889	3.5
11. Provided an opportunity for interaction with healthcare professionals	881	3.4

From McMillan SC, Tittle MB, Hill D: *Oncol Nurs Forum* 20:455-461, 1993.
*Scores ranged from 1 ("strongly disagree") to 4 ("strongly agree").

itation, and reinforcement were used as learning principles. Behavioral objectives included demonstrating knowledge of the seven warning signals of cancer and the symptoms of breast cancer; knowing the American Cancer Society's recommendations for screening for breast cancer; demonstrating proper technique for BSE as evidenced by ability to find the lumps in the silicone breast and by answering questions correctly; and knowing where to go for a professional examination if they found suspicious lumps in their breasts.

NATIONAL STANDARDS AND TESTED PROGRAMS

The Oncology Nursing Society has for some time had national standards of oncology education, including patient and family education, as well as public education (see Appendix D).

In addition, the American Cancer Society has offered the "I Can Cope" educational program since 1979. This program is currently available at nearly 1000 locations and is open to persons with cancer, their families, and friends. A national survey of participants[14] provided evaluative data about the degree to which participants agree that the program had met its objectives; results may be seen in Table 5-1.

SUMMARY

Goals in education for patients with cancer include helping the patient adjust to the course of the disease, carrying out self-care and prescribed regimens, recognizing and controlling side effects, achieving a sense of participation in and control over care, and normalization of lifestyle and interactions[25]—all discussed in the preceding examples of educational interventions in institutional and community settings and with varied populations. It is important to note that far more research and educational program development seem to be focused on breast and, to a lesser extent, cervical cancer than on other equally important neoplastic diseases, although

the general principles of screening, self-care, coping, and family support are applicable to all.

❓ STUDY QUESTION

1. A breast- and cervical-cancer screening program was set up at several sites to serve low income African-American women attending public clinics in Chicago. Part of the intervention was an educational program aimed at increasing knowledge about screening, which was evaluated by the classroom survey instrument, which appears in the accompanying box. Provide a critique of this instrument.

◼ CLASSROOM SURVEY INSTRUMENT
(REQUIRES TRUE OR FALSE ANSWERS)

1. Women who have had multiple sexual partners increase their risk of cervical cancer.
2. Bumping or bruising your breasts can cause breast cancer.
3. Shortness of breath is not a warning sign for breast cancer.
4. A chest X-ray can not help discover breast cancer early.
5. Women over 40 should have a breast exam about once every 3 years.
6. All women, regardless of age, should have an annual mammogram.
7. All women, regardless of age, should have an annual Pap smear.
8. Diets high in fat may increase a woman's risk for breast cancer.
9. If you have a lump in your breast, it is likely to be cancer.
10. Pain is usually a symptom of early breast cancer.
11. Pain in both breasts which comes and goes is normal for women even after menopause.
12. An experienced physician can diagnose breast cancer by feeling a lump.
13. When you are examining your breasts, you should always use the palms of your hands.

From Ansell D and others: *Pub Health Rep* 109: 104-111, 1994.

REFERENCES

1. Ansell D and others: A nurse-delivered intervention to reduce barriers to breast and cervical cancer screening in Chicago inner city clinics, *Public Health Rep* 109:104-111, 1994.
2. Ehmann JL: BSE rap: intergenerational ties to save lives, *Oncol Nurs Forum* 20:1255-1259, 1993.
3. Ferrell BR, Rhiner M, Ferrell BA: Development and implementation of a pain education program, *Cancer* (Suppl) 72:3426-3432, 1993.
4. Fife BL: The measurement of meaning in illness, *Soc Sci Med* 40:1021-1028, 1995.
5. Fletcher SW and others: How best to teach women breast self-examination, *Ann Intern Med* 112:772-779, 1990.
6. Greene PE: America responds to cancer pain; a survey of state pain initiatives, *Cancer Practice* 1:65-71, 1993.
7. Gregg J, Curry RH: Explanatory models for cancer among African-American women at two Atlanta neighborhood health centers: the implications for a cancer screening program, *Soc Sci Med* 39:519-526, 1994.
8. Gustafson D and others: Development and pilot evaluation of a computer-based support system for women with breast cancer, *J Psychosocial Oncol* 11(4):69-93, 1993.
9. Hileman JW, Lackey NR, Hassanein RS: Identifying the needs of home caregivers of patients with cancer, *Oncol Nurs Forum* 19:771-777, 1992.
10. Janz NK and others: Interventions to enhance breast self-examination practice: a review, *Public Health Rev* 17:89-163, 1991.
11. Mahon SM, Casperson D: Teaching women about mammography through use of a brochure, *Oncol Nurs Forum* 18:1375-1378, 1991.
12. Manfredi C and others: Patient use of treatment-related information received from the Cancer Information Service, *Cancer* 71:1326-1337, 1993.
13. Maung ZT and others: Patient education for self-referral and on-demand treatment for herpes zoster in lymphoma patients, *Leukemia Lymphoma* 11:447-452, 1993.
14. McMillan SC, Tittle MB, Hill D: A systematic evaluation of the "I Can Cope" program using a national sample, *Oncol Nurs Forum* 20:455-461, 1993.
15. Meyer TJ, Mark MM: Effects of psychosocial interventions with adult cancer patients: a meta-analysis of randomized experiments, *Health Psychol* 14:101-108, 1995.
16. Northouse LL, Peters-Golden H: Cancer and the family: strategies to assist spouses, *Semin Oncol Nurs* 9:74-82, 1993.
17. O'Malley MS: Cost-effectiveness of two nurse-led programs to teach breast self-examination, *Am J Prev Med* 9:139-145, 1993.
18. Peterson R: A nursing intervention for early detection of spinal cord compressions in patients with cancer, *Cancer Nurs* 16:113-116, 1993.
19. Pillon LR, Joannides G: An 11-year evaluation of a living with cancer program, *Oncol Nurs Forum* 18:707-711, 1991.
20. Pinto BM: Training and maintenance of breast self-examination skills, *Am J Prev Med* 9:353-358, 1993.
21. Rimer BK, Kedziera P, Levy MH: The role of patient education in cancer pain control, *Hospice J* 8:171-191, 1992.
22. Sharp E and others: A teaching tool for patients receiving continuous IV infusion recombinant interleukin-2 therapy, *Oncol Nurs Forum* 21:911-914, 1994.
23. Sheridan-Leos N: Women's health Loteria: a new cervical cancer education tool for Hispanic females, *Oncol Nurs Forum* 22:697-701, 1995.
24. Stewart DE and others: The effect of educational brochures on follow-up compliance in women with abnormal Papanicolaou smears, *Obstet Gynecol* 83:583-585, 1994.
25. Villejo L, Meyers C: Brain function, learning styles, and cancer patient education, *Semin Oncol Nurs* 7:97-104, 1991.
26. Ward S, Griffin J: Developing a test of knowledge of surgical options for breast cancer, *Cancer Nurs* 13:191-196, 1990.
27. Whitaker VB, Aldrich L: A breast self-examination program for adolescent special education students, *Fam Community Health* 16(2):30-40, 1993.

6 Cardiovascular and Pulmonary Patient Education

CARDIOVASCULAR PATIENT EDUCATION

General Approach

The effects of cardiovascular disease are immense. Each year about 1.25 million Americans suffer a myocardial infarction. Depending on the criteria, 30% to 40% of adult Americans may be hypertensive. More than 20 million are currently in treatment at a cost of $8 to $9 billion.[1] Reported educational programs in the cardiovascular area deal with topics that involve alteration of risk factors, decrease in time delay until treatment, implementation of cardiac rehabilitation after myocardial infarction or cardiac surgery, regimen maintenance, and management of sickle cell disease.

In the 1970s and 1980s several countries, including the United States, invested in large-scale clinical research trials designed to decrease cardiovascular risk factors—high blood pressure, smoking, high blood cholesterol levels, excess weight, and lack of exercise—by facilitating adoption of health practices in entire communities. The interventions lasted 5 to 8 years and frequently used a theoretical framework based on principles of behavioral change. Interventions focused on changing the community environment, training of indigenous leaders, educational self-help, and diffusion of the innovation through social networks in the community, in part to provide people with social support to maintain the initial action.

Multimedia campaigns were aimed at large audiences and were carefully segmented to influence individuals toward behavioral change by using clear, repetitive messages. Summaries of what has been learned from this research are presented in the next section. Although the popularity of large community studies has waned, community-based education is still used to decrease risk factors and patient delay to treatment and is very important for population subgroups that have not been reached successfully (e.g., ethnic minority groups, adults with low literacy levels, older women).[37]

Educational Approaches and Research Base

One meta-analysis[26] summarizes 18 controlled studies of cardiac patient education. The programs provided in these studies demonstrated a measurable impact on blood pressure (effect size 0.51), mortality (effect size 0.24), exercise (effect size 0.18) and diet (effect size 0.19). An effect size can be interpreted as the change (in standard deviation units) attributable to the experimental intervention. Stated another way, the patient education interventions in these studies showed a 28% increase over control subjects in effect on blood pressure and a 19% improvement in survival. Many of the interventions were relatively intensive, with frequent contact and high total contact. Exploration of less intensive interventions would be helpful to assess the amount of investment in education that is required to obtain optimal outcomes. No significant difference was found between didactic and behaviorally focused interventions.

Although morbidity and mortality data have not been reported for the U.S. community-based studies cited at the beginning of the chapter, aggregate risk-factor changes show net improvement in treatment cities over control cities to be modest, generally limited in duration, and usually within chance levels. Other national campaigns on cardiovascular risk factors were changing the environment everywhere, thus washing out differences between experimental and control cities.[37]

At present, two national campaigns are ongoing—the National High Blood Pressure Education Program and the National Cholesterol Education Program. These are not controlled studies; rather, they are health education activities in the form of campaigns, distributing their messages through the mass media and print advertising. In the two decades that the National High Blood Pressure Education Program has been active, there is evidence of change in public knowledge about high blood pressure, and these changes have occurred concurrently with a decrease in age-adjusted stroke mortality. In 1971, 51% of the hypertensive population were aware of their problem and 36% were treated; in 1991, 84% were aware of their problem and 73% were treated. In 1972, only 24% of the public knew the relationship between high blood pressure and stroke and 24% knew of its relationship to heart disease; in 1985, 77% and 92% of the public knew the relationship of high blood pressure to stroke and heart disease, respectively.[31]

The National Cholesterol Education Program has used two strategies to promote lowering of the blood cholesterol distribution of the entire population: a patient-based or clinical approach for those with hypercholesterolemia and a population-based approach. The program is showing limited efficacy of routine dietary education for promoting dietary changes, and many health personnel have a lack of experience and enthusiasm for nutritional interventions.[34] The public education approach is associated with improvements in cholesterol-related knowledge and behaviors and plasma cholesterol levels in the studied communities.[13] Risk-factor reduction is also a significant part of clinical patient education.

Understanding patient delay in seeking care after symptoms of acute myocardial infarction (AMI) or stroke has long been a high priority. Since the mid-1980s, several large-scale studies

have demonstrated that thrombolytic therapy can significantly reduce AMI mortality; the shorter the interval, the better the outcome. Yet over the past three decades, there has been little success in reducing delay time.

The phenomenon of delay needs to be understood before design of education and counseling strategies to reduce delay. Approximately one third of patients do not report an abrupt onset of symptoms and frequently have difficulty identifying the time of onset. These patients may report a prodrome of vague symptoms or symptoms that wax and wane over time, sometimes disappearing completely. Knowledge of the symptoms of AMI does not ensure that a patient will recognize or acknowledge his or her own AMI symptoms and does not reduce delay in seeking medical care.[11] Many subjects reported that they had expectations about the symptoms of heart disease that focused on location, intensity, associated symptoms, and quality. Expectations did not match the symptom experience of 74% of subjects, and these individuals delayed significantly longer before seeking treatment than did subjects whose expectations did match their experience. The longest phase is the time it takes individuals to interpret their symptoms as cardiac and decide to seek medical attention.[19]

Thus, despite widespread educational campaigns through public media, patient delay may not be affected because there is no uniform presenting syndrome for patients with AMI[19]; therefore the educational content provided to patients may not have been accurate for them.

Preparing patients for invasive tests such as cardiac catheterization is reviewed in Chapter 10 (see discussion of preparation for procedures). In general, studies have addressed the kind of information that is most helpful to those with various coping styles and the usefulness of opportunities for modeling.

Studies in the coronary care unit (CCU) suggest that among patients' perceived educational needs, risk factors, anatomy and physiology, medications, when to call a physician, and signs and symptoms of angina and AMI are among the most important. As CCU patients improve, they are transferred to a postcoronary care unit, where motivation level rises as anxiety level decreases. As a consequence, patients are better able to learn and retain information pertinent to their health status and self-care needs. These patients needed to have information from the CCU repeated.[36]

The next phase of care, cardiac rehabilitation, also contains an educational component for risk-factor reduction and development of self-efficacy. In the United States 10% to 15% of people who survive AMI will subsequently participate in supervised outpatient cardiac rehabilitation. Clinical benefits include a 25% reduction in mortality. For patients with mild to moderate anxiety and/or depression, rehabilitation is also cost-effective.[28]

Teaching tools for cardiovascular patient education are commonly available. Materials offered by the American Heart Association are listed in Appendix E. An example of a teaching tool—patient instructions for elective cardioversion—is presented in the accompanying box. Cardioversion has become a standard treatment for certain arrhythmias in which antiarrhythmic drugs have failed to convert the heart back to normal sinus rhythm. Because electrical cardioversion is non-invasive and relatively simple compared with other cardiac procedures, patients sometimes receive only a brief overview of what is going to happen. Yet the application of electric shock to the heart seems anything but simple and routine to patients and their families.[12]

Unlike teaching tools, tools for assessment and evaluation are far less available and tend to be fo-

---

■ PATIENT INSTRUCTIONS: ELECTIVE CARDIOVERSION

Your doctor has scheduled you for cardioversion because your heart is beating in an abnormal rhythm that should be returned to normal. The procedure will help decrease any breathing difficulties you've been having. It will also reduce your chances of suffering heart failure or stroke in the future.

Most patients scheduled for cardioversion have many concerns. The following are some of the questions most frequently asked by patients and their families. We hope the explanations will be helpful to you, but feel free to ask your nurse or doctor if there's anything else you want to know.

What is cardioversion?

The procedure involves delivery of a small electrical impulse to the heart. Your cardiologist or the nurse will place paddles or pads on your chest. They'll be connected to a small machine at your bedside, and, when activated, will deliver the electrical impulse to your heart. One impulse is usually effective in returning the heart to its normal rhythm. Occasionally, though, one or more additional, slightly stronger impulses are needed.

Where is the procedure done?

If you're a hospital inpatient, the procedure will be done in your room or in the ICU or CCU. For Ambulatory Services patients, the procedure is done in a special room in the outpatient department. It usually takes from 15 to 30 minutes.

What preparation is needed beforehand?

You will usually be asked not to eat or drink anything after midnight the night before the procedure, but you will be allowed to take your medications with small sips of water. You will be given a consent form to sign and an intravenous line will be started in your arm. Just before the procedure, the nurse will attach you to a heart monitor at your bedside, and all other necessary equipment will be brought into the room.

Who will be there during the procedure?

Your cardiologist, a nurse, and a respiratory therapist or anesthesiologist will be present. Your cardiologist will perform the procedure. The nurse will prepare you and monitor your blood pressure and heart rhythm. The respiratory therapist or

From Dunn D, Corrubia NM: *RN* 56(1):45-48, 1993.

Continued.

PATIENT INSTRUCTIONS: ELECTIVE CARDIOVERSION—cont'd

anesthesiologist will monitor your breathing. There may be other people in the room to assist as needed.

Will I be awake during the procedure?
Usually yes, but you will be given a sedative through your intravenous line. The medication will make you relaxed and very drowsy for a brief period of time. Sometimes, though, the cardiologist decides that a patient will do better under general anesthesia. If that's to be the case, you'll be notified in advance.

What will I feel?
Some patients say they feel a *very brief* sharp stabbing sensation in the chest when the electrical impulse is delivered. Frequently, however, the sedative eliminates any memory of the procedure. There are usually no aftereffects, except maybe a slight redness or soreness of the chest.

Are there any complications?
Although the risk is very small, complications—more serious heart rhythm irregularities, breathing difficulty, or stroke—can occur. For this reason, there's always emergency equipment in the room to deal with any problems. The risk of serious complications is low—probably less than one in 100. With your heart irregularity, you have a small risk of stroke whether you have the cardioversion or not. To minimize that risk, you may be given heparin or Coumadin before the procedure to thin the blood.

What if the procedure isn't successful?
Occasionally, it is not possible to correct the irregular heart rhythm. Although it is desirable to return your heart to a completely normal rhythm, most people are able to function well with an irregular rhythm as long as the heart is not beating too quickly. If the procedure is unsuccessful, the physician will probably prescribe medication to keep your heart rate in an acceptable range.

What happens after the procedure?
You will be able to drink and eat as soon as your nurse feels that you are fully awake after the procedure. Your family will be able to visit immediately.

When can I go home?
Those who are having cardioversion done on an outpatient basis usually remain in the hospital for three to four hours after the procedure. That's because we have to monitor your heart rhythm to be sure it remains stable. Hospitalized patients are often discharged the next day. The timing of your discharge, however, will depend on your condition. Because each patient's situation is different, each patient's length of stay differs. It is important to discuss this with your doctor.

cused on simpler learning activities. A knowledge questionnaire for hypertension is shown in the box on p. 123. Evaluate this tool. Should the score on this tool predict compliance with the regiment for treating hypertension?[6]

A similar questionnaire for knowledge about cholesterol is presented in Table 6-1. Inasmuch as most Americans can reduce their serum cholesterol levels by 10% through dietary modification, this is important information. Among people at high risk for coronary heart disease, modest reductions in serum cholesterol level are associated with an increase in life expectancy of up to 1 year. The percentage of responses in this study come from patients drawn from cardiology practices in New England, Southern California, and the Midwest.[30] The items on the questionnaire were designed to probe a variety of practical questions confronting persons who wish to follow a heart-healthy diet. All questions were pilot-tested for clarity and answers independently confirmed by two registered dietitians. When these patients are taken as a group, their knowledge of nutrition is marginal; mean scores on the quiz did not exceed

---

■ HYPERTENSION QUESTIONNAIRE
(TRUE / FALSE)

1. Hypertension is usually caused by nerves.
2. Hypertension treatment does not prolong life but it does make you feel better.
3. Both hypertension and cigarette smoking greatly increase the risk of heart attacks and strokes.
4. Hypertension is uncommon in our community (less than 1 adult in 100).
5. Less salt in your diet can cause hypertension.
6. Hypertension makes you more likely to have a stroke later in life but not a heart attack.
7. A heavy alcohol intake can cause hypertension.
8. Most headaches are caused by hypertension.
9. Drug therapy for hypertension must cause bothersome side-effects to be effective.
10. Proper control of hypertension can prolong life.
11. Most people with hypertension do not know they have it.
12. Hypertension can often be cured after a few courses of tablets.
13. Obesity (overweight) is a common cause of hypertension.

From Carney S and others: *J Human Hypertens* 7:505-508, 1993.

---

chance levels and were consistent with other surveys of nutrition knowledge.

Some cardiac patients fear resumption of physical activity until long after it is safe to do so, whereas others overestimate their capability. Providers have an important role in assisting patients in correct interpretation of their physical abilities and in providing instruction about home, social, and work activities. Gulanick, Kim, and Holm[15] developed a home activity assessment tool to guide discharge planning for these patients. Table 6-2 shows two scales, which test confidence (self-efficacy) in stair climbing and walking performance. These and others scales can be used as a basis for teaching patients with low confidence to perform activities as their recovery allows.

Finally, identifying the needs of patients and spouses after an acute cardiac event is an important step in the development of nursing interventions to facilitate couples' psychosocial adaptation. A study of 49 such couples found that both patients and spouses identified the need for information as being the most important compared with all other needs.[23] Understandably, patients and spouses identified different needs as important; unfortunately, many of the needs that both patients and spouses ranked as being important or very important were perceived as unmet in 40% to 70% of the cases. Table 6-3 provides a listing of the needs and the percentage of patients and spouses indicating the need was not met either before or after discharge from the hospital. Apparently, information was not consistently delivered to the participating patients and spouses, or it was delivered at a time when patients and families were unable to absorb it. The findings show that patient and spouse need to be assessed both separately and as a dyad. The need to be prepared to deal with emergencies ranked highest among spouses and was most often unmet. For many family members the possibility of a future cardiac event can be a significant concern.

Community-Based Education and Education of Special Populations

As already indicated, much of the activity in cardiovascular education has focused on risk-factor reduction in the community. In addition, considerable need exists for home-based teaching, ranging from defibrillation by a caregiver at home with direction from a hospital[21] or teaching families cardiopulmonary resuscitation (CPR) to routine home monitoring of blood pressure and long-term management of chronic cardiovascular diseases. At present, few family members receive CPR instruction, even though many of the attacks occur at home and the incidence of sudden death can reach as high as 50% in patients with advanced congestive heart failure. The concern of physicians that family members may feel burdened by this responsibility has

Table 6-1   Percentage of respondents answering true, false, and not sure on each item of the nutrition quiz (N = 606)

QUIZ ITEM	TRUE (%)	FALSE (%)	NOT SURE (%)
Ounce for ounce, chicken contains roughly the same amount of cholesterol as beef.	7.3*	78.6	14.1
Hydrogenated vegetable oil increases cholesterol levels more than nonhydrogenated vegetable oil.	38.9*	23.0	38.1
If a 100-calorie portion of food contains 4 g fat, more than 30% of its calories are from fat.	36.6*	17.7	45.7
No foods from animal sources contain dietary fiber.	36.6*	32.7	30.7
Two eggs overlight contain more cholesterol than the daily limit recommended by the government.	55.6*	21.3	23.1
To reduce your cholesterol level, it is more important to reduce the amount of saturated fat you eat than the amount of dietary cholesterol.	65.6*	13.7	20.7
Plant foods contain no cholesterol.	43.6*	31.7	24.7
An ounce of Corn Flakes cereal contains more sodium than an ounce of potato chips.	14.7*	63.1	22.2
Two percent of the calories in 2% milk comes from milk fat.	49.7	22.7*	27.6
A 3-oz serving of lean ground beef contains fewer grams of fat than a 3-oz serving of chocolate ice cream.	48.8	26.0*	25.3

From Plous S, Chesne RB, McDowell AU: *J Am Diet Assoc* 95:442-446, 1995.
*Correct answer.

Table 6-2   Confidence levels in stair climbing and walking

	SELF-EFFICACY FOR STAIR CLIMBING					WALKING PERFORMANCE SCALE					
	DEFINITELY CANNOT DO			DEFINITELY CAN DO			DID NOT TRY			DOING REGULARLY WITHOUT DIFFICULTY	
1. Climb 1 flight*	1	2	3	4	5	1. Walk 2 blocks†	1	2	3	4	5
2. Climb 2 flights	1	2	3	4	5	2. Walk 4 blocks†	1	2	3	4	5
3. Climb 3 flights	1	2	3	4	5	3. Walk 8 blocks (1 mile)†	1	2	3	4	5
4. Climb 4 flights	1	2	3	4	5	4. Walk 2 miles†	1	2	3	4	5
5. Climb 5 flights	1	2	3	4	5	5. Walk 4 miles†	1	2	3	4	5

From Gulanick M, Kim MJ, Holm K: *Prog Cardiovasc Nurs* 6:21-27, 1991.
*1 flight = 12 stairs.
†Without stopping.

Table 6-3   Patient and spouse needs ratings and percentage of subjects reporting needs not met*

NEED STATEMENT	% PATIENT NEEDS NOT MET	% SPOUSE NEEDS NOT MET
To know specific facts about my (the patient's) condition	26.1	20.8
To have honest explanations given in understandable terms	17.4	27.7
To talk to an M.D./R.N. about problems I or my family member may be facing	30.2	35.6
To know the expected course of the disease process	43.5	42.6
To receive specific instructions about care	25.5	25.5
To feel hope that I (my family member) will have a high quality of life	27.3	15.2
To receive information about what to do in an emergency	72.7	70.2
To receive information about expected physical course	26.7	31.9
To receive information about how to go about making life-style changes	42.2	47.6
To feel appreciated/valued by my family member	28.6	28.3
To receive information about life-style changes	46.5	38.3
To have my spouse assist me (be able to assist the patient) in making life-style changes	21.4	34.0
To feel as if others have my welfare in mind	5.0	39.0
To be able to talk with my family member about his/her concerns	35.7	26.7
To receive specific instructions about the return to sexual activity	46.2	48.8
To be able to talk with my family member about my fears/concerns	16.7	4.2
To receive information about expected psychological course	62.5	60.9
To talk to someone about my feelings	37.5	50.0
To have help with financial concerns	36.4	46.7
To receive information about feelings and emotions my spouse (I) may have during my (the patient's) recovery	19.3	69.3
To talk to someone about anger/frustration I may be experiencing	48.7	51.4
To talk to someone about my fears	52.5	52.6
To be told about other people or groups who can help with problems	59.0	59.5
To have time alone for myself	17.5	58.8
To be away from family member without worrying	36.8	41.0
To feel that others are going through the same things, that my experience is not unusual	25.0	35.7
To talk to others going through the same things	51.4	53.8
To have someone run errands or help with the house and/or cooking	11.1	50.0
To be able to offer meaningful assistance to the patient	n/a	28.3

Modified from Moser DK, Dracys KA, Marsden C: *Int J Nurs Stud* 30:105-114, 1993.
*Wording in parentheses is that directed specifically to the spouse.

been shown by some studies to be groundless.[10,22]

Management of hypertension has become a major reason for using ambulatory care facilities. Yet two recent studies[25,33] found that patients could play a much larger role in monitoring their own blood pressure, resulting in improved management of the hypertension, decrease in body weight, and diminished use of antihypertensive drugs. In one model a structured treatment and patient education program was introduced into a general practice.[25] In the other,[33] patients were trained to measure their own blood pressure and return readings by mail, and they were given a standard procedure to follow in case of unusually high or low readings at home. For men in this study, management of uncomplicated hypertension through physician visits and periodic home blood pressure measurement was equal or superior to management by more frequent office visits alone and at a lower cost.

Self-management of chronic heart disease refers to those tasks individuals and families must undertake to maintain optimum health states and reduce the impact of disease on daily life, including handling clinical aspects of disease away from the hospital or physician's office. The "take PRIDE" program was organized around self-regulation processes: *P*roblem selecting, *R*esearching the daily routine, *I*dentifying a heart self-management goal, *D*eveloping a plan to reach the goal, and *E*stablishing a reward for reaching it.[8] The program's group-meeting format allows exchange of ideas and encourages role modeling among the participants. The provider's role is to introduce accurate information, suggest strategies and provide feedback to encourage new behavior, and enhance feelings of self-efficacy through praise and encouragement. A videotape is used, in which a model self-manager, who describes how she previously experienced fear and uncertainty, now demonstrates the PRIDE process. Participants use this process to establish a specific behavioral goal, write a contract, and gain skills in self-management.

Educational materials for sickle cell disease, which predominantly affects African-Americans, are not widely available.[4] Patients need education and support for managing disabling pain, and parents must be taught to recognize the danger signals that indicate need for immediate treatment.

PULMONARY PATIENT EDUCATION
General Approach

Almost all the work in pulmonary patient education focuses on asthma education despite the fact that many people suffer with other pulmonary diseases such as chronic obstructive pulmonary disease (COPD). Morbidity and mortality from asthma have increased over the past decade despite improved understanding and advances in medical therapeutics. Over the past decade several centers have developed effective, tested asthma self-management programs, although none has been demonstrated to have superiority. These programs, designed to help families learn how to become active partners in managing the disease, have been developed with patients and families of different social, educational, and economic backgrounds. It is important to note that no study evaluating these programs has shown an increase in morbidity as a result of patients or parents accepting more responsibility for their care. Those who have participated in such courses did not overtreat at home or delay seeking appropriate medical care.[17]

In 1988 the National Heart, Lung, and Blood Institute of the National Institutes of Health initiated the National Asthma Education Program. One of its goals is to encourage education as a routine part of medical care.

Educational Approaches and Research Base

A meta-analysis was completed of 11 randomized clinical trials (RCTs) that evaluated the impact of interactive self-management teaching programs on the morbidity of pediatric asthma.[3] The overall pooled effect size remained below 0.2—a small effect size—meaning that these programs seem to have little influence on morbidity outcomes. Generally, studies restricted to school-age children showed a more significant reduction of morbidity during the year after the teaching intervention. It is suggested that studies need to be stratified according to severity of the disease and that control groups be limited to very brief instruction on medications and how to use them properly.[20] It is possible that these two changes in study design would result in raised effect sizes.

A summary of studies that evaluated the cost of asthma education programs for children showed that savings resulted from fewer hospitalizations and emergency department visits.[32] There also seemed to be improvements in attitude, self-management skills, and school absenteeism. Economic benefits of an educational program for patients with COPD also showed reduction in consumption of health services.[35] This program followed a pattern similar to that of asthma, assisting patients with knowledge of their disease and medications and teaching skills in handling exacerbations, peakflow meters, and inhalation technique. Another review of the 14 separate asthma education programs for children verified these outcomes and notes that little work has been done to describe problems of asthma management for families of infants and toddlers.[7] Education for health professionals also must be greatly strengthened and expanded.

Although studies of adults with asthma are limited, several investigations have shown decreases in hospitalization and absence from work associated with adherence to maintenance drug therapy and improvement in management skills after an educational program,[24] as well as reduced use of health care facilities after a brief single-session education program.[38] A written patient education program, personalized from a computer database and with interactive aspects, was followed by significant reduction in hospital admissions.[29]

Because asthma is a highly variable disease among patients and in the same patient over time, it is impossible for providers to discuss every contingency when instructing patients. This means that patients and parents must learn to make key observations and exercise considerable judgment in taking the appropriate action in a wide variety of circumstances. To prevent the onset of an attack, a person must recognize the early signs of asthma, act on these signs in appropriate ways, identify and avoid triggers to wheezing, and take prescribed medications properly and on time. Attack management involves efforts to rest and stay calm in the face of symptoms, maintain adequate hydration, use medications, and seek assistance if necessary. Social skills involve interaction with health care providers, as well as in school, home, and work environments. Poorly controlled asthma can have a significant negative impact on a child's self-image, activity level, fitness, and relationships. It is often helpful to send grandparents and other members of the extended family to an asthma education program.[17]

It is extremely useful to understand, from the patient's perspective, the experience of having asthma.[2] Until recently psychological factors were thought to play a major role in asthma, a notion that served to discredit it as a "real illness." The medical notion that a chronic illness can be controlled is a common theme in American medical practice; yet the limits of control are not commonly discussed, placing the patient in the position of feeling responsible for control. This disease is characterized by stable periods punctuated by unpredictable flares. Health professionals may assume that persons with asthma who frequent emergency services are not taking proper preventive measures and therefore are at fault for their asthma being out of control.

Many patients feel that they walk a "tightrope" between delaying formal medical intervention and seeking treatment too soon. In addition, they face uncertainty about the quality and speed of care they are likely to encounter in an emergency room, which affects their feelings of being able to control their illness. Experienced physicians have been found to underestimate the severity of symptoms. Thus these patients walk a fine line in attempting to fulfill practitioners' expectations about how they should manage their asthma and, given the nature of the disease, ascertain what seems actually to be possible.

Difficulties with learning the metered-dose inhaler technique have been noted; this technique is used both with COPD and with asthma. There is evidence that most patients have poor technique and therefore are not receiving optimal drug therapy.[18] Among a group of adults, problems included actuation of the canister before or at the end of inspiration, halt of inspiration after the release of the aerosol into the mouth, breath-hold of less than 5 seconds, and actuation of the canister more than once during the same inspiration. Older adults have been found to have more difficulty; education and re-education are vital. Spacers, which cause a delay between activation of the device and inhalation by the patient, may be helpful.[9] There is some question about whether health care providers know what to teach. In one study, more than half of house staff members and 82% of nurses were judged poor in their ability to use the inhaler.[18]

Community-Based Education and Education of Special Populations

Most of the education programs already described provide general guidelines; home management plans tailored to the needs of the individual child and family should be developed with them.

Teaching approaches can include camps for children that offer puppets, games, crafts, songs, and experiential learning. In one such camp each child took corrugated tubing with a compressed sponge rolled up inside to simulate airway linings and then breathed through it. Dipped into water, the sponge swelled to take up most of the internal diameter of the tubing, and children breathing through it experienced the differences in resistance. The box on p. 129 provides a script for Waldo the puppet. Such teaching-learning activities offer an excellent example of active teaching, well-planned for the developmental levels of the children, and clearly focused on the important outcomes of skill in performing self-care and development of feelings of self-efficacy.[5]

The mortality from asthma is particularly high among racial and ethnic minorities, as compared with whites.[18] In comparison with other patient groups, adults with asthma who have less education and lower income are likely to receive care that has less continuity and is less intensive after hospital discharge. These patients also have worse health and lower levels of physical and pulmonary function.[16] Asthma education programs frequently require multiple patient education sessions and extensive use of written materials, which may create impossible or difficult learning conditions for these patients. On the other hand, a nurse outreach worker assigned to families from a health maintenance organization (HMO) with a 70% black inner-city population achieved a marked reduction in the rate of pediatric hospitalization and emergency ward utilization for asthma.[14] This method of delivering education may be better suited to the needs of this population.

National Standards and Tested Programs

Citations to evaluations of asthma self-management programs are available (see Table 1 in reference 7); see also the box on p. 131.[27]

SUMMARY

The most structured areas of cardiovascular patient education are reduction of risk factors and cardiac rehabilitation; for pulmonary education, they comprise self-management programs for asthma. The cardiovascular field has invested in large-scale community trials and educational campaigns. Pulmonary patient education has invested primarily in tested programs of instruction for families of children with asthma, perhaps because approximately 10% of residents in the United States have asthma or wheezing at some time. Cardiovascular and pulmonary diseases are major health problems. Lack of standardized program development in the many other areas in which patient education could be helpful is unfortunate.

■ SCRIPT FOR A PUPPET SHOW

Session 1

Waldo, a puppet with asthma, speaks with the children. He first introduces them to his lungs when they are symptom free. He shows them his trachea and then his airways as they gradually narrow to end in air sacs. He points out how the tubes are all wide open and how easily his lungs fill with air and then empty. Waldo gets exposed to a trigger and starts to wheeze. He then introduces them to his lungs during an asthma episode. He shows them how the muscles wrapping his lungs get tight and squeeze his airways and describes how the linings of his airways swell and take up too much space making it really hard to move air. He uses an inhaler, carefully demonstrating good technique, and soon is breathing easier. His inhaler demonstration includes asking the audience to help him count while he holds his breath and while he waits between puffs.

Session 2

The Doc interacts first with the audience asking if they know what triggers are and responds to the audience's answers. He discusses a bit about triggers and invites the audience to watch while his patient, Cleveland, encounters many triggers during his day. Cleveland starts his day sleeping. While he sleeps, Might Dust Mightious sneaks in and causes Cleveland to have an asthma attack. Dust Mightious talks about how Cleveland can keep him away if he finds out who causes his problems when he sleeps. Cleveland then wakes coughing and wheezing. His mother gives him his inhaler and, with the help of the audience, coaches him to use it correctly. She then sends him out to play.

A mouse comes on the scene and interacts with the kids. He compliments them on their great assistance so far and invites them to help Cleveland stay out of trouble. Cleveland goes for a walk in the neighborhood and walks past a smoking cigarette, which he knows could trigger a wheeze. He quickly gets away from it explaining that since he just used his inhaler, getting away will be enough. He then passes a truck and again has to

get away quickly. He decides to go for a walk in the woods away from all those terrible triggers.

Mouse returns to chat with the children about how Cleveland did, what a great help they are and what problems they think Cleveland might encounter in the woods. The mouse again asks the children in the audience to help Cleveland avoid his triggers or do the right thing if he is exposed to triggers.

Cleveland walks in the woods and encounters a flock of birds, which drop feathers on him. This is another trigger and with the children's advice, he runs off again (still protected by his inhaler). He then sees flowers growing by the path, stops to sniff them, and gets a face full of pollen. With the audience's advice, Cleveland runs sneezing away from the flowers. He decides next to go to the pond where he thinks he will be safe from triggers. There he meets an alligator who scares him so badly that he wheezes until he can calm down. Cleveland decides to just go back home and on the way he gets rained on. He knows that wet weather often triggers his asthma so he hurries on home. He also knows that it has been hours since his inhaled reliever medicine and he knows with all those triggers he should not be out without his medicine.

Mouse comes back to tell the children what a super job they did helping Cleveland make good decisions. He also points out that most people don't have so many triggers and should do a better job of recognizing and avoiding them.

Session 3

Waldo and Jake have been playing soccer. Jake is wheezing and is short of breath. Waldo discerns that Jake didn't use his preventer medicine before soccer and encourages him to use his inhaler. Jake does so but with terrible technique. Waldo points this out and with the help of the audience, he coaches Jake through correct use. They go back out for the second half of their soccer game and when it is over, Jake is again having trouble breathing. Waldo encourages him to go see his mother.

From Capen CL and others, *Pediatr Nurs* 20:231-237, 1994.   *Continued.*

■ SCRIPT FOR A PUPPET SHOW—cont'd

The mouse comes in to ask the kids their opinions about Jake and Waldo's approaches to Jake's problems breathing. They discuss correct inhaler use.

Jake finds his mother in the garden and tells her he is having trouble breathing. She asks if he used his inhaler. He says yes, and she immediately gives him a nebulizer treatment. During this, she tells him what a good thing he did to use his inhaler first and come right to her when it didn't work. The nebulizer treatment doesn't help. They check Jake's peak flow and it is very low. Jake's mother calls the doctor, and they arrange to go to the office.

The mouse returns to chat with the audience about the decisions Jake and his mother made.

Nurse Dawn talks to Jake and his mother about what a good job they did. She describes The Doc's plan to start Jake on a daily medication that he must take twice each day without fail. She helps him figure out a way to do this by keeping his medicine with his toothbrush. She describes the use of prednisone just for five days and why it is necessary. She also talks about using his inhaler before he exercises. She then tells him to keep using his peak flow meter and to always call if his number is too low.

Ideas for Props

Rain: A squirt gun can be fired from behind the theater.

Smoke/car exhaust: A nebulizer behind the scenes produces a nice mist.

Pollen: Yellow paper punches dropped into silk flowers can be shaken out to simulate pollen.

Lungs: Felt-covered cotton cording of different sizes is glued into the shape of airways with cotton balls, or small Styrofoam balls glued in clusters on the ends. Branches are wrapped with red ribbon (tightly on the wheezy set). Everything below the trachea is placed into clear plastic bags with one end of a piece of tubing inserted into each bag. Behind the scenes air can be blown in or sucked out of the bags.

Holding objects up without being seen can be accomplished by making mittens out of the leftover sheet (they are too long and need to be cut off) so the hand holding the object "disappears" into the background.

■ PATIENT EDUCATION AND MANAGEMENT OF ASTHMA

Patient education is a powerful tool for helping patients gain the motivation, skill, and confidence to control their asthma.[1,2] Patient education should begin at the time of diagnosis and be integrated with continuing care. All members of the health care team should participate in the process.

Building a partnership

Much of the day-to-day responsibility for managing asthma falls on the patient and the patient's family. Active participation by the clinician, the patient, and the patient's family in a partnership can improve patient adherence to the treatment plan and stimulate improvements in asthma management.[3,4] The partnership concept includes open communication, joint development of a treatment plan by the clinician and patient, and encouragement of the family's efforts to improve prevention and treatment of the patient's symptoms. An important step in building the partnership is to ask questions early in each patient visit to identify the patient's main concerns about and expectations for treatment. Patients can focus fully on the clinician's recommendations only after these have been addressed.[5]

The content of teaching

Patient education involves helping patients understand asthma, helping patients learn and practice the skills necessary to manage asthma, and supporting patients for adopting appropriate asthma management behaviors and adhering to the treatment plan. Providing information contributes to but is not enough by itself to accomplish these objectives. Developing the patient's asthma management skills as well as the patient's confidence that the patient can control asthma is also required.

The full report, *Guidelines for the Diagnosis and Management of Asthma*, presents a complete discussion of suggested patient education programs and provides sample handouts. Areas and topics to be considered in patient education for asthma include:

- *Definition of asthma:* With an emphasis on the chronic nature of asthma and goals of therapy.
- *Key points about signs and symptoms of asthma:* The main symptoms of acute asthma episodes, the variability of symptoms among patients, the need to recognize and treat even mild symptoms, the importance of PEFR measurements in detecting early symptoms.
- *Characteristic changes in the airways of asthma patients and the role of medications:* Inflammation, bronchospasm, and excessive thick mucus; inhaled steroids, cromolyn, and bronchodilators.
- *Asthma triggers and how to avoid or control them:* Allergens and irritants, viral respiratory tract infections, and exercise.
- *Treatment:* The need for individualized continuing care, adverse effects and how to reduce them, the need for preventive treatment, the importance of early treatment of acute episodes.
- *Patient fears concerning medication:* Responses to common fears include the following: inhaled steroids are safe and efficacious; toxicity effects can be minimized by reducing the dosage; asthma medications are not addictive; continuous use does not reduce effectiveness.
- *Use of written guidelines:* Including medication plans for maintenance therapy and managing exacerbations as well as criteria for detecting onset of symptoms, initiating treatment for acute episodes, seeking emergency care, and recognizing when long-term treatment is less than optimal.
- *Use of written diaries:* To record asthma triggers, symptoms, actions taken, and PEFR in order to see patterns and report to the clinician.
- *Correct use of inhalers.*
- *Criteria for premedicating to prevent onset of symptoms:* Before exercise, before exposure to allergens, cold air, or irritants.
- *Optimal use of home peak expiratory flow rate monitoring:* To help decide when to initiate or

From National Asthma Education Program: *Guidelines for the diagnosis and management of asthma*, Bethesda, Md, 1991, National Heart, Lung, and Blood Institute.
PEFR, Peak expiratory flow rate.   *Continued.*

■ PATIENT EDUCATION AND MANAGEMENT OF ASTHMA—cont'd

terminate treatment, when to seek emergency care, or when to consider additional chronic treatment because of, for example, high variability in PEFR readings or evening dips below morning PEFR levels.

- *Evaluation of results of treatment plan:* Review whether the goals of therapy are being achieved; identify any adherence problems in order to overcome barriers or to negotiate changes in the treatment plan. Adherence to the treatment plan is enhanced when the plan is simplified as much as possible and when the plan considers both the patient's ability to afford the medications and the payment method.
- *Fears and misconceptions:* Asthma is not caused by psychological factors; most deaths are related to undertreatment and are rare in children; people with asthma should live full and active lives; with proper treatment asthma does not lead to permanent lung disability.
- *Family understanding and support:* Need for family education about asthma, need for help in managing an acute exacerbation.

- *Communication with the child's school:* By parents and by the clinician.
- *Feelings about asthma:* Need for acknowledging negative feelings and their validity; possible need for obtaining referrals to self-management programs, counseling, and social services.

REFERENCES

1. Feldman CH, Clark NM, Evans D: The role of health education in medical management in asthma. *Clin Rev Allergy* 1987; 5:197-205.
2. Mellins RB: Patient education is key to successful management of asthma. *J Rev Respir Dis* 1989; S47-S52 (Suppl).
3. Schulman BA: Active patient orientation and outcomes in hypertensive treatment. *Med Care* 1979; 17:267-280.
4. Clark NC: Asthma self-management education: research and implications for clinical practice. *Chest* 1989; 95:1110-1113.
5. Korsch BM, Gozzi EK, Francis V: Gaps in doctor-patient communication. I. Doctor-patient interaction and patient satisfaction. *Pediatrics* 1958; 42:855-871.

REFERENCES

1. Alderman MH, Lamport B: Labelling of hypertensives: a review of the data, *J Clin Epidemiol* 43:195-200, 1990.
2. Becker G and others: The dilemma of seeking urgent care: asthma episodes and emergency service use, *Soc Sci Med* 37:305-313, 1993.
3. Bernard-Bonnin A-C and others: Self-management teaching programs and morbidity of pediatric asthma: a meta-analysis, *J Allergy Clin Immunol* 95:34-41,1995.
4. Bird ST and others: Patient education for sickle cell disease: a national survey of health care professionals, *Health Educ Res* 9:235-242, 1994.
5. Capen CL and others: The team approach to pediatric asthma education, *Pediatr Nurs* 20:231-237, 1994.
6. Carney S and others: Hypertension education: patient knowledge and satisfaction, *J Human Hypertens* 7:505-508, 1993.
7. Clark NM, Gotsch A, Rosenstock IR: Patient, professional, and public education on behavioral aspects of asthma: a review of strategies for change and needed research, *J Asthma* 30:241-255, 1993.

8. Clark NM and others: Self-regulation of health behavior: the "take PRIDE" program, *Health Educ Q* 19:341-354, 1992.
9. Daniels S, Meuleman J: Importance of assessment of metered-dose inhaler technique in the elderly, *J Am Geriatr Soc* 42:82-84, 1994.
10. Dracup K and others: Is cardiopulmonary resuscitation training deleterious for family members of cardiac patients? *Am J Public Health* 84:116-118, 1994.
11. Dracup K and others: Causes of delay in seeking treatment for heart attack symptoms, *Soc Sci Med* 40:379-392, 1995.
12. Dunn D, Corrubia NM: Patient teaching: cardioversion, *RN* 56(1):45-48, 1993.
13. Frank E and others: Improved cholesterol-related knowledge and behavior and plasma cholesterol levels in adults during the 1980s, *JAMA* 268:1566-1572, 1992.
14. Greineder DK, Loane KC, Parks P: Reduction in resource utilization by an asthma outreach program, *Arch Pediatr Adolesc Med* 149:415-420, 1995.

15. Gulanick M, Kim MJ, Holm K: Resumption of home activities following cardiac events, *Prog Cardiovasc Nurs* 6:21-27, 1991.

16. Haas JS and others: The impact of socioeconomic status on the intensity of ambulatory treatment and health outcomes after hospital discharge for adults with asthma, *J Gen Intern Med* 9:121-126, 1994.

17. Howell JH, Flaim T, Lung CL: Patient education, *Pediatr Clin North Am* 39:1343-1361, 1992.

18. Interiano B, Kalpalatha K, Guntupalli K: Metered-dose inhalers; do health care providers know what to teach? *Arch Intern Med* 153:81-85, 1993.

19. Johnson JA, King KB: Influence of expectations about symptoms on delay in seeking treatment during a myocardial infarction, *Am J Crit Care* 4:29-35, 1995.

20. Kesten S: Asthma education: a time for reappraisal, *Chest* 107:893-894, 1995.

21. Kuhrik N and others: Defibrillation over the phone, *Am J Nurs* 92(11):28-31, 1992.

22. McLauchlan CAJ and others: Resuscitation training for cardiac patients and their relatives—its effect on anxiety, *Resuscitation* 24:7-11, 1992.

23. Moser DK, Dracup KA, Marsden C: Needs of recovering cardiac patients and their spouses: compared views, *Int J Nurs Stud* 30:105-114, 1993.

24. Muhlhauser I and others: Evaluation of a structured treatment and teaching programme on asthma, *J Intern Med* 230:157-164, 1991.

25. Muhlhauser I and others: Evaluation of a structured treatment and teaching programme on hypertension in general practice, *Clin Exp Hypertens* 15:125-142, 1993.

26. Mullen PD, Mains DA, Velez R: A meta-analysis of controlled trials of cardiac patient education, *Patient Educ Couns* 19:143-162, 1992.

27. National Asthma Education Program: *Guidelines for the diagnosis and management of asthma,* Bethesda, Md, 1991, National Heart, Lung, and Blood Institute.

28. Oldridge N and others: Economic evaluation of cardiac rehabilitation soon after acute myocardial infarction, *Am J Cardiol* 72;154-161, 1993.

29. Osman LM and others: Reducing hospital admission through computer-supported education for asthma patients, *Br Med J* 308:568-571, 1994.

30. Plous S, Chesne RB, McDowell AV: Nutrition knowledge and attitudes of cardiac patients, *J Am Diet Assoc* 95:442-446, 1995.

31. Roccella EJ and others: Changes in hypertension awareness, treatment, and control rates: 20-year trend data, *Ann Epidemiol* 3:547-549, 1993.

32. Rutten-Van Molken MPMH, VanDoorslaer EKA, Rutten FFH: Economic appraisal of asthma and COPD care: a literature review 1980-1991, *Soc Sci Med* 35:161-175, 1992.

33. Soghikian K and others: Home blood pressure monitoring; effect on use of medical services and medical care costs, *Med Care* 30:855-865, 1992.

34. Southard DR and others: Increasing the effectiveness of the National Cholesterol Education Program: dietary and behavioral interventions for clinical settings, *Ann Behav Med* 14:21-30, 1992.

35. Tougaard L and others: Economic benefits of teaching patients with chronic obstructive pulmonary disease about their illness, *Lancet* 339:1517-1520, 1992.

36. Wang WWT: The educational needs of myocardial infarction patients, *Progr Cardiovasc Nurs* 9(4):28-36, 1994.

37. Winkleby MA: The future of community-based cardiovascular disease intervention studies, *Am J Public Health* 84:1369-1371, 1994.

38. Yoon R and others: Controlled trial evaluation of an asthma education programme for adults, *Thorax* 48:1110-1116, 1993.

7 Diabetes Self-Management Education

GENERAL APPROACH

Diabetes education is the most fully developed of all the fields of patient education practice and among the oldest, having begun in the 1930s. It has adopted nationally accepted standards for accreditation of programs of diabetes education, as well as certification for an interdisciplinary advanced-practice role of certified diabetes educator (CDE). In addition, a large randomized clinical trial from the Diabetes Control and Complications Trial (DCCT) Research Group provides new guidance for successful management of insulin-dependent diabetes mellitus (IDDM).[15]

Approximately 13 million people in the United States have diabetes, of which 300,000 have IDDM; the cost of their care is $20 billion annually. Numerous studies have shown that education and self-care programs lead to reduced costs associated with diabetes. Because successful management is so dependent on the patient's own efforts, the American Diabetes Association has taken a position that all persons with diabetes must have access to affordable patient education.[1]

Estimates of the availability of diabetes education show a wide gap from this goal, which appears to be widening. A study of diabetes care and education by primary care physicians in Michigan communities from 1981 to 1991 found that the proportion of patients with non-insulin-dependent diabetes mellitus (NIDDM) who were referred for at least one session of formal diabetes education decreased from 70% to 58%. For patients with NIDDM not using insulin, the proportion was only 41%. Glucose monitoring by the patient has become standard,

at least for insulin-taking patients, although there is little information about how patients use these results. There was also a sharp decline in primary diabetes admissions to the hospital.[3]

A nationwide study found that of all persons with diabetes, 35% had attended a class or program at some time during the course of their disease. Younger age, African-American race, residence in the midwest region of the United States, higher level of education, presence of diabetes complications, and being treated with insulin were consistently associated with the person having had diabetes education. Thus a large proportion of patients with diabetes has never received education. The average number of hours of instruction received was 12.[11]

EDUCATIONAL APPROACHES AND RESEARCH BASE

Several meta-analyses of studies on the effectiveness of diabetes education have been completed. A summary of 82 such studies showed a high effect for increase in patient knowledge, medium-sized effects for dietary compliance and urine-testing skill, and lesser-sized effects for glycosylated hemoglobin and blood sugar.[7] Most of the studies did not provide in-depth descriptions of the interventions that were used. A reanalysis of 73 of these studies found that patient education appeared to be more effective in younger patients.[8] For all patients glycosylated hemoglobin levels improved between 1 and 6 months postintervention but decreased to 1-month levels after 6 months. Length of the educational intervention did not appear to influence outcomes. An independent meta-analysis found an effect size of 0.68 for diet instruction, with positive effects decreased but retained at 6- and 12-month follow-up, excepting weight loss.[29]

The DCCT showed that for most patients with IDDM aged 13 to 39 years, intensive treatment can substantially delay the onset and slow the progression of diabetic complications.[15] This intensive treatment attempted to achieve glycemic control as close to the nondiabetic range as possible. It included flexible adjustment of insulin dose, frequent monitoring of glucose levels (a minimum of four times per day) and diet, and diet and exercise instruction at entry to the study, as well as frequent counseling and dietary adjustments. These patients were hospitalized for 2 to 4 days to teach the elements of self-management, and they were seen weekly until they were comfortable with or confident about the regimen. In contrast, conventional therapy attempted to eliminate symptoms of high or low blood glucose levels and did not have specified blood glucose targets.

Table 7-1 compares the conventional and intensive treatment approaches carried out in the DCCT.[23] Note how educational care was intensified, as were other elements of care.

Studies of diabetes self-management education often include only a single measure in each of two categories: a measure of patient knowledge and a measure of the glycosylated hemoglobin level. The box on p. 136 outlines a full range of variables that should be considered, with asterisks indicating variables that have been underresearched. For example, much of the variance in the outcomes of diabetes education programs eventually can be understood by careful analyses of social-environmental factors. The rate of participation among eligible patients often is not reported, and the characteristics of those electing versus declining to participate are seldom available. Many studies have adopted a knowledge-

Table 7-1   Conventional and intensive treatment of IDDM patients in the DCCT

CONVENTIONAL TREATMENT	INTENSIVE TREATMENT
Patient-care team: diabetologist, diabetes nurse-educator, dietitian, behavioral scientist	Patient-care team: diabetologist, diabetes nurse-educator, dietitian, behavioral scientist
Prompt referral to specialists for treatment of complications	Prompt referral to specialists for treatment of complications
Clinic visit quarterly	Clinic visit once per month; frequent (daily/weekly) telephone contact to review and adjust regimens; admission to hospital as needed to achieve blood glucose control
One or two injections of insulin daily; adjustments in insulin dose as needed to eliminate symptomatic hypoglycemia or hyperglycemia	Three or more injections of insulin daily or insulin pump; frequent (even daily) adjustments in insulin dose to achieve target blood glucose level based on the results of self-monitoring
Self-monitoring, usually fingerstick blood glucose but could use urine testing, usually once per day	Four or more fingerstick blood glucose tests daily; blood glucose tests at 0300 [3 AM] weekly; glycohemoglobin measured at every clinic visit, blood glucose measured at quarterly clinic visits
Education about diet and exercise at entry to study; reviewed annually	Diet and exercise instruction at entry to study; frequent counseling and dietary adjustments

From Harris MI, Eastman RC, Siebert C: *Diabetes Care* 17:761-764, 1994.
IDDM, Insulin-dependent diabetes mellitus; *DCCT,* Diabetes Control and Complications Trial.

■ RELEVANT VARIABLES WITHIN EACH ASSESSMENT CATEGORY

Environmental and social context
Social support
Living situation
Health insurance status*
Practices of clinic or organization*
Time, cost, and location of meetings*
Community resources to support diabetes care**

Process and mediating variables
Knowledge
Attitudes
Self-efficacy or sense of control*
Health beliefs
Personal models*
Problem-solving or coping skills*
Intentions
Social support

Short-term health outcomes
GHb
Blood glucose variability*
Hypoglycemic episodes*
  Cholesterol level*
  Blood pressure
  Smoking*
  Weight
Quality of life**
  Functional limitations*
  Psychological*

Patient characteristics
Target population
Demographics, medical history

Cognitive functioning/impairment*
Comorbidity*
Participation rate**
Representativeness of participants**
Attrition rate*
Representativeness of final sample*

Diabetes management
Lifestyle change
  Dietary intake
  Eating behavior*
  Exercise
Medical self-care
  Glucose testing
  Medication adherence
  Insulin self-regulation*
  Foot care and safety
Patient-provider interaction**
  Patient activity level*
  Degree of patient-provider congruence

Long-term health outcomes
Complications*
  Retinopathy/impaired vision*
  Neuropathy*
  Renal failure
  Sexual dysfunction*
  Stroke*
Mortality*
  Diabetes-related
  All causes

Cost-effectiveness**

From Glasgow RE, Osteen JL: *Diabetes Care* 15:1423-1432, 1992.
*Variables that have not been studied sufficiently.
**Variables that have been studied even less often—and that are particularly important to assess.

attitude-behavior measurement when changes in self-efficacy or problem-solving coping skill are likely to be as important or more important. Although glycemic control is clearly relevant, patient functioning and quality of life also are.[19] Indeed, one study has found that quality of life and glycemic control are unrelated. Because good control does not enhance quality of life in the short term, patients may be unwilling to follow complex and intrusive regimens that do not appear to improve their health status.[33]

Modern diabetes self-management programs reflect a movement away from a goal of regimen compliance to a goal of patient empowerment. Such programs include a strong emphasis on self-efficacy, as well as the impact of diabetes on the totality of a person's life. Goals include enhancing the ability of patients to identify and set realistic goals, to apply a systematic problem-solving process, to manage the stress caused by living with diabetes, and to identify and obtain appropriate social support.[4] There is, however, evidence that the philosophy contained in the empowerment approach is not yet the norm.

One study of explanatory models of diabetes focused on difficulties in the patients' lifestyle and relationships; however, staff members viewed diabetes primarily as a pathophysiologic problem.[10] Among these highly educated patients, the restrictions required to manage diabetes were seen as major obstacles to social relationships, causing such things as divorce, loss of jobs, sexual problems, the death of newborn children, and difficulty traveling. What patients viewed as fears, professionals discussed as difficulties, without the same depth of turmoil that patients felt. Staff members did not elicit patients' perspectives on their illness, and major difficulties for patients were unknown to the staff.

Studies of learning conditions for persons with diabetes show that poor glycemic control in older persons with NIDDM is associated with decreased cognitive functioning, including verbal learning and memory, and the worse the control, the greater the impairment.[21] One experiential model of learning how to manage diabetes

reflects a rich series of sequential stages, including the following[30]:

- Trying out the regimen with rigid adherence
- Making regimen modifications that are more compatible with daily schedules or that ameliorate untoward and often frightening body responses
- Experimenting with effects of foods, activities, and circumstances, such as stressful situations, on blood glucose levels in an effort to find a regimen that would work for these patients
- Settling into a basic routine if the patient could recognize a predictable response pattern

Eventually, patients were able to apply their basic routines to new situations such as travel, illness, or change in work schedule; this adaptation sometimes required them to return briefly to trial-and-error activities. This approach allowed patients to tailor the regimen to their preferred lifestyles and perceived selves.

In this experiential model body listening was interpreted as a crucial source of information and became more important to these patients than did monitoring from health providers and significant others.[30] In fact, a special form of training, called *blood-glucose awareness training* (BGAT), has been effective in teaching individuals with insulin-requiring diabetes to improve their ability to better recognize blood-glucose fluctuations, although it is still less accurate than actual measures—self-monitoring of blood glucose (SMBG)—and quite variable across patients. Patients use both internal cues (body feelings) and external cues (timing, type and amount of insulin, food, and exercise). Blood glucose estimates made by adults in this way have been found to be accurate about 50% of the time but dangerously inaccurate 15% of the time, failing to detect hypoglycemia and hyperglycemia.

The data suggest there are no symptoms consistently associated with hypoglycemia or hyperglycemia for all patients. Most patients appear to have one or more symptoms that are highly idiosyncratic, varying from patient to patient, and they are unaware of which symptoms are actually predictive in their own case. BGAT involves teaching patients how to identify symptoms sensitive and specific to their hypoglycemia and hyperglycemia. At an average of 4.9 years after training, these patients had improved glycosylated hemoglobin levels and fewer automobile accidents than did control subjects who received routine diabetes education. Booster training (periodic brief retraining) was important. This work suggests that teaching classic signs or symptoms of hypoglycemia or hyperglycemia may be seriously misleading. Only one symptom (feeling shaky) was predictive of hypoglycemia for more than half of those studied, and in some cases the same symptom predicted hyperglycemia for one patient and hypoglycemia for another. Postintervention levels were still far from ideal.[12,28]

Teaching materials and approaches must reflect the fact that diabetes involves a complex regimen and often necessitates lifestyle changes on the part of the patient and family. One survey showed that individual education and counseling were the teaching methods most frequently used by diabetes educators and were identified as most educationally effective by them. The educators believed that videotapes, booklets, and slide/tape programs were both educationally effective and cost-effective. Many educators use free or self-developed materials, in part because of limitations on reimbursement of these programs. Very few computer-assisted programs were used, and they were rarely believed to be effective educationally or in cost.[16]

Games and active learning are excellent ways to teach both motor and cognitive skills to children. They provide learning conditions that are motivating and highly repetitive so that the knowledge is retained. Table 7-2 summarizes games used to teach children ages 7 to 12 years at the International Diabetes Center.[6] Assessment and evaluation tools are also important. Readers will recall that in Chapter 2 the transtheoretic model was described as useful for assessing whether patients were ready for behavior change. In the boxes presented on p. 142 are sample questions for such an assessment of persons with diabetes; similar tools should be used for each important self-care behavior such as glucose testing or weight loss.[31] The outcomes of such an assessment allow the educator to match much more specifically the education to the patient's stage of readiness and to prioritize which of multiple target behaviors are most amenable to change.

An intervention designed to reduce serious foot lesions in persons with diabetes portrays the kind of multiple-pronged intervention necessary to create improved outcomes. Approximately 20% of all diabetic patients hospitalized in the United States are admitted because of foot complications; yet it has been estimated that one half of the amputations in patients with diabetes are preventable. Although simple preventive strategies on the part of the health care provider or patient can reduce the likelihood of amputation, many of these procedures are not being systematically applied.[25]

In one study, patients were questioned about their regular foot-care routine and were asked to show how they examined their feet.[25] During this self-examination, nurse-clinicians observed whether patients scrutinized the toenails, the soles of the feet, and the area between the toes. Musculoskeletal and dermatologic abnormalities were assessed, pulses palpated, and lesions noted. In a clinical setting patients received education about how to assess their feet, signed behavioral contracts, and received telephone and postcard reminders; the records of these patients were placed in colorful folders marked with foot decals, which prompted providers to perform foot examinations and provide foot-care education at each visit. Serious foot lesions decreased, and some appropriate foot care behaviors increased.

Diabetes education is the area of practice most likely to have formal programs, especially in hospitals. Lowe, Hogue, and Delcher[26] write of the program of diabetes education at Georgia Baptist Medical Center, whose educational opportunities are broad-based and multiple and include

Table 7-2   Games from the Children's Classweek Curriculum

GAME	OBJECTIVES	EQUIPMENT	INSTRUCTION
What is Diabetes?	To identify body parts, to define diabetes and discuss possible causes, to demonstrate how food is digested	Brown wrapping paper (large roll, 3 ft wide, cut into pieces corresponding to children's height), paper cutouts of body parts (pancreas, heart, lungs, stomach, heart, brain), "What causes diabetes?" flashcards, models of stomach, sample breakfast foods (juice, milk, cereal, etc.)	Children trace an outline of each other on brown paper and then paste body parts to the corresponding area. Discussion involves defining each body part and its function. Using the diabetes flashcards, children work in small groups to decide which do/do not cause diabetes. Then the entire group reconvenes and discusses causes of diabetes. Each child is given a model stomach to fill with breakfast foods. Children's hands are used to simulate "digesting" food and the group discusses how food turns into blood sugar.
A Hanging Drop and Other Blood Sugar Mysteries	To state reasons for self blood glucose monitoring (SBGM), to describe/explain hemoglobin A_{1c}, to discuss steps necessary to get an accurate blood test using a meter, to describe pattern control, to describe ketone testing and its purpose	HbA_{1c} puppets, one apple, toothpicks, marshmallows, SBGM concentration gameboard and cards, various meters and equipment for demonstration, four colored pens, diabetes record book, Ketostix, life-size duplicate of a Ketostix, and color-code chart	Children act out the way hemoglobin and glucose function. Instructor demonstrates by placing marshmallows on toothpicks and sticking them into an apple (higher A_{1c} = more marshmallows). The class is divided into two or more teams for a concentration game. Each team member takes a turn to get a match on the board and after each match the team member must say whether the step is required for an accurate blood test. For the four-colored pen game each child is given a pen and record book. Children are told to circle morning regular insulin and lunch blood sugar in red, morning NPH and evening meal blood glucose in green, evening meal regular and bedtime blood glucose in blue, and evening meal NPH and morning blood glucose in black. Discussion is then held regarding the relationship between these insulins and tests and how adjustments might be made. In the Ketostix game children pick a Ketostix and match it to the area/color on the color-code chart.

Continued.

From Barry B: *Diabetes Educ* 21:27–30, 1995.
NPH, Neutral protamine Hagedorn; *CHO*, carbohydrate.

Table 7-2   Games from the Children's Classweek Curriculum—cont'd

GAME	OBJECTIVES	EQUIPMENT	INSTRUCTION
Eating Right = Feeling Great and In Control	To understand the importance of consistency for blood sugar control and good nutrition for growth and development, to understand carbohydrate choices at meals and snacks, to learn what is included in each exchange list and what constitutes a portion	Writing board, erasable markers, examples of each type of macronutrient (eg, sugar and starch for carbohydrate, egg white for protein, margarine or oil for fat), Exchange Lists handout, large picture of Food Pyramid, supplies for Guess the Exchanges game	The class begins with a description of the macronutrients and micronutrients in foods. The food pyramid then is discussed and the components of each group are described. The exchange lists are compared with the food pyramid by listing similarities and differences. Discussion is held about carbohydrate, protein, and fat, and their effects on blood sugar, emphasizing that CHO has the greatest impact. The concept of starch, fruit, and milk affecting blood sugar the most also is discussed. Examples of each nutrient can be demonstrated. To help visualize portions, children play the Guess the Exchanges game. They go to different stations where a food is shown in two portions (one correct/one incorrect) and they are told to pick which portion is correct. The class then discusses the answers as a group.
Exchange Relay	To learn what foods are in each exchange group	Pictures of foods	The class is divided into two or more teams. Each person on the team is assigned one of the six exchange groups and must retrieve a food from that group from a large pile of pictures at the other side of the room. The first team to get all of the required foods wins the game. To reinforce learning, the foods chosen then are reviewed at the end of each race.
Weak and Wobblies, Trick or Treat 'Em	To define hypoglycemia, to describe how it feels to be hypoglycemic, to name at least three treatments for hypoglycemia and what supplies should be carried, to identify causes of hypoglycemia, to determine one's individual blood glucose target range	Targeting Blood Glucose game contents (board, markers, Nerf brand dart gun, hypoglycemia treatment center)	A general discussion of hypoglycemia is conducted in a group setting and each of the objectives is addressed. The game, Targeting Blood Glucose, then is played to reinforce proper treatment of hypoglycemia.

	Objective	Materials	Description
Shop 'N Bop	To identify the main components of the new nutrition label, to identify guidelines for fat and sugar content when choosing foods, to demonstrate how to use the nutrition labels for doing carbohydrate counting	Nutrition Facts Label handout, grocery store	The Nutrition Facts Label handout is discussed in class, and children are told to highlight/circle serving size, total fat, and total carbohydrates. The class discusses how much fat to eat in one serving of food (<3 to 5 grams). The class goes to a grocery store and the children are given assignments to look for the carbohydrate content on breakfast cereals and the grams of fat in snack foods.
Sick Days Rummy	To identify the steps necessary to prevent diabetic ketoacidosis (DKA) when ill	Sick Days Rummy cards	The class discusses the proper steps to take for sick-day management and each step is listed on the board and reviewed. Sick Days Rummy is played by dividing the class into groups, each receiving a deck of cards. The object of the game is to collect the cards that contain all of the proper steps to follow for sick-day management.
Be the Teacher	To demonstrate to the class and instructors a topic learned during the children's classweek	Various diabetes teaching aids used during the week or a container filled with papers on which various diabetes topics are written	The class is divided into groups and each group is given a topic to present. They are allowed to use any prop or tool they have seen used for teaching in the past week. Each group has at least 1 hour to prepare and must present for at least 10 minutes. This game also can be played by placing in a container papers on which topics are written and having each child draw a topic. The child then has 1 minute to describe the topic, give examples, etc. The "teaching" by children can be videotaped to show to parents later.
Diabetes Hangman	To help teach concepts related to diabetes and management	Chalkboard or dry erase board, markers	This game is played just like regular hangman, except that diabetes-related words are used and the person who guesses the word must also give a definition of that word.
Exchange Bingo	To help teach about foods and portions from the exchange lists	Exchange Bingo cards, cover chips	This game is played just like regular bingo, except that the names of the six exchange groups are printed across the top of each card and below each name is a food and one serving/portion size. The object of the game is to cover six squares in a row, horizontally, vertically, or diagonally. Other options include covering the four corners or a coverall.

■ SAMPLE STAGING QUESTIONS

Glucose self-monitoring: *Do you always check your blood sugar (glucose) in the way you were instructed to?*
____ Yes, I have been for more than 6 months *(maintenance)*
____ Yes, I have been but for less than 6 months *(action)*
____ No, but I plan to in the next month *(preparation)*
____ No, but I plan to in the next 6 months *(contemplation)*
____ No, and I do not intend to in the next 6 months *(precontemplation)*
If you answered no above, how often do you check your blood glucose?
____ Never
____ Rarely
____ Sometimes
____ Often
____ Usually

Diet: *Do you always follow your special diet in the way you were instructed?*
____ Yes, I have been for more than 6 months *(maintenance)*
____ Yes, I have been but for less than 6 months *(action)*
____ No, but I plan to in the next month *(preparation)*
____ No, but I plan to in the next 6 months *(contemplation)*
____ No, and I do not intend to in the next 6 months *(precontemplation)*
If you answered no above, how often do you follow your diet?
____ Never
____ Rarely
____ Sometimes
____ Often
____ Usually

From Ruggerio L, Prochaska JO: *Diabetes Spectrum* 6:22-24, 1993.

■ SAMPLE DECISIONAL BALANCE QUESTIONS

How important is each of the following in deciding whether to take care of your diabetes as recommended?

Pros
When I follow my diet, there is less chance that I will have serious health problems.
When I test my glucose, I feel more in control of my life.
When I exercise, I see myself as a "healthy person."
When I take my insulin as recommended, I feel more responsible.

Cons
Following my diabetes diet gets in the way of other people's plans.
Testing my blood glucose makes me feel different.
My exercise routine interferes with other activities.
Injecting myself with insulin is painful.

From Ruggerio L, Prochaska JO: *Diabetes Spectrum* 6:22-24, 1993.

■ SAMPLE SELF-EFFICACY QUESTIONS

How confident (sure) are you that you would continue to follow the . . . aspect of your diabetes regimen in each of the following situations?

Diet: When I am on vacation.
Self-monitoring of blood glucose: When my fingers hurt from the last monitoring.
Exercise: When I am tired.
Insulin use: When I am with other people.

From Ruggerio L, Prochaska JO: *Diabetes Spectrum* 6:22-24, 1993.

Table 7-3   Diabetes patient educational opportunities at Georgia Baptist Medical Center

SOURCE	SERVICE
Literature	Diabetes starter kits with educational materials on diabetes, insulin, diet, and exercise
Video learning series or Closed circuit TV	Presentation of: 1. Diabetes information and essential components of treatment 2. "A Positive Approach to Diabetes" (video)
Bedside teaching by nurse	1. Insulin injection 2. Emphasis on signs/symptoms of hypo/hyperglycemia 3. Other survival skills as appropriate
Patient care assistant	Demonstration of fingerstick technique for blood glucose monitoring
Inhouse classes	Multidisciplinary teaching each Thursday, 2 to 3 PM; subject and location announced prior to presentation.
Diabetes nurse consultant	Consultation by request (provide appropriate extension)
Diabetes resource nurse	Unit nurse liaison
Pharmaceutical services	Bedside teaching on therapeutic effect of insulin and oral agents for all new prescriptions
Nutritional services	Bedside assessment and teaching of appropriate diet prescriptions
Blood glucose monitoring	Delivery and instructional use of blood glucose monitor (optional service offered to GBMC patients)
Home health follow-up	Provided as appropriate (per physician order) for a minimum of two visits regarding compliance, safety, or other self-care deficits
Skin consultation	Skin and foot assessment with review of skin care
Chaplain	Assessment of psychosocial/spiritual needs
Preventive medicine	Supplemental literature on exercise

From Lowe DH, Hogue JK, Delcher HK: *Diabetes Educ* 20:199-203, 1994.

continuous staff development (Table 7-3). The role of diabetes nurse coordinator is described in the first box on p. 144 and includes clinical practice, case management, consultation, and staff education and extends into home care. The critical path for newly diagnosed patients with IDDM could be strengthened by adding patient outcomes (see the second box on p. 144)

COMMUNITY-BASED EDUCATION AND EDUCATION OF SPECIAL POPULATIONS

Because diabetes requires lifelong self-management, education must be ongoing and available from a variety of sources in the community.

In Michigan a survey found that many patients were not referred for diabetes education or received only a few minutes of it from the office nurse at each visit. A newsletter, costing about 25 cents per person, was sent to 7000 of these individuals to provide diabetes care information.[4] On evaluation it was rated as most helpful by those who did not have the financial means to acquire comprehensive diabetes education through either programs or written materials. The box on p. 145 shows a sample newsletter, and the box on p. 146 lists newsletter topics.[2]

Community walking groups and support groups provide important normative models and resources for patients who do not receive much formal diabetes education, especially older persons. These groups also offer the social support necessary to cope with the disease. Indeed, community-wide interventions are increasingly important alternatives or additions to the usual model of formal instruction for diabetes.[18]

■ DIABETES NURSE COORDINATOR ADVANCED PRACTICE ROLE DELINEATION

- Assesses physical, psychosocial, economic, and spiritual responses of patients, families, and significant others to actual/potential diabetes health-related problems.
- Determines with healthcare team the appropriate interventions for clinical problems and case-management issues based on needs assessment.
- Develops and coordinates continuous quality improvement systems based on patient outcome criteria.
- Develops practice standards for diabetes patient education.
- Functions as a liaison between patients, families, physicians, healthcare team members, and the Diabetes Advisory Committee (DAC), facilitating communication and quality patient care with regard to the diabetes patient population.
- Develops, plans, and implements diabetes programs based on assessment of patient/physician population.
- Serves as a consultant to healthcare professionals who request information, assistance, etc in diabetes and diabetes-related healthcare issues.
- Maintains a level of clinical and theoretical expertise necessary to provide consultation to the healthcare team members.
- Develops and evaluates critical pathways for diabetes management.
- Utilizes knowledge base concerning reimbursement issues whereby cost-effective diabetes patient care is identified.
- Supports, initiates, participates, and/or facilitates formal and informal research and relates findings to clinical practice and home health services.

From Lowe DH, Hogue JK, Delcher HK: *Diabetes Educ* 20:199-203, 1994.

■ CRITICAL TEACHING/LEARNING PATH FOR NEWLY DIAGNOSED PATIENTS WITH INSULIN-DEPENDENT DIABETES

Day 1
1. Review contents of diabetes kit, emphasize diary.
2. Patient acknowledges he/she is challenged with diabetes.
3. Patient views video learning programs.
4. Patient observes fingerstick.
5. Patient observes nurse administering insulin.

Day 2
1. Patient does fingerstick.
2. Patient demonstrates eye estimation of blood glucose.
3. Patient documents in blood glucose diary.
4. Patient is assisted with insulin administration.
5. Nutrition Service visits with patient.

Day 3
1. Patient assesses and identifies trends in blood glucose (see diary).
2. Patient demonstrates insulin administration and verbalizes rationale for insulin.
3. Review with patient the signs and symptoms of hypo/hyperglycemia.
4. Pharmacist consultation.
5. Diabetes nurse consultant visits with patient (optional).

Day 4
1. Blood glucose monitoring instruction.
2. Patient identifies trends in blood glucose (see diary).
3. Nurse explains glycosylate hemoglobin assay.
4. Patient verbalizes actions needed for high and low blood glucose.
5. Patient verbalizes diabetes education resources (eg, ADA).

From Lowe DH, Hogue JK, Delcher HK: *Diabetes Educ* 20:199-203, 1994.
ADA, American Diabetes Association.

THE EYES HAVE IT!

Sometimes people are surprised to find out that diabetes can affect their eyes—especially if they find out after damage has been done! One of the major dangers of diabetic eye disease is that it can cause serious damage to the eyes before either the patient or the doctor finds out about it. The time to think about diabetes and eye disease is before problems occur.

Diabetic retinopathy is the name for the eye disease caused by diabetes. Retinopathy affects the small blood vessels in the back of the eye (retina). As time goes on, these blood vessels get weaker and may break. Diabetic retinopathy can cause vision problems and even blindness if not treated. In fact, it is the major cause of new blindness among adults in the United States. The sad thing is that much of this blindness could be prevented if the eye disease was found and treated in time. Laser therapy is used to treat retinopathy. Thin beams of light are used to seal the broken blood vessels. Laser treatment is safe and fairly painless.

You can do three important things to preserve your eyesight. First, have your eyes checked once a year by a medical doctor who specializes in eye care (an ophthalmologist). This will ensure that any eye disease is found and treated in the early stages.

Second, if you have high blood pressure (hypertension), make sure your blood pressure stays near the normal range—120/80. Take your medicine as prescribed and check your blood pressure often. High blood pressure can cause narrowing of the blood vessels in the eye. This can speed up the onset of diabetic eye disease.

Third, keep your blood sugar levels as close to normal as possible—70 to 120 mg/dL. High blood sugar is known to play a role in diabetic eye disease.

Diabetes can cause damage to the eyes, but vision loss and blindness can be prevented if found and treated early. See your ophthalmologist each year and keep your blood pressure and blood sugar in good control.

Question to ask your doctor

- Can you refer me to an eye doctor (ophthalmologist) who can check my eyes each year for diabetic eye disease?

From Anderson RM and others: *Diabetes Educ* 20:29-34, 1994.

There are many populations that require special education in diabetes. For example, urban African-Americans without sufficient access to adequate medical care have particular problems, including limited resources, insufficient access to health care, marginal education, and health beliefs that are barriers to improved health care. These problems are associated with a higher risk of chronic complications than the white population faces. Musey and others[27] found that half of these patients stopped taking insulin because of reported lack of money, and 14% did so because they did not know how to manage diabetes on sick days. Symptoms of metabolic decompensation were recognized by patients in only 43% of episodes; 64% of their hospital admissions should have been preventable. Self-monitoring of blood glucose was limited by the availability of supplies (glucose testing strips and meters) and access to health care providers. Many of these problems could be solved by education.

A group of children 14 to 15 years of age from poor, single-parent families with limited social support were found to have repeated hospital admissions because of diabetic ketoacidosis as a result of missed insulin injections.[20] An aggressive management program that included education reduced these admissions 47%. It involved a sequence of steps, utilized until the goal was reached: first, filling knowledge gaps, then confronting the parents and encouraging them to take responsibility; second, sending home care nurses to give the insulin if the parents did not do so; and if all else failed, obtaining a court order.

Culturally relevant educational interventions, which have been tested for their effectiveness, are

---

■ NEWSLETTER TOPICS

1. The importance of diabetes patient education.
2. The importance of testing blood sugar levels each day.
3. Exercise in the treatment of diabetes.
4. High blood pressure and diabetes.
5. Foot care.
6. The seriousness of diabetes as a disease and the importance of taking care of it.
7. Maintaining good blood sugar control.
8. Eating a balanced diet.
9. Weight loss.
10. Making large behavior changes one step at a time.
11. Definition and use of the glycosylated hemoglobin test.
12. Importance of yearly eye exams.
13. The value of multiple insulin injections.
14. Sick-day care.
15. Balancing food, exercise, and medicine.
16. Self-assessment of level of diabetes care.
17. Smoking cigarettes and diabetes.
18. Cholesterol and diabetes.
19. Keeping a record of your diabetes tests.
20. A reminder sticker of important tests and exams for diabetic patients to be given by their doctor.
21. The activated patient newsletter philosophy.

From Anderson RM and others: *Diabetes Educ* 20:29-34, 1994.

extremely important. Such a program was developed by Brown and Hanis[9] in a Texas-Mexico border community, in which 50% of the Hispanic population over the age of 35 years either had diabetes or were the first-degree relative of someone with diabetes. Spanish-language videotapes were used. Religious leaders were present to convey the belief that assuming responsibility for one's health is not interfering with the will of God. Eight weekly meetings were designed as social activities, with demonstrations of preparing healthy foods, to capitalize on the value that Mexican-Americans place on social events involving family and friends. Statistically significant

improvements were observed in diabetes knowledge, fasting blood sugar levels, and glycosylated hemoglobin levels.

Cerebrovascular accident (CVA) occurs more frequently in persons with diabetes, resulting in cognitive, perceptual, communicative, and motor disturbances, making it difficult to learn and carry out aspects of diabetes care. The most common disturbances that occur are memory difficulties, diminished sensation, depression, and inappropriate behavior. Persons with brain damage have difficulty in applying what was learned in one setting to another situation. The box on p. 147 describes the kinds of altered functioning these patients may have and presents strategies for promoting independence when memory impairment is involved. Additional strategies useful for the other disturbances these patients have include teaching in a quiet environment with no distractions, using demonstrations and visual aids to assist the hearing impaired, and giving frequent encouragement for taking on learning tasks.[24]

NATIONAL STANDARDS AND TESTED PROGRAMS

The first diabetes education programs accredited by the American Diabetes Association were recognized in 1987, with more than 375 programs approved since then. The standards against which programs are judged (see Appendix D) are primarily process standards; the usual expected content to be taught may be found in standard 12. In addition, several states have developed mechanisms to approve programs that meet the National Standards for Diabetes Patient Education Programs. Inasmuch as there are no reported studies that compare programs that meet the standards with those that do not, the impact of the standards on the quality of diabetes education remains undocumented. There is a trend toward referring to diabetes education programs as self-management education training programs.[17]

In addition to accreditation or recognition of diabetes education programs, certification is

ALTERED FUNCTIONING ASSOCIATED WITH CEREBROVASCULAR ACCIDENT: CHARACTERISTICS AND COPING STRATEGIES

Strategies for promoting independence in individuals with memory problems

1. Keep messages short and simple.
2. Establish and maintain fixed routines.
3. Present new information one step at a time.
4. Do not proceed to the next step until the client has completed the previous step.
5. Use continuous feedback.
6. Structure the environment so that it is as close as possible to the home situation to which the patient is going.
7. Use memory aids generously (eg, written notes, instruction cards, daily schedules).
8. When teaching new tasks, use familiar objects and old associations to facilitate the instruction.
9. Plan teaching sessions at the best time of day for the client.
10. Teach content that is meaningful to the individual.

Characteristics of right- vs. left-hemisphere damage

Characteristics	Left-hemisphere CVA	Right-hemisphere CVA
Affected body side	Right hemiplegia/paresis	Left hemiplegia/paresis
Effects on visual/perceptual abilities		Spatial/perceptual deficits, unawareness or minimization of deficits, dressing apraxia
Effects on speech/language abilities	Aphasia, verbal apraxia	
Effects on decision-making abilities	Slow and anxious decision making	Impulsivity
Effects on emotions	Depressive affect, exaggerated emotional response	Emotional lability, indifferent emotional state

Modified from Hernandez C, Grinspan DR: *Diabetes Educ* 20:311-316, 1994.

available to diabetes educators. The scope and standards of practice for certified diabetes educators (CDEs) are shown in Appendix D. The role is continuing to evolve and now encompasses management, as well as counseling of persons with diabetes. In some instances it has expanded into a true advanced-practice role, including the ordering and interpretation of laboratory tests, dietary assessment, and prescription and medication adjustments. Table 7-4 shows activities that registered nurses (RNs) and registered dietitians (RDs) indicate they perform either frequently or always. These activities reflect the evolving and broadening scope of practitioners in diabetes education.[13]

It is apparent that educational resources and standards are better developed for diabetes education than for any other area of practice. The American Diabetes Association has constructed a Diabetes Index, which assesses key resources of providers, including CDEs, specialized facilities, educational programs, financing arrangements and reimbursement, and state legislation and policy. Reimbursement has been a problem for the field. This index reveals that in more than 30 states, Medicaid does not pay for outpatient diabetes education and will not pay for outpatient nutrition counseling in 40 states; private insurance is even less supportive. Five states mandate statewide public education programs, with 11 funding diabetes outreach programs to high-risk and culturally diverse populations.[14] Reimbursement is generally available only for complete programs and for those that are recognized or approved. The Medicare coverage policy has recently been amended to include coverage of outpatient diabetes education programs. Services must be furnished under a physician's order, and patients must be newly diagnosed and/or unstable or have a change in treatment plan.[5]

Table 7-4   Percent of registered nurses and registered dietitians who indicated they frequently/always performed specified educator and medical management roles

ROLES	% OF RNs (N = 74)	% OF RDs (N = 25)
Educator		
Teach foot care	80.8	04.0
Teach general diabetes information	86.5	76.0
Teach diabetes emergency information	86.5	52.0
Teach insulin injection	79.5	0
Teach blood glucose monitoring	78.1	28.0
Teach urine glucose monitoring	19.0	04.0
Teach urine ketone monitoring	59.5	16.7
Develop diabetes education program	65.3	45.8
Develop quality assurance protocols	50.0	24.0
Medical management		
Perform physical examination	8.1	0
Prescribe medications	9.7	0
Adjust insulin	41.9	8.0
Adjust oral hypoglycemic medications	20.6	0
Prescribe diet	26.4	64.0
Prescribe exercise	32.1	29.1
Order laboratory tests	37.5	4.0
Follow-up on abnormal lab tests	68.1	54.2
Assess complications by physical exam	24.3	0

From Cypress M and others: *Diabetes Educ* 18:111-114, 1992.

Two examples of statewide diabetes management programs, including education, are instructive. In Maine a network of health care providers collaborated on the development and adoption of three patient care guidelines that address preconception counseling, prenatal care, and contraception for women with established diabetes.[34] For women with diabetes whose pregnancies are appropriately managed, the perinatal mortality rate approaches the corresponding rate for the nondiabetic population, and the rate of malformations can be decreased.

The Maryland Medicaid Diabetes Care Program incorporates payment for preventive services to control the long-term effects of the disease and hospitalization.[32] The program requires physician education in diabetes management, outpatient educational programs in self-management, and increased accessibility of specialty services such as ophthalmologists, nutritional counseling, therapeutic footwear, and blood glucose monitors and supplies. Table 7-5 shows how the Diabetes Care Program builds on the Maryland Medicaid program.

National standards for diabetes self-management programs may be found in Appendix D.

SUMMARY

Perhaps more than any other area of practice, diabetes has demonstrated what can be accomplished with research, policies, standards, and services in support of self-management education. Yet large numbers of persons with this disorder are still not reached.

❓ STUDY QUESTION

1. Read the article by Hardway, Weatherly, and Bonheur,[22] which provides an excellent example of one institution evaluating its diabetes education practice and revising it. Make a list of the learning principles that strengthen the process undertaken by this institution.

Table 7-5   Managed care program characteristics

MARYLAND ACCESS TO CARE (MAC)	DIABETES CARE PROGRAM (DCP)
Managed care program for the general Medicaid population.	Managed care program for Medicaid's diabetes population.
Enrollment is *required* for all recipients unless they are enrolled in one of Maryland Medicaid's specialized managed care programs. Those enrolled in specialized managed care may not be enrolled concurrently in MAC.	Enrollment is *optional*. Any recipient who has been hospitalized with a diabetes-related diagnosis may enroll. Enrollment in DCP voids enrollment in MAC.
Patient selects a primary care provider from among practitioners who have agreed to participate in the Medicaid program.	Patient selects a primary care provider from among practitioners who have agreed to participate in the Medicaid program *and* attend a five-hour diabetes management course.
Recipient's selected primary care provider provides or preauthorizes all care including specialty care.	Recipient's selected primary care provider provides or preauthorizes all care including specialty care. *In addition,* provider serves as a diabetes case manager and develops a network for making diabetes specialty care referrals as needed.
Fee-for-service reimbursement.	Fee-for-service reimbursement. *Plus* a $20/month case management fee for which the provider is expected to promote preventive strategies, including timely referrals for specialty care.
Comprehensive Maryland Medicaid benefit package.	Comprehensive Maryland Medicaid benefit package. *Plus* reimbursement for outpatient diabetes education, nutrition counseling, therapeutic footwear, blood glucose monitors, and supplies for non–insulin-dependent diabetes patients.

From Stuart ME: *Milbank Q* 72:679-704, 1994.

REFERENCES

1. American Diabetes Association: Third-party reimbursement for outpatient diabetes education and counseling, *Diabetes Care* 18(Suppl 1):45, 1995.
2. Anderson RM and others: Evaluation of an activated patient diabetes education newsletter, *Diabetes Educ* 20:29-34, 1994.
3. Anderson RM and others: The diabetes education experience of randomly selected patients under the care of community physicians, *Diabetes Educ* 20:399-405, 1994.
4. Anderson RM and others: Patient empowerment; results of a randomized controlled trial, *Diabetes Care* 18:943-949, 1995.
5. Baker SB and others: Medicare reimbursement guidelines for a diabetes and training program in a public healthcare setting, *Diabetes Educ* 21:139-144, 1995.
6. Barry B: Games and activities to teach children about diabetes and nutrition, *Diabetes Educ* 21:27-30, 1995.
7. Brown SA: Studies of educational interventions and outcomes in diabetic adults: a meta-analysis revisited, *Patient Educ Counsel* 16:189-215, 1990.
8. Brown SA: Meta-analysis of diabetes patient education research: variations in intervention effects across studies, *Res Nurs Health* 15:409-419, 1992.
9. Brown SA, Hanis CL: A community-based, culturally sensitive education and group-support intervention for Mexican Americans with NIDDM: a pilot study of efficacy, *Diabetes Educ* 21:203-210, 1995.
10. Cohen MZ and others: Explanatory models of diabetes: patient practitioner variation, *Soc Sci Med* 38:59-66, 1994.
11. Coonrod BA, Betschart J, Harris MI: Frequency and de-

terminants of diabetes patient education among adults in the U.S. population, *Diabetes Care* 17:851-858, 1994.

12. Cox DJ and others: Long-term follow-up evaluation of blood glucose awareness training, *Diabetes Care* 17:1-5, 1994.

13. Cypress M and others: The scope of practice of diabetes educators in a metropolitan area, *Diabetes Educ* 18:111-114, 1992.

14. Dawson LY: The Diabetes Index: a national study of diabetes resources, *Diabetes Spectrum* 6:138-142, 1993.

15. Diabetes Control and Complications Trial Research Group: Implementation of treatment protocols in the Diabetes Control and Complications Trial, *Diabetes Care* 18:361-376, 1995.

16. Funnell MM and others: Perceived effectiveness, cost and availability of patient education methods and materials, *Diabetes Educ* 18:139-145, 1992.

17. Funnell MM, Haas LB: National standards for diabetes self-management education programs, *Diabetes Care* 18:100-116, 1995.

18. Glasgow RE: A practical model of diabetes management and education, *Diabetes Care* 18:117-126, 1995.

19. Glasgow RE, Osteen VL: Evaluating diabetes education, *Diabetes Care* 15:1423-1432, 1992.

20. Glasgow AM and others: Readmissions of children with diabetes mellitus to a children's hospital, *Pediatrics* 88:98-104, 1991.

21. Gradman TJ and others: Verbal learning and/or memory improves with glycemic control in older subjects with non-insulin-dependent diabetes mellitus, *J Am Geriatr Soc* 41:1305-1312, 1993.

22. Hardway D, Weatherly KS, Bonheur B: Diabetes education on wheels, *J Nurs Staff Dev* 9:122-126, 1993.

23. Harris MI, Eastman RC, Siebert C: The DCCT and medical care for diabetes in the U.S., *Diabetes Care* 17:761-764, 1994.

24. Hernandez C, Grinspun DR: The challenges of teaching clients with cerebrovascular accidents to manage their diabetes, *Diabetes Educ* 20:311-316, 1994.

25. Litzelman DK and others: Reduction of lower extremity clinical abnormalities in patients with non-insulin-dependent diabetes mellitus, *Ann Intern Med* 119:36-41, 1993.

26. Lowe DH, Hogue JK, Delcher HK: Evolution of a progressive self-directed diabetes education model, *Diabetes Educ* 20:199-203, 1994.

27. Musey VC and others: Diabetes in urban African-Americans. I. Cessation of insulin therapy is the major precipitating cause of diabetic ketoacidosis, *Diabetes Care* 18:483-489, 1995.

28. Nurick MA, Johnson SB: Enhancing blood glucose awareness in adolescents and young adults with IDDM, *Diabetes Care* 14:1-7, 1991.

29. Padgett D and others: Meta-analysis of the effects of educational and psycho-social interventions of management of diabetes mellitus, *J Clin Epidemiol* 41:1007-1030, 1988.

30. Price MJ: An experiential model of learning diabetes self-management, *Qualitative Health Res* 3:29-54, 1993.

31. Ruggiero L, Prochaska JO: Introduction, *Diabetes Spectrum* 6:22-59, 1993.

32. Stuart ME: Redefining boundaries in the financing and care of diabetes: the Maryland experience, *Milbank Q* 72:679-704, 1994.

33. Weinberger M and others: The relationship between glycemic control and health-related quality of life in patients with non-insulin-dependent diabetes mellitus, *Med Care* 32:1173-1181, 1994.

34. Willhoite MB and others: The impact of preconception counseling on pregnancy outcomes; the exerpience of the Maine Diabetes in Pregnancy Program, *Diabetes Care* 16:450-455, 1993.

8 Education for Pregnancy and Parenting and Education of Children

EDUCATION FOR PREGNANCY AND PARENTING

General Approach

Education for pregnancy and parenting and education of children are established fields of practice in patient education. Although many of the goals remain the same, prenatal education has become more varied philosophically. All three fields reflect dramatic shifts in the way health is delivered and the tremendous increase in self-management currently expected of patients and families.

Educational Approaches and Research Base

Ideally, prenatal education should begin before pregnancy, with formal classes starting early in pregnancy and extending across the childbearing year, from conception to 3 months after delivery. In actuality, formal early-pregnancy education has been neglected; formal midpregnancy education classes are not widely available, and most prenatal teaching that takes place during the third trimester prepares for birth. A frequently used format is weekly classes in a community setting, in which the following topics are addressed[29]:

- *Health maintenance:* Prevention of urinary tract infections, Kegel exercises and exercise in general, smoking and alcohol ingestion, medication use, and nutritional intake
- *Management of pregnancy and birth:* Signs of complications, discomforts of pregnancy, potential complications of pregnancy, the birth plan, recognition of labor and preterm labor and preparation for it
- *Parenting, as well as postpartum and infant care:* Prebirth preparation for parenting,

preparation for infant feeding, including breastfeeding, circumcision and cord care, and other topics

The box on p. 152 provides an outline for prenatal education that includes both preconception and the trimesters. In addition, special classes may be held for pregnant adolescents, for first-time mothers over 35 years of age, for adoptive parents, for those who have a scheduled cesarean section or a vaginal birth after cesarean, for siblings, for grandparents, and others.[29]

There is some evidence that postpartum women have transient deficits in cognitive function, particularly in memory function and attention. This finding would, of course, have major implications for informed consent, discharge planning, and instructions as to subsequent care of the newborn. There is strong support for the conclusion that this is not a side effect of intrapartum narcotic medication but rather is due to the stress of labor and delivery. In one study the women's scores on cognitive tests had returned to normal by the second postpartum day, although other studies have found them to be altered for a longer duration.[11] Equally interesting is the finding that maternal self-efficacy in coping with labor, which can be a goal of pregnancy education programs, significantly contributes to a lessened perception of pain during labor. Recall from Chapter 2 that development of self-efficacy may occur through previous experience with significant pain, watching others perform successfully, verbal persuasion, and knowledge that develops during childbirth-preparation classes.[21]

Several excellent meta-analyses of studies of prenatal education have been completed, al-

■ Outline for Prenatal Education

At the earliest contact between client and nurse, a teaching plan is developed. This reflects the unique learning needs of each client and incorporates information that health care providers identify as essential for all pregnant women to know and information that clients identify as learning priorities. The outline is reviewed with the client and updated whenever necessary. Client referral to individuals or organizations sponsoring childbirth education can also be appropriate for meeting overall learning objectives.

Preconception

How pregnancy occurs (menstrual cycle)
Lifestyle factors with potential impact on becoming pregnant and on early pregnancy: drugs such as alcohol, nutritional status, general health, occupational and environmental considerations
Alternatives in childbirth settings and in obstetric caregivers
Pregnancy tests
Myths about conception and pregnancy

First trimester

Feelings about pregnancy, ambivalence, developmental tasks of early pregnancy, age-related issues
Family reactions to pregnancy, first-trimester emotional responses of expectant fathers
Early-pregnancy physical changes
Sexuality during the first trimester
Lifestyle factors with potential impact on early pregnancy: drugs such as alcohol, nutrition (including prescribed vitamin and iron supplements), general health, exercise, rest, occupational and environmental considerations
Warning signs of early pregnancy
Fear of miscarriage (suggested presentation as a topic in a group setting)
First-trimester diagnostic tests for maternal/fetal well-being (as appropriate)
Client expectations for pregnancy and childbirth
Options available to client within the selected prenatal and delivery setting, tour of birthing facility

Anticipatory guidance regarding what to expect at prenatal visits
Sibling concerns, telling other children about pregnancy
Resources within the caregiving agency or private practice and within the community (including relevant literature)

Second trimester

Feelings about pregnancy, acceptance of pregnancy, developmental tasks of midpregnancy, age-related issues
Family responses to progressing pregnancy, second-trimester responses of expectant fathers
Fetal growth and development
Midtrimester physical changes, relief of discomforts associated with enlarging fetus and physical changes
Sexuality during the second trimester
Lifestyle factors with potential impact on midpregnancy: drugs such as alcohol, smoking, nutrition (including prescribed vitamin and iron supplements), general health, exercise, body mechanics, rest, occupational and environmental considerations, stress
Changes in activities of daily living related to midtrimester
Warning signs of midpregnancy
Diagnostic tests for assessment of maternal/fetal well-being (as necessary)
Client's expectations for pregnancy and birth
Client's fears and anxieties related to second trimester
Sibling concerns
Client expectations for pregnancy and childbirth, confirmation of registration for third-trimester prenatal classes

Third trimester

Feelings about pregnancy, developmental tasks of third trimester
Preparation for labor, delivery, and parenting (Content may be given by health care providers during prenatal visits or can be offered in greater depth during a series of prepared childbirth classes.)

From Sherwen LN, Scoloveno MA, Weingarten CT: *Nursing care of the childbearing family*, ed 2, Norwalk, Conn, 1995, Appleton & Lange.

■ OUTLINE FOR PRENATAL EDUCATION—cont'd

Client expectations for labor and birth, progress of prepared childbirth classes

Family reactions to advanced pregnancy; third-trimester emotional responses of expectant fathers; sibling preparation

Late-pregnancy physical changes, management of discomforts related to late pregnancy

Sexuality during the third trimester

Lifestyle factors with potential impact on late pregnancy: drugs such as alcohol, nutrition (including prescribed vitamin and iron supplements), smoking, general health, exercise, body mechanics, rest, occupational and environmental considerations

Signs of labor, "true" labor versus "false" labor, physiology of labor and delivery, passenger, passage, powers, and psyche in labor

Positioning in labor

Techniques useful during labor and delivery (e.g., psychoprophylactic method, Bradley method)

Analgesia and anesthesia during labor and delivery, medications used during labor and delivery

Technology and childbirth, assessment of fetal maturity, potential for induction or augmentation of labor, potential use of electronic fetal monitoring, intravenous infusions, and so on

Variations in labor

The high-risk experience: potential for operative obstetrics (e.g., forceps, episiotomy, cesarean childbirth); potential for transfer from birthing center, home, or birthing room because of obstetric complications; potential for family-centered birth despite operative obstetrics

Warning signs of late pregnancy, signs and symptoms of premature labor

Review of birth plan, anticipatory guidance regarding what can be expected within the selected labor and delivery setting

Discussion of fears and concerns related to late pregnancy, labor and delivery, or postpartum

Tour of labor and delivery setting

Preparations for client's stay in hospital or birth center, preparations for a home birth

Preparations for other family members during client's birthing experience and immediate recovery (e.g., child care for siblings)

Preparations for the newborn, selection of a pediatric caregiver (may include a prenatal introductory meeting)

Infant nutrition, preparation for breastfeeding or bottle feeding

Early parenting

What to expect from caregivers and the health care system during labor, delivery, and postpartum

Anticipatory guidance for postpartum (includes physical and emotional changes, family changes, and strategies for coping)

Resources available during third trimester and postpartum

---

though two were published long enough ago to need updating. Jones' summary of 27 studies completed through the early 1980s found a moderate-effect size as a result of childbirth education: parents were more attentive and responsive to their infants, more satisfied with the behavior of the infants, and spent more time playing with and cuddling their infants.[17] Few negative effects were found. Larger-effect sizes were obtained for middle-income parents (0.40) as compared with parents of low income (0.16). A research summary of adolescent pregnancy education programs found average effect sizes of 0.35.[20]

Finally, an analysis of 11 randomized trials of prenatal smoking cessation interventions found a 50% increase in smoking cessation.[24] Although there was a high rate of return to smoking among women who were abstinent during pregnancy, approximately one third stopped smoking permanently. Interventions that were more intensive, with multiple contacts, multiple formats, and some form of follow-up, were more effective. The outcomes these programs can effect are important because maternal smoking causes an estimated 20% to 30% of the low birth weight rate and 10% of infant mortality in the United States.

■ QUESTIONS FOR THE PHYSICIAN AND
PARENTS IN THE NEONATAL
INTENSIVE CARE UNIT SETTING

1. How do you understand Billy's medical problems?
2. Has anything like this ever happened to you before?
3. What do you feel may have contributed to Billy's illness?
4. Is there anything that we are doing or not doing to Billy that is worrying you?
5. Do both of you see Billy's medical problems and the decision that we are facing in the same way? Do either of you see anything differently?
6a. Have you been able even to consider that Billy, being this ill, is in danger of not getting better or actually dying?
6b. Just as we fear not being able to save every child, we also fear going too far, even worsening their suffering, when our efforts are futile. Do you think that this could happen to Billy?
6c. If I am sure that certain treatments will cause suffering for Billy without really helping him then I won't be able to do those things. We always tell parents when we think this time is approaching. [Initially] For Billy things have not reached this point and we hope they do not. [Later] For Billy we could be there in a matter of hours. (A brief period of silence will allow parents to respond.)
7. Do you feel I'm helping or guiding you too much or too little?
8. How do your religious or cultural values influence this decision?
9. What was your main reason for deciding the way you did?
10. How do you feel about holding the baby when the machines are removed?

From Jellinek M and others: *Pediatrics* 89:119-122, 1992.

A special current area of concern is patient education to aid in the early detection and treatment of preterm labor, which is part of a larger program of management. Of all preterm births, about 80% are the direct result of preterm labor, defined as the presence of uterine contractions with progressive cervical dilation or effacement, or both, occurring before 37 weeks' gestation. Programs for prevention have had inconsistent results in decreasing overall preterm birth rates, in part because risk-scoring systems still fall short of identifying most patients who experience the problem.[12] Another study[26] has shown that women found the symptoms ambiguous in that they were subtle, lacked a pattern, and unpredictably waxed and waned. Thus these symptoms were confused with the expected discomforts of pregnancy. Yet a recent large prospective trial incorporating education and increased visits for a largely Hispanic population did show a significant reduction over the control group in preterm birth rates.[13]

After birth some parents of gravely ill infants face difficult decisions about withdrawal of the neonate's life supports and limiting resuscitation efforts in the neonatal intensive care unit (NICU). Education is almost always necessary to help them cope and be full participants. The accompanying box describes questions for the physician and parents; these same questions and their answers are also highly relevant for caregiving by other staff members. These questions are meant to assess parent understanding, as well as guilt they may be feeling, their worries about painful procedures, and how to deal with the ambiguity that is frequently a part of these situations.[15]

Likewise, the transition from NICU to home is stressful for parents and requires concentrated instruction to become competent and confident in the care of the infant. Prematurity may have been the reason for NICU treatment; such infants are often less responsive and more difficult to care for than are healthy full-term infants. They have less effective care-eliciting behavior and may not cry to signal need for care; feeding is often characterized by slow food intake and excessive body movements or frequent spitting up; and they are more likely to have residual medical problems that require treatment at home.

Parents need to be taught basic caregiving, regulation of temperature, growth and development, and infant stimulation, and they must learn to recognize the signs and symptoms of illness, including abnormal breathing patterns. Despite agreement as to the discharge preparation needs, there is little evidence to indicate whether parents are currently being well-prepared for their infant's discharge. Table 8-1 provides a list of the topics thought to be important, the staff and parents' perception of importance (on a scale of 1 as very unimportant to 5 as very important), and whether the topic was discussed.[28] Note the significant discrepancies between parents and staff members on some items. Parents who receive inadequate discharge preparation may not feel competent or confident in their ability to care for their newborn. If you were working in this NICU, what would you do with the results of this survey?

It has been shown that child abuse is more prevalent among parents of children with a subtle handicap, and preterm infants are highly represented in this group of abused children. Although abuse has many causes, a teaching approach to help parents recognize their preterm infant's behavioral cues and to develop confidence in the infant's competence is a way of building self-efficacy. Some care providers involve the parents in the process of evaluating the behavior of their preterm infant through use of formal assessment tools. For example, a neurobehavioral assessment of the preterm infant is an instrument that measures the differential maturity of preterm infants and provides specific information in several domains, including motor development and vigor, alertness and orientation, irritability, vigor of cry, and percentage of time asleep.[10] The scores can be compared with normative guidelines, and serial assessments of the infant can be made to document change. The provider teaches while making the assessment, confirms observations parents have already made, and helps parents become more aware of their infant's abilities.

Children or infants who have been critically ill may be at increased risk for a respiratory or cardiac event at home. The box on p. 158 provides a description of emergency skills education for parents.[23] In addition to the class content outline, it would have been extremely useful to see outcome objectives and measures to determine how well they were being met. Construct objectives you think would be required.

Community-Based Education and Education of Special Populations

To improve the outcomes of pregnancy and to prevent child abuse, at least 24 states have begun to increase their support of nurse home-visitation services to pregnant women and parents of young children. One study showed that the nurses helped women improve their infant caregiving, promoted positive health-related behaviors, and reduced family stress by improving the social and physical environments in which families live.[25] Those who received visits by a nurse during pregnancy reduced the number of cigarettes smoked, improved the quality of their diets, had few kidney infections, and experienced greater support from family members and friends. Smokers visited by the nurse bore 75% fewer preterm infants, and young adolescents visited by a nurse bore infants who were 395 grams heavier at birth than infants of their counterparts in the comparison group.

Among poor unmarried teenagers, the incidence of state-verified child abuse and neglect during the first 2 years after delivery was 19% in the comparison group and 4% in the group that received both prenatal and infancy nurse-visitation.[25] Such programs can also affect maternal employment and subsequent pregnancies. Those that are successful focus their services on families at greater need for the service and use nurses who visit frequently, beginning during pregnancy and continuing at least through the second year of the child's life.

Table 8-1   Results of staff discharge teaching survey and comparable items from the parent retrospective transition interview

QUESTIONNAIRE ITEM	IMPORTANCE		WAS TOPIC DISCUSSED?	
	STAFF	PARENTS	STAFF (%)	PARENTS* (%)
Feeding				
1. How much and how often to feed baby	4.9	4.7	100	96
2. What to do if baby isn't eating enough	4.9	4.3	94	24
3. Help if I wanted to breastfeed	4.8	3.4	97	56
4. What to do if baby sleeps through feedings	4.4	4.1	91	64
Bathing				
5. How to bathe and how often	4.3	4.4	97	93
6. How to keep baby's hair clean	4.1	4.1	100	73
Sleeping				
7. How long baby should sleep at one time	3.8	3.7	68	20
8. How often baby should nap	3.5	3.6	56	14
9. How to tell if baby is sleepy	3.1	3.3	44	14
10. What to do when baby won't sleep	3.9	4.0	67	22
Crying				
11. How much baby might cry	3.5	3.8	47	13
12. What to do when baby cries	4.2	4.4	88	49
13. What to do if baby cries too much or not enough	3.9	4.0	67	9
Playing				
14. How to encourage baby to interact with mom	4.3	4.2	88	38
15. How to tell when baby is ready to play	3.4	3.8	44	9
16. Tricks to keep baby involved in play	3.2	3.6	32	2
17. How to make or find interesting things to put in baby's crib	3.7	4.0	74	47
Baby's unique characteristics				
18. Baby's personality/temperament	4.0	4.2	85	53
19. How baby lets his/her needs be known	4.2	4.3	94	59
20. Baby's response to handling	4.1	4.4	82	47
Monitoring baby's health				
21. How to recognize differences between normal breathing patterns and those that indicate illness	4.8	4.4	91	38
22. How to recognize the difference between spitting up and vomiting	4.4	4.4	77	38
23. How to recognize the difference between regular stools, diarrhea, and constipation	4.6	4.6	82	58
24. How to get in touch with the NICU staff	4.6	4.8	100	100

From Sheikh L, O'Brian M, McCheskey-Fawcett K: *Children's Health Care* 22:227-239, 1993.
*Parent data represent percentage of those who responded to the question; when a topic was not relevant for a particular mother and infant, it was recorded as not applicable.

Table 8-1   Results of staff discharge teaching survey and comparable items from the parent retrospective transition interview—cont'd

QUESTIONNAIRE ITEM	IMPORTANCE		WAS TOPIC DISCUSSED?	
	STAFF	PARENTS	STAFF (%)	PARENTS* (%)
Taking care of baby's health				
25. How to give medications	5.0	4.8	100	100
26. How to take baby's temperature	4.9	4.6	100	98
27. How to use a bulb syringe	4.9	4.4	100	84
28. What to do if someone living at home gets sick	3.9	4.3	42	27
29. How to give CPR	4.9	4.8	100	64
Medical care				
30. How soon to schedule a visit with baby's primary care physician	4.8	4.8	100	93
31. How baby's medical records are transferred	3.3	4.1	38	27
32. How to get help in an emergency	4.9	4.7	94	64
33. How to pay for the hospital stay	3.8	4.1	71	42
Learning more about prematurity				
34. How to get in touch with other parents of preemies	3.4	3.6	47	5
35. Books or pamphlets about prematurity	4.1	4.5	97	46
36. Where to get preemie diapers and clothing	3.6	3.9	82	47
37. Awareness of normal and delayed growth and development	4.2	4.5	67	38
38. Suggestions on ways to encourage baby's growth and development	4.1	4.4	68	22
39. When to schedule baby for developmental follow-up	4.2	4.6	85	73
With family and friends				
40. Who should hold and handle baby	3.4	3.5	68	33
41. How relatives and friends might react to the baby	3.3	3.3	32	7
42. Whether it is okay to leave the baby with another caretaker	3.6	3.6	53	38
43. How much clothing baby needs indoors and outdoors	4.1	4.1	82	47

In a study of interventions provided by clinical nurse specialists who followed very low birthweight infants from hospital to home, 68% were teaching interventions.[7] Before discharge, parents were required to demonstrate satisfactorily the basic caretaking skills (such as bathe, handle, feed and soothe; take the infant's temperature; provide skin care; prevent infection) and a basic knowledge of any medications or special procedures required in the infant's care. It was important to teach adaptations of basic care due to pre-maturity of the infant, including use of "preemie" nipples, problems of reflux, and frequent feeding problems caused by diminished or weaker sucking and reduced gastric capacity. The need to maintain warmth because of less advanced neurologic development, less adipose tissue, and thinner, more fragile skin was taught. Infant stimulation and how to gauge developmental milestones were also addressed.

Management of chronic illness in children requires a special approach to education frequently

---

■ EMERGENCY SKILLS EDUCATION PARENT CLASS CONTENT OUTLINE

Introduction: Purpose and organization of the class

Emergency Medical Services System: Access and use
  a. "911"
  b. Other

Causes and prevention of injury

ABC's of lifesaving

Management of foreign body airway obstruction:
  Conscious victim
  a. Lecture: Assessment of airway obstruction in the conscious victim and actions to relieve the obstruction
  b. Demonstration of skills needed to relieve the obstructed airway
  c. Mannequin practice and skills demonstration by participants

Management of foreign body airway obstruction:
  Unconscious victim
  a. Lecture: Assessment of airway obstruction in the unconscious victim and actions to relieve the obstruction
  b. Demonstration of skills needed to relieve the obstructed airway
  c. Mannequin practice and skills demonstration by participants

Rescue breathing
  a. Lecture: Assessment of the need for rescue breathing
  b. Demonstration of rescue breathing techniques

Cardiopulmonary resuscitation
  a. Lecture: Assessment of pulselessness to determine the need for CPR and determination of the effectiveness of CPR when given
  b. Demonstration of CPR skills
  c. Mannequin practice and skills demonstration by participants

Closing
  a. Questions and answers
  b. Refer participant to CPR courses in their communities for further information and reinforcement of skills

From Moynihan P, Naclerio L, Kiley K: *Nurs Clin North Am* 30:231-241, 1995.

---

difficult to deliver in acute care settings. For example, McCrindle and others[22] provide recent data on an old problem that could be solved with appropriate education. Most children with heart murmurs are found to have no significant heart disease; yet many parents believe a heart murmur to be an actual heart lesion. Restrictions and emotional distress may therefore be imposed on the child in spite of the absence of significant heart disease. The data in this study show that 1 month after assessment, 10% of parents continued to believe that their child had a heart problem, although none could describe or specify a lesion.

Advances in the treatment of childhood diseases have created a population of technology-dependent and medically fragile children whose life expectancy is unknown and whose future quality of life is unpredictable. The family has, of course, to cope with the uncertainty. As much as the family may understand what can be known about their child's condition, certain triggers heighten awareness of the uncertainty concerning the child's survival. Triggers are routine medical appointments; body variability inasmuch as the initial presenting symptoms frequently were not seen as harbingers of a serious illness; key words and provocative questions such as "remission"; changes in therapeutic regimen, including a therapeutic success; evidence of negative outcomes; new developmental demands; and nighttime. The responsibility for management of this chronic uncertainty has been largely left to the ingenuity of the parents, without much deliberate assistance from health care providers. Cohen[9] reports that parents who are trying to attain some degree of family normality by consciously controlling the awareness of the seriousness of their child's illness are thwarted by health professionals who mistakenly assess their behavior as denial.

Although there will always be triggers, attending to them has the potential to reduce some of the stressful events experienced by these families. For example, when a child is seen for a routine medical appointment, there should be no time lag between the physical examination and the explanation of the findings to the parents. Anticipatory guidance that will enable parents to recognize normal or common behavioral and physiologic alterations has the potential to reduce uncertainty for parents who may lack plausible alternative explanations for the variation in their child's usual behavior or who may be unsure of how to change their own behavior in relation to the child's changing needs. The simple act of teaching parents to use a stethoscope to recognize abnormal breath sounds has been shown to be a significant factor in reducing uncertainty about the status of a child who had cystic fibrosis.[9] It gave the parents immediate feedback and some sense of control to be able to distinguish an actual problem from a false alarm.

An excellent theoretically based intervention program for self-management of a chronic childhood illness has been developed by Bartholomew and others[3]—the Cystic Fibrosis (CF) Family Education Program. Self-management behaviors to be attained by children of various ages and their parents are shown in the box below. Use of social learning theory means that goal setting, self-monitoring, modeling (use of models who are positively coping), skill training

---

> ### ■ SELF-MANAGEMENT BEHAVIORS FOR CYSTIC FIBROSIS
>
> **Medical self-care**
> Manage lower respiratory infection
> Manage respiratory obstruction
> Manage malabsorption
> Maintain adequate nutritional status
>
> **Adjustment**
> Use coping strategies to manage problems in CF
> Communicate effectively in the context of self-managing CF
> Engage in developmentally appropriate activities
> Utilize health care services

From Bartholomew LK and others: *Health Educ Q* 18:429-443, 1991.

tailored to fit into the family's lifestyle, and positive reinforcement are important intervention strategies (see Chapter 2 for a review of this theory). The self-paced print program format is composed of modules that include a parent core, as well as cores for each child developmental stage.[3]

In general, although the prenatal and parenting educational needs of special populations have not had high priority, some excellent programs exist. Research has shown that poor women in Tijuana, Mexico, tended to delay or avoid seeking prenatal care, and they were not aware of symptoms that could warn of pregnancy complications.[1] These women believed that prenatal care was unnecessary if the mother felt well, and some avoided prenatal care because they experienced embarrassment in medical offices or hospitals. On the basis of an ethnographic study, culturally appropriate messages were developed about health services use, weight gain, and nutrition and anemia. The material was developed in terms of sound educational principles: being specific about symptoms of high-risk complications during pregnancy and actions that should be taken, and the messages were delivered through media the women experienced in their daily lives—posters, calendars, and radio.

Because some adolescents encounter problems in their parenting roles, this group is also considered to be a special population for prenatal and parenting education. These mothers have been observed to have difficulty in interactions with their infants, tending to use less praise and more physical punishment than did adult mothers, perhaps related to their own developmental stage and lack of familiarity with child developmental norms.[19] Most programs provide basic instruction in caretaking skills and infant safety. It is also important to foster maternal behaviors to assist in the social and cognitive development of children, such as offering praise and encouragement. Videotapes of standard problem situations, as well as parents interacting with their own children, serve as effective teaching materials.

Developmentally disabled parents also have special needs in learning parenting skills—recognizing and meeting the medical, nutritional, so-cial, emotional, developmental, and cognitive needs of their children, including appropriate stimulation for normal growth and development.[18] The usual parenting and childbirth education classes and books are frequently not accessible to these parents, and they often face isolation from extended family, lack of a support network, and poverty-level income. Neglect of their children is one of the most common problems found among mentally retarded parents. The parents may have difficulty in identifying and providing for the needs of the children, such as for adequate fluid and nutrition or medical needs. Although most injuries have predictable causes, these parents may show inadequate judgment or lack the skills to predict possible outcomes. Teaching of safety must be linked with the normal stages of development, interwoven with age-appropriate activities and discipline.

Kaatz[18] lists curriculums available throughout the United States that address parenting skills for retarded parents. As learning theory indicates, these parents learn best from hands-on experience. A retarded mother may not understand instructions to give her baby 0.4 ml of medication drops but might be able to understand instructions to give an amount up to "here" when the dropper is marked with a piece of tape. Teaching bonding skills and use of supportive resources is also important.

National Standards and Tested Programs

Both childbirth educators and lactation consultants can be certified through international associations.

EDUCATION OF CHILDREN
General Approach

Theory and research about how children learn is presented in Chapter 2. In addition, several earlier chapters include examples of education for health problems, such as asthma, that heavily affect children. Some earlier sections of this chapter that focus on education for parenting also include an educational component for children. This section provides examples of how patient education services primarily focused on children are being offered in communities and health care institutions.

A distinct philosophy guides educational programs for children. It is articulated in a statement by the American Academy of Pediatrics on child life programs.[2] The statement notes that these programs have become the standard in pediatric settings to address the psychosocial concerns that accompany hospitalization and medical care. Child life specialists facilitate coping and adjustment of children and families by providing play experiences, presenting information about events and procedures, and establishing supportive relationships to encourage family involvement in each child's care. These activities are shared by members of the health care team and the child life specialist.

Play is a central part of child life programs because it sustains normal development and because play episodes allow children to process their concerns and cope with health treatments. Clinical data support the value of play in reducing the emotional disturbance of children in hospitals and clinics. Preparation programs that introduce children and their families to the circumstances and procedures they will encounter also reduce emotional disturbance. Family resource centers that make educational materials available can assist in the goal of helping to reduce parental anxiety, which can be transmitted to children.[2]

Educational Approaches and Research Base

Although not all education of children takes place as part of a formal child life program, there is general acceptance of the need to design education according to the developmental levels of recipients and with the essential involvement of families.

Of the four summaries of research on patient education for children shown in Appendix C, none is recent. Those that use techniques of meta-analysis generally provide a more reliable summary of the research available a few years before the time they are published. Broome, Lillis, and Smith[6] found that pain-management programs for children resulted in at least a 30% reduction in their distress responses.

Because an understanding of internal anatomy is useful to much health teaching, it is helpful to have available a summary of research about children's knowledge of internal body parts. Preschool-age children, who may be in the preoperational stage of cognitive development, have only a vague idea that something is going on inside their bodies. Internal body image is not a significant part of children's body image until age 5 to 6 years. They seem to make the most dramatic gains in this knowledge at about age 8 years, corresponding to expected entry into the concrete operational stage of cognitive development. From that age forward, children usually have rudimentary information about the brain, heart, bones, and stomach but only minimal knowledge of the nervous system, parts of the gastrointestinal system besides the stomach, the circulatory system, or the immune system.[16]

Little information is available about possible cross-cultural differences in children's knowledge of internal anatomy or about the mediating effects of altered health status. It is believed that it is not until close to the midteen years that individuals achieve the conceptual-integrative capacity to simultaneously relate the multiple factors involved in understanding diabetes and its control.[16]

Much education for children in medical settings focuses on helping them through procedures; misunderstandings, fears, and fantasies often manifest as overt upset behavior during procedures. Figure 8-1 shows portions of a coloring book about intravenous (IV) therapy for children between the ages of 3 and 11 years. It is expected that after the teaching session, children will be able (1) to explain at least one reason why IV therapy is used, (2) to verbalize two sensations they will see, feel, or smell during IV insertion, (3) to demonstrate their role during the IV insertion, and (4) to describe what they will feel when the IV is removed.[30]

Because children at the preoperational stage are egocentric, the first frame of Figure 8-1 is blank for them to draw a self-portrait. The booklet is designed to be used in conjunction with an IV pump, dolls, syringes, a tourniquet, and alcohol swabs for medical play. This play involves examination of equipment, performing procedures on dolls or puppets, and games or stories. Teaching sessions should take place before the procedure so that children will have time to assimilate the information and feel adequately in control and again after IV insertion, to allow them to talk about the procedure and ventilate their feelings about the experience. It is best to prepare preschoolers shortly before the planned procedure because they become overly anxious if told too far in advance. Evaluation of the intervention usually is based on how the child behaved and felt during the procedure.[30]

Consider children with acute lymphoblastic leukemia (ALL), which typically involves at least 3 years of frequent invasive medical procedures, including intramuscular (IM) and IV injections, lumbar punctures, and bone marrow aspiration. Children between the ages of 2 and 5 years are at the highest risk for developing ALL, and their distress reactions to invasive medical procedures are greater in amount, intensity, and variety than those of children older than 6 years. Interventions focused on training in coping skills have proved effective in decreasing children's behavioral distress. They frequently employ some combination of several treatment strategies, including provision of procedural information, filmed modeling, imagery, breathing exercises, muscle relaxation, positive incentives, and behavioral rehearsal. Parents are also taught coping-promoting skills via modeling, role play, and behavior rehearsal.[27]

Community-Based Education and Education of Special Populations

Summer camps are examples of community-based education for children. They use a variety of teaching approaches. One diabetes education camp used structured fantasy as a way of encouraging

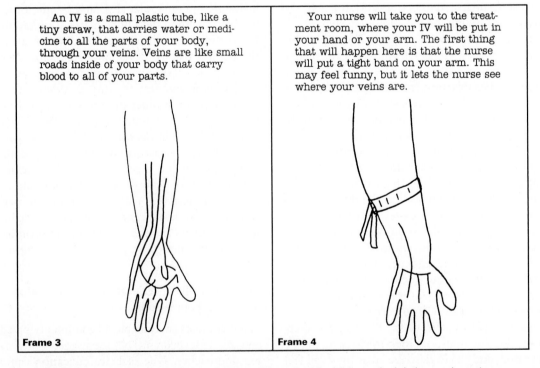

MY COLORING BOOK ABOUT IV THERAPY

Frame 1

Your doctor has decided that you need an IV to help you get better. An IV will give you water when you are too sick to drink for yourself, or it will give you medicine that will help you get better faster.

Frame 2

An IV is a small plastic tube, like a tiny straw, that carries water or medicine to all the parts of your body, through your veins. Veins are like small roads inside of your body that carry blood to all of your parts.

Frame 3

Your nurse will take you to the treatment room, where your IV will be put in your hand or your arm. The first thing that will happen here is that the nurse will put a tight band on your arm. This may feel funny, but it lets the nurse see where your veins are.

Frame 4

Figure 8-1 Sample educational tool designed for use with children scheduled to undergo intravenous therapy. (From Thompson V: An IV therapy teaching tool for children, *Pediatr Nurs* 20:351-355, 1994.)

After we have decided where your IV will go, the nurse will clean off that spot with some alcohol. Alcohol kills germs. The alcohol may feel cold and smell funny, but it will not hurt.

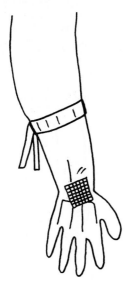

Frame 5

After the vein is picked, and the spot cleaned off, the hard part comes. A needle will be put under your skin and into your vein. This part hurts, but it is a short hurt. Some boys and girls have said that it feels like a hard pinch, or like a bee sting. The nurse will tell you before putting the needle in. It is OK to cry, or squeeze the nurse's hand when it hurts, but it is very important that you hold very still during this part.

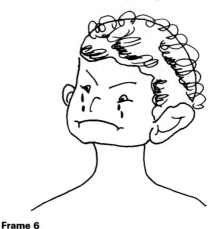

Frame 6

After the IV is in place in your vein, the needle is taken out, and the small plastic tube will stay in your vein. The hurting part is over now. The IV will be taped in place, and you will have a small, soft board taped to your hand or arm. This will help the IV to stay in place while it is needed.

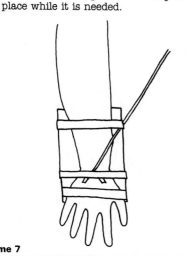

Frame 7

Some patients need to get water or medicine all of the time. The bottle of medicine will hang on a pole that looks like this. You can roll this pole with you wherever you go. You can go to the bathroom, or to the playroom, when you are feeling better. The machine on the pole may beep sometimes. Ask your nurse what it sounds like. Some children think that it sounds like a Nintendo game. When it beeps it means that the nurse needs to look at your IV or that you need a new bottle of medicine.

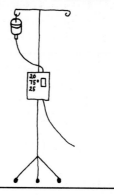

Frame 8

Figure 8-1, cont'd   For legend, see opposite page.

Continued.

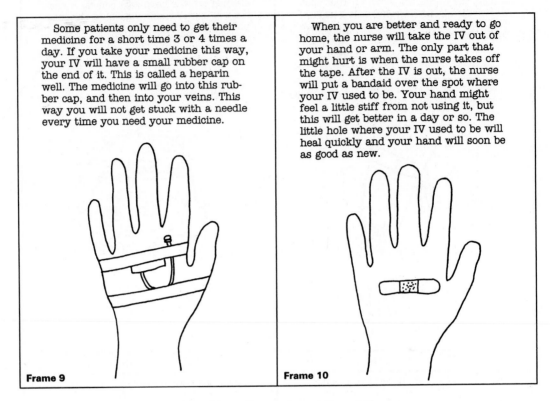

Some patients only need to get their medicine for a short time 3 or 4 times a day. If you take your medicine this way, your IV will have a small rubber cap on the end of it. This is called a heparin well. The medicine will go into this rubber cap, and then into your veins. This way you will not get stuck with a needle every time you need your medicine.

Frame 9

When you are better and ready to go home, the nurse will take the IV out of your hand or arm. The only part that might hurt is when the nurse takes off the tape. After the IV is out, the nurse will put a bandaid over the spot where your IV used to be. Your hand might feel a little stiff from not using it, but this will get better in a day or so. The little hole where your IV used to be will heal quickly and your hand will soon be as good as new.

Frame 10

Figure 8-1, cont'd   For legend, see p. 162.

children to examine their own feelings, issues, and concerns and to express themselves in terms of anger and dependency issues involving parents, medical staff, and occasionally siblings.[4] A group of children created, planned, rehearsed, enacted, videotaped, and then viewed their own improvised dramatic show. For example, one group planned a skit dealing with how to decline foods that everyone else consumed at a social event.

Community-based programs on self-care for children with chronic illnesses are fairly numerous, and some of these children may have no adult supervision on return home from school. Parents report that many after-school day-care programs will not take a child with a chronic illness. Self-care education programs are important and, if the children are ready for them, have potentially positive effects, such as developing maturity, self-reliance, decision-making ability, and

responsibility.[14] Negative consequences of children's self-care are obvious, and parents worry about emergencies and security. Because cognitive, social, and emotional development rates differ with each child, it is best not to identify an exact age at which children with a chronic illness can begin self-care. Instead the provider and parents need to jointly assess the child's maturity levels, knowledge of the illness, and ability to perform medical treatments. The boxes on p. 165 and the box on p. 166 provide assessment tools for this purpose and guidelines for a self-care training program.

The child's motivation is perhaps the most important predictor of success in self-care programs. Children need not only to be comfortable with their ability to perform treatments and to manage the illness but also to know how to follow important rules without testing the limits

ASSESSMENT OF THE CHILD'S READINESS FOR SELF-CARE

1. What is the child's cognitive developmental level? Is the child capable of solving problems in a rational manner? Can this child read well enough to follow written instructions and write well enough to take messages?
2. Is the child able to follow instructions related to aspects of self-care and to record behavior and signs?
3. Is the child socially mature? Can the child demonstrate the ability to judge right from wrong? Can he or she resist peer pressure? Does the child show respect for the rights of others?
4. Is the child overly shy or fearful? Can the child tolerate separations without excessive fear or upset?
5. Does the child have self-discipline?
6. Can the child entertain himself or herself?
7. Does the child take responsibility for home chores?
8. Does the child know basic first aid?
9. Does the child know what to do in case of an emergency (e.g., fire, police)?
10. How well does the child understand his or her illness?
11. Does the child have the knowledge and manual dexterity to safely carry out treatments?
12. Can the child manage during a medical emergency?
13. Can the child distinguish between a real medical emergency and a more trivial problem?
14. Can the child handle unusual and unexpected situations without excessive fear and upset?

From Holaday B and others: *Pediatr Health Care* 7:256-263, 1993.

SELF-ASSESSMENT FOR PARENTS OF CHILDREN IN SELF-CARE

1. How many days per week and hours per day will the child be in self-care?
2. Will the child be able to maintain friendships with other children?
3. Are your health care providers (e.g., physician, nurse) aware of the fact that your child is in self-care?
4. Have you developed clear in-home rules that the child is to follow?
5. Is an older sibling going to care for the ill child? How does the sibling feel about this? Is the sibling prepared to care for the ill child?
6. How do you plan to monitor the child's safety, activities, and status when the child is home alone?
7. Do you have a neighbor who is willing to periodically check on things?
8. Do you have a designated neighbor to help in case of an emergency?
9. Have you purchased any types of special entertainment devices (e.g., VCR, computer, radio) to keep the child entertained while at home alone?
10. Will the child have to prepare a snack or meal? Can the child do this safely?
11. What types of safety devices (e.g., first aid kit, smoke and burglar alarms) have been purchased to protect the child?
12. Have you specified what activities the child is allowed to take part in while home alone?
13. Is the child motivated for self-care?
14. Have you taught your child the self-care skills needed to manage the illness when at home alone? Do you believe your child can correctly and safely perform these activities?
15. Does the child have the necessary support from parents, siblings, or neighbors to carry out a self-care regimen?
16. Have you taught your child what to do in case of an emergency? A medical emergency? Does the child know the role of police, fire fighters, paramedics, and 911?
17. Can the child safely operate household appliances (e.g., stove, microwave, fans, heater)?
18. Does you child know basic first aid?

From Holaday B and others: *Pediatr Health Care* 7:256-263, 1993.

■ GUIDELINES FOR A SELF-CARE
TRAINING PROGRAM

I. Management of chronic illness
  1. Knowledge of disease and its management
    a. Symptom discrimination
    b. Effects and side effects of medications
    c. Treatments
  2. Self-care skills related to disease
    a. Self-monitoring and self-recording of data by child about condition
    b. Processing and evaluating of information the child gathers about himself
    c. Decision making with respect to child's selecting the most appropriate action from among potential solutions
    d. Self-instruction on the use of self-statements by child to prompt, direct, or maintain performance
    e. Panic control
II. Safety
  1. Safety rules and prevention of injury
  2. How to safely use household appliances
  3. Handling household emergencies ranging from power failure to personal injury
  4. First aid for home accidents
  5. Discriminating between safe and unsafe play activities
  6. How to use 911
  7. Traveling safely to and from school
  8. Taking care of the key
  9. Protection from abduction and molestation
III. Self-care/child care
  1. Safe and nutritious snack preparation
  2. Telephone skills
  3. Child care techniques
  4. Family rules
  5. Activities for after school
  6. Time management
  7. Ways to cope with fear

From Holaday B and others: *Pediatr Health Care* 7:256-263, 1993.

and how to get help.[14] Physically, children should be able to safely manipulate medical equipment, avoid injury, manage locks, and operate relevant appliances and equipment. They also need the ability to tolerate separation from adults without loneliness, fear, or self-destructive behavior.

The training program described in the accompanying box should run over a 4- to 5-week period to give children the time to develop required skills. Children learn best from active participation, including skill rehearsal and role playing, rather than from passive observation of adults modeling behaviors. Booster (review) sessions are needed periodically. Providers can also explore other training opportunities in their communities, including whether health information is available over latchkey telephone hotlines.[14]

National Standards and Tested Programs

Certification of child life specialists is available through the Child Life Certifying Commission.

SUMMARY

Pregnancy, parenting, and child development offer many opportunities for teaching that will make a real difference in people's lives. Yet little evidence exists that indicates whether these opportunities are exploited. Much work remains to be accomplished in the development of standards of practice and tested programs.

? STUDY QUESTIONS

1. Because children who have been critically ill may be at increased risk for a respiratory or cardiac event at home, it is important that the parents learn basic life-support skills. What learning conditions are essential so that the parents are competent and feel confident in providing this care for their child?
2. Federal law now requires that health care providers give to parents of children receiving immunizations standardized written informa-

tion about many aspects of the vaccines and the diseases they may prevent. Thus parents are given vaccine information pamphlets (VIPs) that must contain the information necessary to meet statutory requirements, and frequently they are long. Concerns that these VIPs might frighten parents and deter them from having their children immunized proved to be unfounded; however, some parents felt overwhelmed with information.[8] Are you surprised by the concerns of providers? What could be done to make the mandated information more accessible to parents with little formal education?

3. A summary of an article by Brent and others[5] on breastfeeding in a low-income population shows that it is the consensus of the international pediatric community that breastfeeding is the optimal form of infant nutrition. Because women from low-income groups have a much lower incidence of breastfeeding and the rates of infant mortality and morbidity among inner-city poor children are high, the authors believe it is extremely important to reverse this trend. Women who planned to breastfeed were counseled about management; women who planned to bottle-feed were counseled on the benefits of breastfeeding to mother and infant. The program, which used a lactation consultant, was successful in increasing the incidence and duration of breastfeeding in an inner-city, low-income population. Are you surprised by the methods or the findings in this study?

REFERENCES

1. Alcalay R, Ghee A, Scrimshaw S: Designing prenatal care messages for low-income Mexican women, *Public Health Rep* 108:354-362, 1993.
2. American Academy of Pediatrics: Child life programs, *Pediatrics* 91:671-673, 1993.
3. Bartholomew LK and others: Development of health education program to promote the self-management of cystic fibrosis, *Health Educ Q* 18:429-443, 1991.
4. Basso R: A structured-fantasy group experience in a children's diabetic education program, *Patient Educ Counsel* 18:243-251, 1991.
5. Brent NB and others: Breast-feeding in a low-income population, *Arch Pediatr Adolesc Med* 149:798-803, 1995,
6. Broome ME, Lillis PP, Smith MC: Pain interventions with children: a meta-analysis of research, *Nurs Res* 38:154-158, 1989.
7. Brooten D and others: Functions of the CNS in early discharge and home follow-up of very low birthweight infants, *Clin Nurse Specialist* 5:196-201, 1991.
8. Clayton EW, Hickson GB, Miller CS: Parents' responses to vaccine information pamphlets, *Pediatrics* 93:369-372, 1994.
9. Cohen MH: The triggers of heightened parental uncertainty in chronic, life-threatening childhood illness, *Qualitative Health Res* 5:63-77, 1995.
10. Constantinou JC, Korner AF: Neurobehavioral assessment of the preterm infant as an instrument to enhance parental awareness, *Children's Health Care* 22:39-46, 1993.
11. Eidelman AI, Hoffmann NW, Kaitz M: Cognitive deficits in women after childbirth, *Obstet Gynecol* 81:764-767, 1993.
12. Graf RA, Perez-Woods R: Trends in preterm labor, *J Perinatol* 12:51-57, 1992.
13. Hobel CJ and others: The West Los Angeles preterm birth prevention project, *Am J Obstet Gynecol* 170:54-62, 1994
14. Holaday B and others: Chronically ill children in self-care: issues for pediatric nurses, *J Pediatr Health Care* 7:256-263, 1993.
15. Jellinek M and others: Facing tragic decisions with parents in the neonatal intensive care unit: clinical perspectives, *Pediatrics* 89:119-122, 1992.
16. Jones EG, Badger TA, Moore I: Children's knowledge of internal anatomy: conceptual orientation and review of research, *J Pediatr Nurs* 7:262-268, 1992.
17. Jones LC: A meta-analysis study of the effects of childbirth education on the parent-infant relationship, *Health Care Women Int* 7:357-370, 1986.
18. Kaatz JL: Enhancing the parenting skills of developmentally disabled parents: a nursing perspective, *J Community Health Nurs* 9:209-219, 1992.
19. Koniak-Griffin D, Verzemnieks I, Cahill D: Using videotape instruction and feedback to improve adolescents' mothering behaviors, *J Adolesc Health* 13:570-757, 1992.
20. Levy SR, Iverson BK, Walberg HJ: Adolescent pregnancy programs and educational interventions: a research synthesis and review, *J Soc Health* 3:99-103, 1983.
21. Lowe NK: Maternal confidence in coping with labor; a self-efficacy concept, *JOGNN* 20:457-463, 1991.
22. McCrindle BW and others: An evaluation of parental concerns and misperceptions about heart murmurs, *Clin Pediatr* 34:25-31, 1995.

23. Moynihan P, Naclerio L, Kiley K: Parent participation, *Nurs Clin North Am* 30:231-241, 1995.

24. Mullen P, Ramirez G, Groff JY: A meta-analysis of randomized trials of prenatal smoking cessation interventions, *Am J Obstet Gynecol* 171:1328-1334, 1994.

25. Olds DL: Home visitation for pregnant women and parents of young children, *Am J Dis Child* 146:704-708, 1992.

26. Patterson ET and others: Symptoms of preterm labor and self-diagnostic confusion, *Nurs Res* 41:367-372, 1992.

27. Powers SW and others: Helping preschool leukemia patients and their parents cope during injections, *J Pediatr Psychol* 18:681-695, 1993.

28. Sheikh L, O'Brien M, McCluskey-Fawcett K: Parent preparation for the NICU-to-home transition: staff and parent perceptions, *Children's Health Care* 22:227-239, 1993.

29. Sherwen LN, Scoloveno MA, Weingarten CT: *Nursing care of the childbearing family,* ed 2, Norwalk, Conn, 1995, Appleton & Lange.

30. Thompson V: An IV therapy teaching tool for children, *Pediatr Nurs* 20:351-355, 1994.

9 Patient Self-Management for the Rheumatic Diseases

GENERAL APPROACH

A firm theoretical base for patient education in rheumatic disease care has been developed during the past 15 years. Education in self-management has enabled patients to control their symptoms and to become partners in care with their health care providers.[1,2] A large variety of organized programs, planned according to educationally and psychologically valid principles, implemented consistently by trained personnel, have produced desirable changes in knowledge, behavior, and health outcome in patients with arthritis—over and above the medical treatment and incidental education to which they have been exposed. As a result, national dissemination of programs and standards for patient education in arthritis management is in progress.[3] Programs for other rheumatic diseases are following a similar model.

The model for arthritis education and the research base to support it developed largely in the 1980s. Early advances in chronic disease education occurred in diseases with significant mortality and strong links between behaviors and disease outcomes. The preceding chapters on heart disease, asthma, and diabetes describe these developments. The toll of arthritis is found more in disability and discomfort than in death, and most forms of the rheumatic diseases are not preventable and are only partially responsive to treatment. There are 105 recognized rheumatic conditions, many of them rare. Osteoarthritis of the hands, weight-bearing joints, and the back affects 12% of the U.S. population between age 25 and 74 years. The most common symptoms are musculoskeletal pain, loss of function, and consequent decreased ability to perform daily activities and work. The systemic inflammatory diseases affect about 3 million persons; examples include rheumatoid arthritis, systemic lupus erythematosus, and ankylosing spondylitis.[3]

Elements of care include medication for pain and inflammation; prescribed exercise for strength, endurance, and range of motion; rest; joint protection; modalities such as ice, heat, and splints; and in selected cases joint surgery. Outcome goals commonly considered important include improvement or maintenance of function, employability, and psychosocial status and control of pain, symptoms, and disease activity.[3] The patient must learn to constantly readjust the regimen according to changing disease activity. The education programs that most affect health status and behavior emphasize the development of a daily routine of self-management activity and give attention to coping with physical exercise, developing self-efficacy, and achieving success in problem solving.[8] The unpredictable course and varying disease activity may cause patients to view their disease as uncontrollable, which in turn may cause them to experience anxiety and depression, leading to increased perception of pain and decreased efforts to cope. The need to avoid this spiral makes it particularly important that these patients develop self-efficacy.[14]

EDUCATIONAL APPROACHES AND RESEARCH BASE

Behaviors thought to affect the health and psychological status of persons with arthritis include exercise, relaxation, joint protection, and adherence to medication regimens. Educational techniques already tested, with generally positive results, include interactive computer, telephone, and mail versus in-person classes. Almost no study has been undertaken on patient education by direct caregivers within the context of clinical care.[3] Outcome objectives to be met by the completion of a British patient education program are shown in the box below.[15] Note the strong emphasis on development of a sense of control.

The Arthritis Self-Management Program (ASMP) is perhaps the best known model program and one whose effectiveness has been well studied. It is taught 2 hours a week for 6 weeks and includes content on pathophysiology, medications, personal exercise and pain-management programs, nutrition, appropriate use of joints, and communication with physicians. Its iterative development since 1978 has been constantly improved through research and its strong theoret-

ical base. Early studies found that individuals who felt they had control improved.[7] The medical interventions for arthritis have, for the most part, limited benefits. Because of the chronic nature of arthritis, persons with this disease must learn to manage and cope with it on a day-to-day basis. Their ability to succeed in this task commonly differentiates those who are incapacitated from those who continue to lead full and active lives in the face of equal disease severity.[8]

Behavioral learning theory, with its emphasis on self-efficacy, has served as a prime theoretical base for the ASMP. The leaders teaching the course are individuals with arthritis, and thus they serve as models for solving problems. The program also strongly emphasizes successful adoption of new behaviors and provides regular feedback. Skills mastery is aided by contracting for some self-management behavior the patient wants to develop for the following week, with a

---

■ OBJECTIVES OF THE BRISTOL PATIENT EDUCATION PROGRAMME

By the end of the programme the patient will:

Knowlege

1. Describe the variable nature of rheumatoid arthritis.
2. Explain the effects, side effects, and regimens of the drugs they are taking for arthritis.
3. Explain the simple principles of exercise for mobility and strength.
4. Understand that people with arthritis get anxious and depressed, that this is variable, and that there are ways of coping with these feelings.
5. Explain the simple principles of joint protection.
6. Know that there is a list of agencies/individuals to contact for help for their arthritis and related problems.
7. Know the basic principles of relaxation and of hot/cold treatment.
8. Describe the features of a chair most appropriate for their condition.

Skills

9. Demonstrate the use of hot/cold treatment safely.
10. Demonstrate principles of joint protection using a tap, and other everyday objects.
11. Demonstrate exercises for mobility and strength in the knee and one other appropriate joint.
12. Design a daily programme which incorporates rest and activity.
13. Demonstrate correct self-medication.

Attitudes

14. Believe they can reduce their pain by adopting self-help techniques.
15. Believe that adopting changes in their lifestyle and environment will be beneficial.
16. Feel less anxious and depressed.
17. Feel more in control.

From Tucker M, Kirwan JR: *Ann Rheum Dis* 50:422-428, 1991.

minimal confidence level of 70%. The contract script is shown in the box below.[10] Course materials contained in *The Arthritis Helpbook* were written with an emphasis on modeling, showing real persons with whom participants could identify. Participants are taught to use positive self-talk, to identify the negative ways they think about the disease and their self-help behaviors, and then to consciously change these to more positive behaviors.[7] Measurement of progress is

---

■ CONTRACT SCRIPT

I. Deciding what one wants to accomplish
Ask the person, "What will you do this week?" It is important that the activity come from the participant and not you. This activity does not have to be something covered in class—just something that the participant wants to do to change behavior. Do not let anyone say. "I will try . . ." Each person should say, "I will . . ."

II. Making a plan
This is the difficult and most important part of contracting. Part I is worthless without part II.
   The plan should contain all of the following elements:

1. Exactly what is the participant going to do (i.e., how far will you walk, how will you eat less, what relaxation techniques will you practice)?
2. How much (i.e., walk around the block, 15 minutes, etc.)?
3. When will the participant do this? Again, this must be specific (i.e., before lunch, in the shower, when I come home from work).
4. How often will the activity be done? This is a bit tricky. Most participants tend to say every day. In contracting, the most important thing is to succeed. Therefore, it is better to contract to do something four times a week and exceed the contract by actually doing it five times than to contract to do something every day and fail by only doing it 6 days. To insure success, we usually encourage people to contract to do something 3 to 5 days a week. Remember that success and self-efficacy are as important, or maybe even more important, than actually doing the behavior.

III. Checking the contract
Once the contract is complete, ask the participant "Given a scale of 0 to 100, with 0 being totally unsure and 100 being totally certain, how certain are you that you will (repeat the participant's contract verbatim)?"
   If the answer is 70 or above, this is probably a realistic contract and the participant should write it on his or her contract sheet.
   If the answer is below 70, then the contract should be reassessed. Ask the participant: "What makes you uncertain? What problems do you foresee?" Then discuss the problems. Ask other participants to offer solutions. YOU should offer solutions LAST. Once the problem solving is completed, have the participant restate the contract and return to repeat part III, checking the contract.

• • •

NOTE: This contracting process may seem cumbersome and time-consuming. However, it does work and is well worth the effort. The first time you contract with a group, plan 2 to 3 minutes per person. Contracting is a learned skill. Your participant will soon be saying "I will _____ four times this week before lunch and am 80% certain I can do this." Thus, after two or three contracting sessions, contracting should take less than a minute per participant.

From Lorig K, Gonzalez V: *Health Educ Q* 19:355-368, 1992; reprinted from Lorig K: *Arthritis self-management leader's manual*, rev ed, Atlanta, Ga, 1984, Arthritis Foundation.

accomplished in part by the Arthritis Self-Efficacy Scale, which appears in the box on p. 85.

Most research on patient education to date has been undertaken on relatively few of the rheumatic diseases and for populations that are predominantly white and relatively well educated.[3] Several reviews of this literature may be found in Appendix C. The most recent review concludes that medical care, including the use of medications, can offer a 20% to 50% improvement in reported arthritis symptoms. Data from patient education studies suggest that a further improvement of 15% to 30% is attainable through patient education interventions.[5] The one review that provides a meta-analysis summarizes 15 studies and shows moderate effect sizes of psychoeducational interventions on pain, depression, and disability.[11]

Research on ASMP shows the following results.

1. In randomized trials ASMP improves behaviors, self-efficacy, and aspects of health status.
2. Formal reinforcement appears to improve the long-term outcomes of ASMP.
3. The effects of the ASMP last for as long as 4 years without formal reinforcement.
4. The mechanism by which the ASMP affects health status appears to be more closely linked to changes in self-efficacy than to changes in behaviors.
5. The ASMP is an intervention that can be and has been disseminated widely. In 1984 the Arthritis Foundation began to distribute it throughout the United States, and in more recent years its use has been encouraged internationally.[8]

Evidence indicates that 4 years after participation in the ASMP patients' pain declined a mean of 20% and their visits to physicians by 40%, while physical disability increased 9%. Estimated 4-year savings were $648 per person for patients with rheumatoid arthritis and $189 per osteoarthritis patient.[9]

Relapse prevention in patients who are attempting to cope with persistent pain from rheumatoid arthritis should be part of a self-management program. Figure 9-1 provides a model of this process. Early warning signs include an increase in pain, disruption in sleep patterns, and lack of response to a usual medication regimen. Interpersonal situations, such as a visit from out-of-town relatives, and intrapersonal events, such as increased depression or anxiety, may overwhelm the patient's perceived ability to control pain or other symptoms with previously successful coping strategies. To help identify high-risk situations that are likely to lead to relapse, patients can be asked to describe past setbacks. Through self-monitoring and cognitive rehearsal of previous relapse episodes, patients can pinpoint specific early warning signs of relapse and can rehearse how to cope with differ-

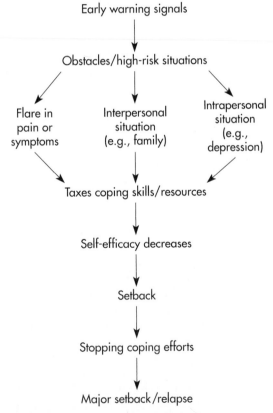

Figure 9-1   Model of relapse process in coping with pain. (From Keefe FJ, Van Horn Y: *Arthritis Care Res* 6:213-222, 1993.)

ent relapse situations. Spousal training should also be studied.[6]

Arthritis self-management education has been used as a model to develop programs for other rheumatic diseases such as fibromyalgia. This syndrome is characterized by widespread musculoskeletal pain and multiple tender points, severe fatigue, sleep disturbance, and stiffness. Because the etiology of fibromyalgia is unknown, treatment is largely symptomatic and unstandardized. These self-management education programs are only beginning to be developed and have yet to be evaluated or widely distributed. Critical elements include information on the fibromyalgia syndrome; physical training; cognitive-behavioral therapy, including self-efficacy training, relaxation, and coping techniques; and communication with providers and family.[2]

For all education in the rheumatic diseases, it is important to note that unless educational treatments attend to creating an appropriate level of self-efficacy, they may increase awareness of the disease process without developing a corresponding confidence to cope with it.[6]

COMMUNITY-BASED EDUCATION AND EDUCATION OF SPECIAL POPULATIONS

The Arthritis Self-Management Program, originally developed at Stanford University, was designed to be community-based—to be held in settings such as libraries, senior centers, churches, and shopping malls.[7] The ASMP is endorsed by the Arthritis Foundation and sponsored by local chapters throughout the country. Some persons either may choose not to participate in ASMP or may not have access to it; however, several home-study programs have been developed and tested.

One home-study program, "Bone up on Arthritis" (BUOA), contains six lessons presented on audiocassette tapes and in booklets, which can be used when and where clients choose. BUOA is intended to be easily implemented within a community, with a community-based intervener acting as facilitator and coordinator. Each BUOA participant is matched with a resource person who teaches classes to small groups or distributes the lessons through the mail and who serves as a local information and referral source. The program has been tested on a rural population that showed improved scores on all outcome measures (self-care behavior, helplessness, pain, dysfunction, and depression.)[4]

Learning About Rheumatoid Arthritis (LARA) is a written individualized instruction program tested on an urban population and shown to be effective.[12] It uses performance measures of outcome, for example, asking participants to drink from a coffee mug, carry a handbag or flight bag (handle over the shoulder or elbow), move a pot with a handle from one flat surface to another two feet away, get up from a chair (use of two hands), and slide objects across the floor instead of carrying them. It will be important to investigate the cost-effectiveness of these various educational programs, as well as to understand their instructional effectiveness and access for persons in various living situations.[12]

Considerable work is required to understand how best to help persons from a variety of special groups attain the benefits of the self-management programs described here. For example, generalizability of self-efficacy theory across cultures still needs further study.[7]

Folk models—the tacit beliefs that are commonly held and communicated among lay members of a group and that are frequently at odds with the expert's set of beliefs—need to be understood for a variety of groups. A study of a folk model of arthritis among middle-class older adults found that commonly mentioned causes of arthritis were damp and cold weather, which was said by some to cause "frozen joints"; a diet of too much calcium, which leads to deposits in joints; and injury, overuse, or misuse of joints.[13] It is important for those who wish to communicate with persons about arthritis to have an understanding of the kinds of knowledge and beliefs individuals have about it.[12] No description of a folk model of arthritis for minorities or low-income groups appears to exist.

NATIONAL STANDARDS AND TESTED PROGRAMS

The Arthritis Foundation has played a major role in this field and has adopted four of the more successful programs and has used trained leaders to disseminate them nationwide.

Patient education standards for the rheumatic disease field are shown in Appendix D. As with the diabetes field, these are essentially process standards—that is, they do not set targeted levels of outcome standards.

SUMMARY

Inasmuch as work on the ASMP has been the most widely available program, it serves as an excellent model of patient education. Well grounded in both theory and research and currently widely disseminated, it is community based, uses trained lay leaders, and is sufficiently standardized to be replicable. It appears that the success of the ASMP depends more on strengthening or changing psychological attributes such as self-efficacy than on the performance of a particular behavior or techniques.[9] Health care providers have also defined patient education standards.

REFERENCES

1. Burckhardt CS: Arthritis and musculoskeletal patient education standards, *Arthritis Care Res* 7:1-4, 1994.
2. Burckhardt CS, Bjelle A: Education programmes for fibromyalgia patients: description and evaluation, *Ballieres Clin Rheumatol* 8:935-955, 1994.
3. Daltroy LH, Liang MH: Arthritis education: opportunities and state of the art, *Health Educ Q* 20:3-16, 1993.
4. Goeppinger J and others: From research to practice: the effects of the jointly sponsored dissemination of an arthritis self-care nursing intervention, *Appl Nurs Res* 8:106-113, 1995.
5. Hirano PC, Laurent DD, Lorig K: Arthritis patient education studies, 1987-1991: a review of the literature, *Patient Educ Couns* 24:9-54, 1994.
6. Keefe FJ, Van Horn Y: Cognitive-behavioral treatment of rheumatoid arthritis pain; maintaining treatment gains, *Arthritis Care Res* 6:213-222, 1993.
7. Lorig, K, Gonzalez V: The integration of theory with practice: a 12-year case study, *Health Educ Q* 19:355-368, 1992.
8. Lorig K, Homan H: Arthritis self-management studies: a twelve-year review, *Health Educ Q* 20:17-28, 1993.
9. Lorig KR, Mazonson PD, Homan HR: Evidence suggesting that health education for self-management in patients with chronic arthritis has sustained health benefits while reducing health care costs, *Arthritis Rheum* 36:439-446, 1993.
10. Lorig K and others: Development and evaluation of a scale to measure perceived self-efficacy in people with arthritis, *Arthritis Rheum* 32:37-44, 1989.
11. Mullen PD and others: Efficacy of psychoeducational interventions on pain, depression, and disability in people with arthritis: a meta-analysis, *J Rheumatol* (suppl 15)14:33-39, 1987.
12. Neuberger GB and others: Promoting self-care in clients with arthritis, *Arthritis Care Res* 6:141-148, 1993.
13. Rice GE, Young LH: A folk model of arthritis, *Health Values* 18(2):15-27, 1994.
14. Taal E and others: Group education for patients with rheumatoid arthritis, *Patient Educ Couns* 20:1677-1687, 1993.
15. Tucker M, Kirwan JR: Does patient education in rheumatoid arthritis have therapeutic potential? *Ann Rheum Dis* 50:422-428, 1991.

10 Other Areas of Patient Education Practice

A number of areas of patient education practice are developing slowly (mental health), are in decline because of philosophical changes (adherence), were developed years ago and are now stable (preprocedure and postprocedure preparation), or are predominantly dealt with in public health education interventions (AIDS education). There are many other areas in which patient education practice could be helpful to patients but that have not been developed with a research base and a body of literature that describes assessment, intervention strategies, and programs of education in the field. For example, there is very little focus on men's health outside of major disease categories, and the same is true for older adults, especially those with chronic illness.

Homeless populations could benefit tremendously from community-based education focused on staying well and dealing with the problems associated with their lifestyle. May and Evans[23] describe education provided by volunteers, including nurses, in 13 urban shelters. Health problems, for which education was provided, included mental health, alcohol and drug concerns, injuries, skin disorders, high blood pressure, infection, and dental health. Human immunodeficiency virus (HIV)–risk reduction, prevention of pregnancy, parenting skills, and instruction in first aid would also have been helpful.

Patient education of older adults offers several obvious challenges but as yet has not developed into a full-fledged field of practice in terms of a research base and standards of practice. Much of the existing literature has focused on issues regarding learning, especially deficits in memory, increased cognitive response time, and sensory function decline with age. Perhaps an equally relevant focus should be on empowerment and self-management of disability. Researchers have reported significant correlations between autonomy, active involvement, achievement motivation, and health.[26]

Yet there is an inclination on the part of some professionals to use a paternalistic approach to care, thereby undermining older adults' autonomy. Older adults with a positive mindset (characterized by optimism, positive attitudes about self and self-care, and determination to remain independent) have been noted to remain independent despite the severity of their medical problems. The more paternalistic and biomedically oriented the professional, the greater the patient's perception of being misunderstood, which in turn undermines his or her self-confidence. On the other hand, one study shows that the health care professionals involved believed they had fulfilled their goals for care despite the patient's experience of threatened autonomy and undermined care goals.[26]

Clark and others[6] present another perspective on the educational tasks before older adult patients. Many older adults face the need to successfully self-manage chronic illness, to make decisions about their care, to perform activities aimed at management of their condition, and to apply skills to maintain adequate psychosocial functioning. All these behaviors are aimed at decreasing the impact of the disease on daily life. Table 10-1 shows typical self-management tasks for five common chronic illnesses.

Very little empirical data are available that detail learning needs for older adults in managing multi-

Table 10-1   Common self-management tasks for five chronic diseases

TASKS	HEART DISEASE	ASTHMA	ARTHRITIS	COPD	DIABETES
Recognizing and responding to symptoms, monitoring physical indicators, controlling triggers to symptoms	X	X		X	X
Using medicine	X	X	X	X	X
Managing acute episodes and emergencies	X	X	X		X
Maintaining nutrition and diet	X		X	X	X
Maintaining adequate exercise/activity	X	X	X	X	X
Giving up smoking	X	X	X	X	X
Using relaxation and stress-reducing techniques	X	X	X		
Interacting with health care providers	X	X			X
Seeking information and using community services		X	X		X
Adapting to work	X	X	X		
Managing relations with significant others	X	X	X	X	
Managing emotions and psychological responses to illness	X	X	X		X

From Clark NM & others: *J Aging Health* 3:3-27, 1991.
COPD, Chronic obstructive pulmonary disease; *X,* reported in a study of self-management.

ple comorbidities and frequently present contradictory or confusing management advice. For example, a postcoronary walking program may conflict with management of arthritic hips and knees. Is the patient to aggravate one condition or avoid managing it? Multiple conditions can deplete physical and mental energy for coping. Little is known about how older adults are able to access and use large, complex health care systems.

Other examples of areas of patient education practice that require developing are readily available. An initial study of education for patients with Parkinson's disease focused on improving functional outcomes by using an educational strategy that sought to improve self-efficacy and optimism.[27] Results showed decreases in visits to physicians, hospital days, and sick days, as well as stabilization of symptoms in the intervention group. The literature documents that in many chronic diseases long-term patient outcomes are affected by such factors as exercise, lifestyle, risk factors, side effects of medications and their management, interaction with comorbid disease conditions, social and spousal support, depres-

sion, and self-efficacy. Many of these are potentially amenable to patient education interventions and have been successfully altered in other disease states and in normal subjects.

In another area of obvious need for eduction, fewer than half of burn-rehabilitation services indicated they provide inpatient education.[9] Such evidence shows that even though licensure and accreditation standards include patient education, it is not yet universally available to many for whom it is reasonable to believe significant benefits would be provided, as well as potentially result in cost savings.

This chapter describes four fields of patient education practice that are in various stages of development.

MENTAL HEALTH
General Approach

The mental health field has developed what it calls "psychoeducation," which refers to the training of individuals in psychological knowledge or skills. A component of the learning pro-

---

■ TOPICAL OUTLINE FOR PATIENT AND FAMILY PSYCHOEDUCATION

Both patients and family	Patients	Family
Nature of illness, etiology, treatment	Monitoring stress; balancing stimulation with caution about adding stressors	Maintaining simple, structured, consistent environment
Relationship of illness and stress	Self-regulation of specific symptoms of illness	Management of specific behavioral problems
Identification of early symptoms of acute episodes of illness	Learning to understand others; empathy development	Importance of low-key, non-critical attitude and communication
Medications—their purpose, importance	Developing social and leisure skills; balancing with constructive activity	Including the patient in activities
Aftercare visits—using staff for consultation on problems	Learning to live with stigma	Importance of developing own life
Communication and problem-solving skills	Self-help groups for the mentally ill	Support groups for families; advocacy for mentally ill

From Holmes H and others: *Issues Ment Health Nurs* 15:85-104, 1994.
NOTE: Education is tailored to the needs of the individual patient and family but includes information in these topical areas when they are assessed as appropriate.

---

cess in therapy,[21] it is also used to refer to programs that in other fields would be called patient education. Originally used with persons with schizophrenia, this model is now applied to individuals with depression, to the seriously mentally ill, to those with obsessive-compulsive disorder, and to persons with addiction disorders.

Educational Approaches and Research Base

Psychoeducation provides knowledge and skill development and support for individuals with psychiatric illness, as well as for the families. The family is especially important because the environment it creates can influence the course of illness and recovery of the patient and because family members themselves need help in coping with the negative effects of the illness. The purposes of patient and family psychoeducation include ameliorating symptoms of the illness, reducing family burden and stress, helping participants acquire new coping skills that will improve their quality of life, enhancing treatment compliance, and relapse prevention and warning.[10]

Much of the body of literature on patient psychoeducation programs implies that a group format is the most beneficial structure. In some in-

stances, however, patients are so severely impaired that they may require individual sessions because the group may be overstimulating and disorganizing for them or because they may disrupt the group. Typical program topics include specific mental illness diagnosis and causes, symptoms, medications, stress management, goal setting and self-esteem, and highly structured problem solving. A topical outline of one program is shown in the box above.[19]

It is important not only to provide information but to teach and model specific management skills for dealing with the illness. The group leader for a psychoeducational group needs to be able to tolerate the slow pace and frequent repetitions of content as well as the patients' internal states of depression.

Psychoeducation can help families move beyond shame and stigma and develop the skills and knowledge to meet professionals on an equal footing.[18] This change in relationship with families may be difficult for the providers. It is important to note that especially in some settings psychoeducation focuses heavily on teaching basic life skills that patients need to negotiate day-to-day living. Many patients have problem-solving as well as self-care deficits, skills not addressed in the traditional treatment programs.

A sufficiently large, accumulated research base for psychoeducation could not be located, although McFarlane and others[25] cite studies that show decreased relapse rates in medicated patients receiving psychoeducation in the community. The studies were conducted under special circumstances rather than ordinary clinical situations. Some research addresses elements commonly found in psychoeducation. For example, studies have shown that individuals with schizophrenia can and do identify indicators that relapse is beginning, frequently depression or anxiety, and that these indicators are somewhat stable.[17] Other research has shown that it is common for mental health patients not to know the names or doses of prescribed medications. Not only does this situation raise concerns about patients' ability to identify adverse effects and do something about them; serious questions must also be raised about the adequacy of informed consent when difficult benefit-risk issues, such as the link between tardive dyskinesia and benzodiazepine dependence, are involved. Thus medication instruction is universally important.[8]

Community-Based Education and Education of Special Populations

Much of the education just described occurs at least partially in community settings, and clearly its goals for at least some patients are strongly oriented to the development of competencies so that patients can function in the community.

For the severely demented population, such as those with Alzheimer's disease (AD), educational support groups have long been available for caregivers. During the early stages of dementia caregivers are more likely to benefit from a structured, time-limited educational group—to gain the information necessary to provide care. They need to understand the functional impact of dementia; the need to accommodate care to the receiver's cognitive, emotional, and behavioral dysfunction; caregiver self-care; legal and financial planning; and community support groups. In later stages of the illness caregivers may prefer to participate in an ongoing support group.[13]

Recent research findings seem to indicate that the causes of death for persons with AD vary with the level of cognitive impairment close to the time of death. Illnesses potentially amenable to treatment caused death at all levels of disease but more so early in the course of AD. Cognitive impairment may make patients less able to recognize and report symptoms of medical problems, which means that caregivers must be well educated to note these problems early.[21]

Older women with depression are a special population for whom education is useful in conjunction with other therapies. Not only can knowledge and skills be taught that can prevent depressive symptoms from becoming severe enough to require hospitalization but education can also function as a tool for perspective transformation. Participants learn that they are not the problem but that they suffer from a role-determined social-identity deficit, which can be altered. Education has been incorporated into traditional therapeutic interventions to overcome self-destructive thinking habits and to develop communication skills, particularly assertiveness. Education is also a primary intervention tool, including the use of stimulation to avoid boredom, learning why and how social deficits can cause depressive symptoms, and how to construct a satisfactory social self.[4]

Maynard[24] describes content and sequence for psychoeducational group meetings for women with depression (Table 10-2). The program is based on the belief that attaining skills to better manage life events can help prevent depressive symptoms from becoming severe enough to require hospitalization. Note that, as with other examples common in the literature, the content and sequence should be preceded by a clear set of behavioral outcome goals.

ADHERENCE TO PRESCRIBED REGIMENS
General Approach

Adherence to a regimen prescribed by a provider has been a prevailing goal of patient education in the past. Previously referred to as "compliance," the concept itself came under attack as moralistic and inappropriate in some patient care

Table 10-2   Content and sequence for psychoeducational group meetings

MEETING NO.	TOPIC	CONTENT
1	Depression	Do get-acquainted exercises; provide overview of the sessions; state group objectives and ground rules; discuss the holistic approach to depression; give information about depression (i.e., nature of depression, symptoms of depression, causes of depression, differences in depression in women and men, and social factors related to depression in women); and give information about medication for depression (i.e., benefits and side effects, limitations of medications, and how to talk with the physician about medications).
2	Relationship of thoughts to depression	Discuss the role of thoughts in feelings, particularly depression; discuss irrational beliefs and steps in changing cognitive patterns; identify personal negative self-statements and irrational beliefs; and discuss the theory of learned helplessness.
3	Role of social factors in depression	Discuss how current social expectations of women influence feelings; discuss realistic and unrealistic expectations women have of themselves; discuss the concept of multiple roles and identify number of roles each woman has; discuss expectations others have for women; identify factors in society that are oppressive for women and discuss how they affect their lives; identify which factors can be changed; and discuss marital and parenting relationships.
4	Goal setting	Share importance of goal-setting and steps in goal-setting; share steps to take in setting goals; and discuss types of goals.
5	Self-esteem	Share goals set over previous week; teach information related to self-esteem, including the nature of self-esteem, factors in development of self-esteem, and self-ideal; and share techniques for improving self-esteem based on awareness of self and self-messages, affirmations to substitute positive messages, and action to change behavior.
6	Understanding family of origin	Discuss family structure, messages received during childhood, and kinds of relationships between family members; discuss how childhood messages continue to influence adult life; discuss how to give up old messages and old hurts; discuss verbal, physical, and sexual abuse in the family; and discuss consequences and methods of handling abuse.
7	Assertiveness	Give information about characteristics of assertive, passive, and aggressive behaviors; identify and discuss basic rights; and discuss and practice skills for accepting and giving criticism, communicating needs, and saying no.
8	Stress management	Provide information about stress and its role in depression; discuss physiologic and psychologic responses to stress; and teach stress management strategies.
9	Caring for the body	Teach the importance of diet, exercise, rest, and other preventive health practices; give information about such practices as breast self-examination; and discuss relationship of health practices to depression.
10	Review and terminate	Teach role of social support and methods to increase social networks; discuss what each woman has gained from the meetings; discuss long-term goals; and share positive feelings and experiences.

From Maynard C: *J Psychosoc Nurs* 31(12):9-14, 1993.

situations, particularly when the regimen had to be adjusted to fit the patient's changing condition. Errors in taking or not taking prescribed medications have been documented on a widespread basis. In most studies at least one third of patients failed to comply with instructions, and in some the rate is 50% or higher. Both clinical judgment on the part of the provider and self-report on the part of the patient are known to be inaccurate. Clear instructions, simplified regimens, reminder pill containers and calendars, telephone follow-up, tailoring the regimen to the patient's lifestyle, and involving a significant other are all known to be helpful in attaining adherence.[3]

Although the goal of adherence to a prescribed regimen is still legitimate, it is open to several caveats. First, it is not always clear that the regimen will accomplish the benefits expected, even if the patient reliably follows it. Second, judging patients by whether they adhere to medical authority is now widely understood to be paternalistic and assumes an authority providers do not have. At the least, regimens should be jointly developed around treatment goals shared by the patient and the provider and constructed so that they are convenient and reflect the patient's assessment of benefit from and burden of the regimen. Perhaps self-management to a jointly specified set of behaviors and outcomes is a more satisfactory alternate goal.

Educational Approaches and Research Base

The box shown on p. 181 summarizes adherence-enhancing educational and behavioral interventions.

A decade ago Posavac and others[32] reviewed 58 studies evaluating the effectiveness of programs to increase compliance with medical treatment regimens. The mean effect size was 0.47, with lesser impact as the amount of lifestyle changes required by the treatment regimen increased. The most successful interventions involved improving the facility providing care and helping patients to incorporate the treatment regimen into their daily routine. More recently Morris and Schulz[29] completed a nonquantitative review of the patient-compliance literature and concluded that after decades of research very little consistent information is available. One major reason for this lack of understanding is that compliance research has been dominated by the perspective of the health care professional. Future research needs to investigate the patient's decision-making process and the reasons for those decisions. Although the conclusions of the authors of these two reviews differ somewhat, each provides a valid perspective.

Obtaining a more useful body of research for understanding adherence issues is important. In addition to increased costs of treatment and the deaths that might have been delayed, in older adults alone nonadherence has been linked to 23% of nursing home admissions and 10% of all hospital admissions.[29] Outcome-oriented definitions of adherence differ from process-oriented ones. Although it is important to take medication safely (process), it is possible to obtain a satisfactory therapeutic outcome without taking the medication exactly as prescribed.

Community-Based Education and Education of Special Populations

Adherence education takes place wherever care is given, including in ambulatory and community settings.

Cultural issues clearly play a role in adherence. An interesting study of Cambodian adults with minimal formal education, who were receiving public assistance and utilizing an ambulatory clinic in Seattle, found two thirds of the group to be noncompliant with their medications.[34] Some of this resistance can be attributed to concern about the effects of Western medication on "internal strength" and Cambodian ideas about pharmacokinetics—in other words, culturally conceived compliance. These individuals made considerable effort to comply with therapy but did so in a manner consistent with their underlying understanding of how medicines and the body work. They believed that Western drugs were "strong medicine" (in comparison with herbal medicine) and might interfere with the

■ ADHERENCE-ENHANCING INTERVENTIONS

Educational strategies to enable patients to implement and maintain regimen

- Provide verbal instruction in small amounts, specific to activity; deliver over time
- Dispense limited amounts of printed instructions to reinforce verbal information
- Use material at patient's reading/comprehension level
- Dispense materials over time
- Assess level of patient's understanding; encourage questions
- Focus on activities of the regimen, not on the disease
- Augment verbal instructions with demonstrations
- Utilize other instructional media (e.g., videotapes, interactive computer programs)
- Provide opportunities for practice and return demonstration (e.g., counting pulse, taking nitroglycerin, selecting foods from a menu)
- Refer to community resources for additional skill development (e.g., YMCA for exercise class, American Heart Association for food shopping tours, hospital for cooking classes)

Behavioral strategies to enhance adherence

- Modeling of behavior via word, action, video; reference model must be similar in ability (e.g., demonstrate exercise in cardiac rehabilitation session; select food from a restaurant menu)
- Tailor regimen to fit patient's lifestyle (e.g., develop medication schedule to accommodate work schedule; recommend diet changes with sensitivity to cultural food preferences and available resources)
- Goal setting: Make goals proximal, attainable, very specific (e.g., walk eight blocks three times/week for the next month; reduce milk fat to 1%; reduce meat portion to 4 oz)
- Self-monitoring: Record activities related to goal and review with provider at next visit; use for self-review to identify patterns threatening adherence; use for problem solving
- Reinforcement (administered by provider or patient [self-reinforcement]): Review self-monitor records, provide praise for attempts and progress in meeting goals; patient can use to reinforce self for progress made
- Problem-solving: Review threats to adherence; identify problems; anticipate potential problems; identify solutions; select a solution and test it; rehearse how potential problems might be managed
- Cuing: Set up system of reminders to take medicine, exercise (e.g., set out walking shoes; place a reminder sticker in obvious place about a bedtime medicine)
- Habit building: Pair an activity with an established habit (e.g., place pill bottle next to morning juice glass or toothpaste; bedtime medication by clock radio)
- Contracting: Make a written agreement between patient and provider concerning how/when patient will reach set goal; usually involves a reward when goal is achieved; uses incremental steps in reaching goal; specifics included in contract
- Social support: Enlist assistance of significant support systems at home, work, and social environment; invite attendance at exercise, cooking classes, and follow-up appointment; involve others in behavior change plan
- Self-efficacy enhancing: Provide opportunities for successful performance (performance mastery is most influential); give feedback and praise; use verbal persuasion; instill self-confidence; set short, specific goals; practice self-regulation through continuous or episodic self-monitoring, followed by self-evaluation and self-reinforcement; develop skills and enhance knowledge

From Burke LE, Dunbar-Jacob J: *J Cardiovasc Nurs* 9:62-79, 1995.

body's "internal strength," and so they stopped taking them when they felt weak. For the same reason they feared taking two different medications at the same time. They believed that in some cases higher dosages yielded faster results and that in the absence of symptoms medication should be discontinued. Once these cultural ideas are understood, cultural noncompliance is predictable and can be addressed systematically.

There is also some evidence that certain populations, such as those with diabetes, have a considerably increased rate of depression, which is associated with less adequate adherence to self-care and poorer glycemia control.[15] Because most somatic illnesses are associated with an increased prevalence of depression, treatment of the depression may be an important way to increase adherence.

PREPROCEDURE AND POSTPROCEDURE EDUCATION
General Approach

Preprocedure and postprocedure education encompasses a wide variety of medical treatments, including surgery. A relatively strong research base has developed around the use of sensory information (what the patient will see, hear, feel, smell, and taste) during the procedure and procedural information (description of what will be done during the procedure) to help patients minimize their emotional reactions, increase their coping strategies, and have a better outcome from the procedure. The optimal amount of each kind of information has not been established. Self-regulation theory, a cognitive theory that explains human behavior as an outcome of information processing, is the basis for research on preparatory teaching. A schema (mental image based on prior experience) serves as a framework for organizing input as an experience progresses, and teaching sensory and procedural information helps to develop the schema about the event.

Educational Approaches and Research Base

An example of a preoperative program is the Pre-operative Total Joint Assessment and Education Program at the University of Pittsburgh.[33] Because nearly all these patients are admitted the day of surgery, the program is offered, in conjunction with pretesting for the procedure, on an outpatient basis 2 to 4 weeks before surgery. Content focuses on postoperative care, including exercises, wound care, and pain management. Possible complications and their prevention include the following:

Respiratory problems (coughing, deep breathing, use of spirometer)

Deep vein thrombosis (elastic stockings and a sequential compression device)

Wound care (dressings, signs and symptoms of infection)

Pain management (patient-controlled analgesia, epidural analgesia, and medications as needed)

Comfort meaures (relaxation techniques, breathing exercises)

Antibiotic therapy (including coverage for future invasive procedures)

Patients are provided with the total joint orthopedic clinical pathway, which highlights critical events and corresponding time.[33] Special care related to total knee and total hip arthroplasty surgeries includes hip reflexion precautions, use of adaptive equipment such as an elevated toilet seat, and guidelines for exercise and sexual activity after surgery. Patients see the physical therapist to learn about assistive devices, gait training, and transfer techniques, including appropriate weight bearing, and consult the occupational therapist to help gain independence in activities of daily living. The addition of specific learning objectives would be helpful.

Patient-controlled analgesia (PCA) is a portion of the operative teaching plan. PCA allows patients to receive a continuous or bolus administration of an analgesic and to administer it when they believe it is necessary. This method is also used for obstetric patients and for those with cancer pain. One study found that structured instruction provided a more efficient way to learn about pain management with use of PCA than did an incidental teaching mode[36] (Table 10-3).

Table 10-3   Questionnaire to evaluate PCA instruction

Directions: Please read the following statements and circle the number that best represents your experience after surgery when using the PCA pump. If you agree with the statement, circle (1); if you disagree with the statement, circle (2).

	AGREE	DISAGREE
Part I: use of the PCA pump		
1. I was receiving pain medicine because the PCA pump provides continuous administration of pain medicine.	1	2
2. The only time I received pain medicine was when I gave it to myself.	1	2
3. I knew I could never overdose myself because the PCA pump controls the amount of medicine I receive.	1	2
4. If I didn't get pain relief after I pressed the control button of the PCA pump, I waited 10 minutes before I pressed the button again.	1	2
5. I only received pain medicine when I pressed the button on the PCA pump.	1	2
6. If I didn't get pain relief after many tries at pressing the control button on the PCA pump I waited until my doctor visited to tell him (her).	1	2
7. If I had pain I pressed the control button of the PCA pump to receive additional pain medicine.	1	2
8. If I didn't get pain relief after I pressed the control button of the PCA pump, I called the nurse for a "pain shot."	1	2
9. I know I had to keep the number of times I self-administered pain medicine to a minimum so I wouldn't become sleepy or drowsy.	1	2
10. I didn't press the control button of the PCA pump when I had pain because I was afraid I would overdose myself.	1	2
11. I knew if I used the PCA pump to self-administer pain medicine I would not become drowsy and sleepy.	1	2
12. I knew I had to call a nurse if I didn't get pain relief after many tries of pressing the control button of the PCA pump.	1	2
Part II: management of pain		
1. I never worried about giving myself an overdose when I administered pain medicine using the PCA.	1	2
2. One of the reasons I hated to cough or deep breathe is because I couldn't get optimal pain relief using the PCA pump.	1	2
3. The reason I would use the PCA pump again is because I liked the feeling of control I had over my pain.	1	2
4. I had difficulty keeping free of pain when I used the PCA pump to administer the pain medicine.	1	2
5. One of the reasons I hated to move in bed is because I couldn't relieve my pain using the PCA pump.	1	2
6. I felt drowsy and sleepy when I used the PCA pump to relieve the pain.	1	2
7. I was able to get optimal pain relief using the PCA pump before I coughed and did deep breathing.	1	2
8. If I didn't get pain relief after my first try with the PCA pump, I didn't try again because I was afraid I would overdose myself.	1	2
9. I was able to keep relatively free of pain when I administered the pain medicine when using the PCA pump.	1	2
10. One of the reasons I was able to move freely while in bed is because I was able to reduce my pain using the PCA pump.	1	2
11. I was alert and awake while I used the PCA pump to control my pain.	1	2
12. I would never use a PCA pump again to control my pain.	1	2

From Timmons ME, Bower FL: *Orthop Nurs* 12:23-31, 1993.

Investigators have examined preparation for a variety of stressful events such as gastroendoscopy, orthopedic cast removal, pelvic examination, surgery, radiation therapy, and colposcopy. Conclusions are that (1) the sensory information alone is superior to procedural information alone; (2) either is superior to a control condition; but (3) a combination of sensory and procedural information is the most effective preparatory strategy.

Table 10-4 describes sensations associated with cardiac catheterization as they were experi-

Table 10-4   Procedure for cardiac catheterization with associated sensations

PHASE OF PROCEDURE	SENSATIONS	
	MEDICAL CENTER	RURAL HOSPITAL
Phase 1—Patient is placed on table, undressed, and partially covered with a cloth. Right and left groin are washed with soap and water. Groin area is shaved and swabbed with Betadine.	Coldness in groin area; buzzing and humming (machine noise); seeing tubing, lights, monitors, and clocks; seeing doctors and nurses	Coldness in groin area; wet feeling in groin
Phase 2—Cardiac monitor is attached. Sterile drapes are put down. Physician locates pulse in right groin. Needle is inserted to numb area with Xylocaine.	Burning in groin; needle-stick in groin	Stinging in groin; needle-stick in groin
Phase 3—Small incision is made in the groin and enlarged with hemostats. Physician palpates artery and inserts needle into artery.	Pressure in groin; pain in groin	Pressure in groin
Phase 4—Guidewire is inserted over needle. Dilator is inserted and removed.	Pressure; pushing; pain in groin	Pressure
Phase 5—Sheath is inserted. Physician moves table to see, on fluoroscopy, the location of the tip of the wire. Guidewire is removed and needle flushed with heparin. Catheter is inserted and visualized on fluoroscopy.	Popping, buzzing, clicking (machine noises); seeing knobs, screens (equipment); pressure; pushing	Pressure
Phase 6—Monitor is observed for heart pressures; pressures recorded. Dye is injected using injector machine. Dye transit is observed on fluoroscopy.	Hot, burning feeling (mostly traveling from upper body downward); background talking; seeing camera, lights, monitor	Hot, burning feeling (mostly upper body downward); moist, wet
Phase 7—Guidewire is reinserted, catheter is removed, second catheter is inserted. Catheter insertion visualized on fluoroscopy. Dye is injected by hand. Dye transit is observed on fluoroscopy.		Pain, pressure in chest
Phase 8—Guidewire is reinserted, catheter is removed, third catheter is inserted. Catheter insertion visualized on fluoroscopy. Dye is injected by hand. Dye transit is observed on fluoroscopy. Catheter is removed. Guidewire is removed. Occlusive pressure is applied to groin.	Pain, pressure (chest and back); equipment noise; seeing equipment	Pain, pressure (chest and back)
Phase 9—Sheet is removed, patient is moved to stretcher, and stretcher is moved to hallway. Occlusive pressure is applied for 20 minutes.	Pressure; back pain	

From Cason CL, Russell DG, Fincher SB: *Cardiovasc Nurs* 28:41-45, 1992.

enced by at least 40% of the patients in two different settings.[5] The box below develops a script for preparatory sensory information for cardiac catheterization, which is based on the sensations described in the study.

Some investigators have identified the need to tailor the type and amount of information according to the coping style of the patient, with use of "blunters" for avoiding information that will intensify the psychological impact of the procedure and "monitors" for seeking information.[14] A study of individuals undergoing cardiac catheterization found that a videotape containing procedural and sensory information in a modeling format was better for monitors, whereas a procedural modeling video was the optimal preparatory treatment for blunters (Table 10-5).[11] The effectiveness of preparatory information interventions in reducing anxiety in patients undergoing cardiac catheterization is supported by a number of studies. This intervention enables patients to form accurate expectations about the impending procedure rather than anticipating it in threatening or unrealistic terms.[18]

Summaries of research on procedure/operative teaching were among the first to be completed; six are shown in Appendix C. One reviewer found that offering both procedural information and emotional support was more effective than offering either alone.[30] From nearly 200 studies, Devine[12] found statistically reliable

---

■ PREPARATORY SENSORY INFORMATION FOR CARDIAC CATHETERIZATION

Just before you are taken to the catheterization lab you may be given a sedative. This will relax you, but you will be awake during the procedure. You may also be given an antihistamine to decrease the chance of a reaction to the dye. When you get to the lab, you will see x-ray equipment, monitors, and hospital staff dressed in surgical clothing. The room will be cold and you will hear fans and motors running. You will lie on your back on the examining table during the entire procedure. Because the table is hard, you may feel some discomfort. If you do, tell the doctor. Your clothes will be removed and you will be partially covered with a cloth. The lab technicians will clean the groin with soap and water, shave it, and swab it with Betadine. The Betadine will feel cold and will leave a yellowish color that will wash off your skin. The lab technicians will put patches on your chest and attach wires so they can watch your heart rhythm during the procedure. You will be covered with a special sheet from neck to foot. The doctor will check for a pulse in your groin area and numb the area with Xylocaine. When he or she gives you the Xylocaine, you will feel a needle-stick, followed by a burning or stinging sensation. Once the area is numb, you mainly will feel pressure in the groin as the doctor makes a small incision and inserts the catheter. While the doctor guides the catheter up to the heart, the lights in the room periodically will be turned on and off, and you will hear a popping or clicking noise. The doctor will move the table to see where the catheter is by looking at the monitor. When the catheter reaches the heart, a machine will inject dye through the catheter. You will feel a burning or hot sensation, which you may feel anywhere in your body. Most people feel the burning in their faces, shoulders, chests, and down to their bottoms. Some describe the feeling as a hot flash or as if they had urinated or are sitting in warm water. It lasts only a few seconds. The doctor will then change catheters and inject more dye by hand. You may then feel pressure in your groin and tightness or heaviness in your chest. Some people have chest discomfort. If you do, be sure to tell the doctor. At the end of the procedure, the doctor will remove the catheter and place a bandage on your groin. You will be moved from the examining table to a stretcher and taken to a waiting area for about 20 minutes. The doctor or nurse will hold the bandage to your groin to keep it from bleeding. You will feel pressure in the groin and may feel some discomfort from lying on the table for such a long time. When the doctor is sure that you will not have any problems, you will be taken back to your room.

From Cason CL, Russell DG, Fincher SB: *Cardiovasc Nurs* 28:41-45, 1992.

Table 10-5   Videotapes on procedural modeling and procedural-sensory modeling

PREPARATORY INFORMATION TREATMENT	VISUAL INFORMATION	AUDITORY OR PRINTED INFORMATION
Procedural modeling videotape	Patient is on a stretcher just outside the cath lab. Staff members wheel the patient into the cath lab and (1) cover patient with a drape sheet, (2) remove patient's gown, (3) help patient transfer from a stretcher to x-ray table, and (4) place a pillow under patient's head.	Accompanying "voice-over" by patient: "The staff members assisting with my cath wheeled me into the cath lab next to a narrow bed—called an x-ray table. They covered me with a light sheet to protect my privacy and slipped off my hospital gown. I was helped off the stretcher and onto the cath table and I was asked to lie as still as possible throughout the procedure."
Procedural-sensory modeling videotape	As above.	As above, but with this addition: "When I was on the table I had a chance to look around the room. Next to the table were the x-ray cameras which would photograph the inside of my heart and chest. Overhead were TV screens which would be used to monitor my progress. I also noticed beeping signals, which the doctor said were sounds from the heart monitor. Another thing I noticed was that the staff members were dressed in masks and gowns to prevent the spread of germs. I mentioned to them that I was a bit cool, but the doctor said I'd be warmer in a couple of minutes when they covered me with sterile sheets."

From Davis TMA and others: *Heart Lung* 23:130-139, 1994.

and positive effects of this kind of teaching on recovery, pain, psychological well-being, and satisfaction with care. Positive cost-relevant effects have been obtained across a wide range of patients, treatment providers, settings, and historical periods.

Community-Based Education and Education of Special Populations

Current patterns of practice mean that much preprocedure education occurs in an outpatient setting or at home. Because many procedures are performed on an outpatient basis in a matter of hours, the opportunities for education are limited unless they are specifically created.

HIV-AIDS PATIENT EDUCATION
General Approach

Controlling the AIDS epidemic continues to depend heavily on educating people in ways to avoid becoming infected. Of necessity, this information must be widely available in communities, particularly those with high risk factors. Issues of education and informed consent are extremely important in testing. Much less has been written about educating persons with AIDS (PWAs) in how to take care of themselves when their test results are positive for HIV or after they are sick. The mass media have been very influential in shaping attitudes about AIDS. Table 10-6 presents an analysis of the predominant messages

Table 10-6 Summary of media images

CANCER	HEART DISEASE	AIDS
Moral worth		
Cancer is described as an evil, immoral predator.	Heart disease is described as a strong, active, painful attack.	Little is said about the nature of the disease other than it debilitates the immune system. Much is said about the moral worth of the victims of the disease.
Euphemisms		
Euphemisms such as the "Big C" are used rather than the word *cancer*.	Heart disease, stroke, coronary/arterial occlusion, and all the various circulatory system diseases are usually called the *heart attack*.	Acquired immune deficiency syndrome is called AIDS. The opportunistic diseases that attack the weakened immune system often are not mentioned.
Societal view		
Cancer is viewed as an enemy. Military imagery and tactics are associated.	The heart attack is described as a mechanical failure, treatable with available new technology and preventable with diet and other lifestyle changes.	AIDS is viewed as an overpowering enemy, an epidemic, a scourge.
Location of disease		
The whole self, particularly the emotional style of the person and the disease, is subject to discussion. Because the disease spreads and because the spread often is unnoticed through symptoms or medical perusal, the body itself becomes potentially suspect.	It occurs in a particular part that is indeed interchangeable with other parts located in a specific area.	Is described as affecting the immune system and resulting from mostly immoral behavior—connotes "shameful" sexual acts and drug abuse.
Optimism/pessimism		
Cancer is associated with hopelessness, fear, and death.	There is a degree of optimism about the preventability and the treatability of the disease.	Is associated with fear, panic, and hysteria because it is contagious through body fluids, primarily blood and semen.
Preventability		
Prevention through early medical testing is advised.	The heart attack is described as very preventable. Recurrent specific listings of necessary lifestyle changes are often given.	Prevention through monogamous sexual behavior (or abstinence) and avoidance of unsterilized needles and drug abuse.

From Clarke JN: *Health Commun* 4:105-120, 1992. *Continued.*

Table 10-6   Summary of media images—cont'd

CANCER	HEART DISEASE	AIDS
Causes (specificity)		
There are innumerable potential causes listed. They range from sperm to food-stuffs to the sun.	There is a specific and limited list of putative causes offered again and again.	Initially, the causes for AIDS were very general. Being homosexual, a drug user, or a Haitian was considered risky.
Causes (sociopolitical)		
There is little consideration of the sociopolitical, environmental causes.	There is little mention of sociopolitical causes.	There is little mention of sociopolitical causes.
Causes (uncertainty)		
There is uncertainty about cause.	There is certainty about cause.	There is uncertainty about cause.

on cancer, heart disease, and AIDS that appeared in six major magazines in Canada and the United States.[7]

Educational Approaches and Research Base

As with nearly all other diseases, knowledge alone is insufficient to bring about necessary behavior changes. Most interventions have used social learning theory. Individuals must become skilled in preventive behaviors, and those behaviors must be reinforced by their peers. They must have the materials they need, such as condoms. In addition to education, people must have strong negotiating skills to maintain preventive behavior in pressured social relationships. They must be rigorously tested to learn if they can maintain these behaviors, and they must be confident in their ability to avoid risky behaviors.[1]

A survey of brochures directed at intravenous drug users and their sex partners showed that they failed to provide self-efficacy–information that could convince recipients that they are personally capable of undertaking the recommended actions.[31] Many also failed to provide detailed diagrams that showed how to use bleach to clean needles or how to put on a condom.

Since the AIDS epidemic began, educators have produced thousands of brochures and pamphlets to educate the public. Such material is useful because it is portable and inexpensive, can be shared, and can be referred to repeatedly. However, as with other areas of education, much of this literature is written at a higher reading level than the target population has mastered. For example, distributing brochures in family planning clinics is one viable option for teaching women about HIV prevention. Yet one study showed that the mean reading level of brochures was equivalent to grade 9.9, and the formal education of 18% of the women seen in Virginia family planning clinics fell below this level.[37] Recall that, in addition, most individuals read several grade levels below the last grade they completed. The mean reading level of brochures targeted to adolescents and to minority women was lower than the average. Yet only 16% of adolescents, 6% of minority women, and 12% of women who spoke English as a second language had educational attainment equal to or exceeding the reading level of the brochures targeted for their group. Expert assistance with adult literacy problems can usually be obtained from the local school district office.

When an individual is notified of HIV positivity, counseling and education are crucial. These persons must be helped to cope emotionally and should not be allowed to leave the notification session until they can repeat the information they have been given. They must know how to recognize important symptoms and how to avoid infecting others.

Because 80% of women with HIV are of reproductive age, testing frequently occurs in obstetrical and neonatal settings. Although prenatal treatment is available, a substantial number of urban pregnant women at risk for HIV infection received little or no prenatal care, precluding serostatus determination before they gave birth.[22] The benefits of HIV-antibody screening include treatment for both mother and infant. Yet a positive test result provides inconclusive information about the infant's long-range condition even though it yields information about the woman's HIV status. If there is a loss of confidentiality, serious discrimination in housing, employment, insurance, child care, and family support is quite possible in a group already at risk of discrimination because of race or poverty. In a study in San Francisco, most women understood that they had given permission for the test but did not understand its clinical implications and recalled few risks; 78% of those tested did not return to learn their test results. These findings clearly raise questions about the adequacy of the informed consent obtained.

Community-Based Education and Education of Special Populations

Experience in California[28] shows that the success of a program appears to depend on the staff's ability to locate and gain access to members of the specified target groups, to identify the appropriate type of educational intervention, and to determine whom to hire and how to train them to deliver the education. Gay men were contacted at home-based parties and at gay bars and resorts. However, it is difficult to reach minority gay, bisexual, or closeted men, especially in rural areas. To reach ethnic minorities, it is effective to employ ethnic staff members who understand the social networks in those communi-

ties. Intravenous drug abusers are best served by street outreach programs.

Systems of technology for delivering education on AIDS in the community can be very helpful. A number of AIDS hot lines offer confidential telephone call-in services. One specialized computer network provides nurse-supervised information, decision support, and communication services to home-dwelling PWAs.[2] An electronic encyclopedia, which includes more than 200 pages of information relevant to living at home with AIDS, was designed to help PWAs enhance their self-care, understand illness-specific issues, and promote home-based management of their illness. The decision-support module guided users in an analysis of a self-defined decision problem, helping the user focus on the values and trade-offs that occur during difficult choices. The public communication area functions as a support group. Instructions about self-care or messages encouraging hope can be retained and reviewed for as long as an individual desires. Such a network is an example of how innovative technologies can be used to deliver scarce nursing resources to persons in the community.

Other vulnerable populations may be seen in community-based organizations, such as day hospitals or partial hospitalization programs for individuals with prolonged mental illness.[35] These persons may have cognitive deficits that interfere with acquiring knowledge about HIV and AIDS, as well as impairments in impulse control and judgment that increase their risk of exposure to the disease through intravenous drug use or sexual activity. They are frequently at high risk for the disease and need to be taught preventive behaviors.

Finally, a study of poor African-American women seeking care in an inner-city prenatal clinic found that use of condoms in the previous year was significantly related to perceptions of susceptibility.[16] Items measuring elements of the health belief model are shown in Table 10-7. The findings suggest that messages emphasizing the ubiquity of risk, especially in demographically

Table 10-7   Distribution of responses to the health belief model items

SCALE	% STRONGLY AGREE/AGREE
Susceptibility scale	
You can't get AIDS because your sexual partner(s) is (are) very clean.	25.0
You are not the kind of person who is likely to get AIDS.	25.0
You are less likely than most people to get AIDS.	43.6
Given your lifestyle, there is a chance you could get AIDS.	44.3
You're afraid you could get AIDS from your sexual partner(s).	41.3
Mean = 3.19, *SD* = 0.74, Range = 1 to 5	
Severity scale	
AIDS is a life-threatening disease.	98.6
You are not worried about getting AIDS.	28.2
AIDS is not as bad as venereal disease (VD).	5.5
AIDS can be cured if treated early.	8.3
You are afraid of getting AIDS.	83.6
Your body could fight off AIDS because you are very healthy.	8.3
Mean = 4.08, *SD* = 0.50, Range = 1 to 5	
Barriers scale	
The quality of your sex life would suffer if you did all the things that are important to protect yourself from getting AIDS.	33.2
Protecting yourself against AIDS would be hard to do, given your lifestyle.	10.4
If you tried hard to protect yourself against AIDS, it would be a hassle.	10.6
It would be embarrassing for you if you were to do all the things you have to do to protect yourself from getting AIDS.	11.6
Mean = 2.18, *SD* = 0.69, Range = 1 to 5	
Benefits scale	**% Rated very effective**
Refuse to have sex with casual sexual partners if they don't agree to use a condom (rubber).	81.5
Avoid sex with men who have many sexual partners.	84.8
Refuse to have sex with anyone who is infected with the AIDS virus.	89.2
Refuse to have sex with a man who shoots drugs, because he could have the AIDS virus.	88.0
Mean = 3.75, *SD* = 0.37, Range = 1 to 4	

From Gielen AC and others: *AIDS Educ Prev* 6:1-11, 1994.

high-risk populations, may be particularly appropriate and effective.

A second study of the same population found significant deficits in understanding of treatment, whereas transmission was much better understood.[20] Such a finding should not be surprising because most educational messages from public health sources have emphasized transmission. The knowledge test used in this study can be found in Table 10-8. Although knowledge is only a portion of what is necessary to adopt protective behavior against the AIDS virus, it is important to learn whether basic knowledge is being disseminated to vulnerable populations.

Table 10-8 Knowledge of routes of transmission

Women who have had certain experiences are more likely to be infected with the AIDS virus than other women. But, not everybody agrees on what experiences put women at increased risk of AIDS. For each of the following, please tell me whether you think a woman having had this experience would make her a lot more likely, a little more likely, or no more likely to get AIDS.

	A LOT MORE LIKELY (%)	A LITTLE MORE LIKELY (%)	NO MORE LIKELY (%)	DON'T KNOW (%)
Getting a blood transfusion?	49	40	10	1
Being around someone with AIDS?	6	15	79	<1
Having sex with a lot of different partners without using a condom?	96	4	<1	0
Deep kissing or French kissing a person who has AIDS?	23	31	42	4
Sharing needles when shooting drugs?	99	1	1	0
Having a sexual partner who had frequent blood transfusions?	55	36	6	2
Having anal intercourse?	58	24	8	11
Touching someone with AIDS?	1	8	89	1
Having a sex partner who had AIDS or had a positive test for the AIDS virus?	92	7	1	<1
Having a sexual partner who shoots up drugs?	90	9	<1	<1
Having a sexual partner who was bisexual (he had sex with a man)?	86	11	2	1
Having ever had a disease or an infection spread by sex?	33	41	22	6

	TRUE (%)	FALSE (%)	DON'T KNOW (%)
Knowledge of HIV antibody test			
The AIDS virus test is done by taking a sample of blood.	92	3	6
The AIDS virus test can tell you if you have the disease AIDS.	76	20	4
If an AIDS virus test comes back positive, it means that the person can give AIDS to someone else.	86	11	3
If a person's AIDS virus test comes back positive, it means that the person has been infected with the AIDS virus.	91	6	3
If an AIDS virus test comes back negative, it means the person can never get AIDS.	1	98	1
If an AIDS virus test comes back negative, it means that no sign of the virus has shown up yet.	85	13	3

From Kass NE and others: *Women's Health Issues* 2:17-25, 1992.   *Continued.*

Table 10-8   Knowledge of routes of transmission—cont'd

	TRUE (%)	FALSE (%)	DON'T KNOW (%)
Knowledge of treatments			
Doctors can help people with the AIDS virus feel better and live longer.	40	51	9
There is a drug that a pregnant woman who has the AIDS virus can take to keep her baby from getting the AIDS virus.	4	67	30
There is a drug that can cure babies who get AIDS from their mothers.	5	73	22
Doctors can help babies who have AIDS feel better and live longer.	33	53	14
Knowledge of vertical transmission			
A pregnant woman who has the AIDS virus can give AIDS to her baby.	98	1	1
If a pregnant woman's AIDS virus test comes back positive, it means that her baby will definitely have AIDS.	61	28	11
If a newborn's AIDS virus test is positive it means that the mother must be infected with the AIDS virus.	83	12	5
If a newborn's AIDS virus test is positive it means that the baby's father must be infected with the AIDS virus.	58	31	11
All newborns with a positive AIDS virus test are infected with the AIDS virus.	79	15	6

SUMMARY

This chapter describes four areas of patient education practice that range from those that are just developing to those with a stable research base, the findings of which should be widely applied in practice. Yet there are many other patient problems in which education could be very useful. The postscript that follows Chapter 11 and summarizes Part II of this book further details these opportunities.

REFERENCES

1. Bandura A: Perceived self-efficacy in the exercise of control over AIDS infection, *Eval Program Planning* 13:9-17, 1990.
2. Brennan PF, Ripich S: Use of a home-care computer network by persons with AIDS, *Int J Technol Assess Health Care* 10:258-272, 1994.
3. Burke LE, Dunbar-Jacob J: Adherence to medication, diet, and activity recommendations: from assessment to maintenance, *J Cardiovasc Nurs* 9:62-79, 1995.
4. Burnside B, Hodgins G: The role of education in a program to treat depression in older women, *Educ Gerontol* 18:483-496, 1992.
5. Cason CL, Russell DG, Fincher SB: Preparatory sensory information for cardiac catheterization, *Cardiovasc Nurs* 28:41-45, 1992.
6. Clark NM and others: Self-management of chronic disease of older adults, *J Aging Health* 3:3-27, 1991.
7. Clarke JN: Cancer, heart disease and AIDS: what do the media tell us about these diseases? *Health Commun* 4:105-120, 1992.
8. Clary C, Dever A, Schweizer E: Psychiatric inpatients' knowledge of medication at hospital discharge, *Hosp Community Psychol* 43:140-144, 1992.
9. Cromes GF, Helm PA: The status of burn rehabilitation services in the United States: results of a national survey, *J Burn Care Rehabil* 13:656-662, 1992.
10. Daley DC, Bowler K, Cahalane H: Approaches to patient and family education with affective disorders, *Patient Educ Counsel* 19:163-174, 1992.
11. Davis TMA and others: Preparing adult patients for cardiac catheterization: informational treatment and coping style interactions, *Heart Lung* 23:130-139, 1994.

12. Devine EC: Effects of psychoeducational care for adult surgical patients: a meta-analysis of 191 studies, *Patient Educ Counsel* 19:129-142, 1992.

13. Farran CJ, Keane-Hagerty E: Interventions for caregivers of persons with dementia: educational support groups and Alzheimer's Association support groups, *Appl Nurs Res* 7:112-117, 1994.

14. Garvin BJ, Huston GP, Baker CF: Information used by nurses to prepare patients for a stressful event, *Appl Nurs Res* 5:158-163, 1992.

15. Gavard JA, Lustman PJ, Clouse RE: Prevalence of depression in adults with diabetes, *Diabetes Care* 16:1167-1178, 1993.

16. Gielen AC and others: Women's protective sexual behaviors: a test of the health belief model, *AIDS Educ Prev* 6:1-11, 1994.

17. Hamera EK and others: Symptom monitoring in schizophrenia: potential for enhancing self-care, *Arch Psychiatr Nurs* 6:324-330, 1992.

18. Hayes R, Gantt A: Patient psychoeducation: the therapeutic use of knowledge for the mentally ill, *Soc Work Health Care* 17:53-67, 1992.

19. Holmes H and others: Nursing model of psychoeducation for the seriously mentally ill patient, *Issues Ment Health Nurs* 15:85-104, 1994.

20. Kass NE and others: Pregnant women's knowledge of the human immunodeficiency virus: implications for education and counseling, *Women Health Issues* 2:17-25, 1992.

21. Kukill WA and others: Causes of death associated with Alzheimer disease: variation by level of cognitive impairment before death, *J Am Geriatr Soc* 42:723-726, 1994.

22. Lester P, Partridge JC, Cooke M: Postnatal human immunodeficiency virus antibody testing: the effects of current policy on infant care and maternal informed consent, *West J Med* 156:371-375, 1992.

23. May KM, Evans GG: Health education for homeless populations, *J Community Health Nurs* 11:229-237, 1994.

24. Maynard C: Psychoeducational approach to depression in women, *J Psychosoc Nurs* 31(12):9-14, 1993.

25. McFarlane WR and others: From research to clinical practice: dissemination of New York State's family psychoeducation project, *Hosp Community Psychiatry* 44:265-270, 1993.

26. McWilliam CL and others: A new perspective on threatened autonomy in elderly persons: the disempowering process, *Soc Sci Med* 38:327-338, 1994.

27. Montgomery EB and others: Patient education and health promotion can be effective in Parkinson's disease: a randomized controlled trial, *Am J Med* 97:429-435, 1994.

28. Moore M and others: AIDS community education: the California experience, *AIDS Public Policy J* 4:92-100, 1990.

29. Morris LS, Schulz RM: Patient compliance—an overview, *J Clin Pharm Ther* 17:283-295, 1992.

30. Mumford E, Schlesinger HJ, Glass GV: The effects of psychological intervention on recovery from surgery and heart attacks: an analysis of the literature, *Am J Public Health* 72:141-151, 1982.

31. Perloff RM, Ray GB: An analysis of AIDS brochures directed at intravenous drug users, *Health Communication* 3:113-125, 1991.

32. Posavac EJ and others: Increasing compliance to medical treatment regimens: a meta-analysis of program evaluation, *Eval Health Prof* 8:7-22, 1985.

33. Roach JA, Tremblay LM, Bowers DL: A preoperative assessment and education program: implementation and outcomes, *Patient Educ Counsel* 25:83-88, 1995.

34. Shimada J and others: "Strong medicine": Cambodian views of medicine and medical compliance, *J Gen Intern Med* 10:369-374, 1995.

35. Steiner J, Lussier R, Rosenblatt W: Knowledge about risk factors for AIDS in a day hospital population, *Hosp Community Psychiatry* 43:734-735, 1992.

36. Timmons ME, Bower FL: The effect of structured preoperative teaching on patients' use of patient-controlled analgesia (PCA) and their management of pain, *Orthop Nurs* 12:23-31, 1993.

37. Wells JA and others: Literacy of women attending family planning clinics in Virginia and reading levels of brochures on HIV prevention, *Fam Plann Perspect* 26:113-115, 131, 1994.

11 Patient Education and Health Policy

Over the years patient education has been commonly regarded as a private matter between provider and patient, usually physician and patient, because for many years this was the only relationship acknowledged to have the authority to provide information to patients. This chapter addresses the development of public policy that is increasing pressures on providers to be responsible for delivering information to patients. The policy mechanisms used are varied—incentives, threat of direct regulation if providers do not voluntarily fulfill their role in informing patients, and potential sanctions attached to institutions in which providers practice.

The ultimate question is whether these mechanisms of public policy work to ensure that patients obtain the information and skills they need. These efforts are part of a slow trend toward support of patient autonomy—enabling patients to make their own decisions—and away from the paternalistic culture of the medical profession in which all information flow to patients is controlled according to medical values. Because patient education falls outside the biomedical model, it has been viewed as discretionary and marginal. Increasingly, those who make public policy see it otherwise. Indeed, a growing body of research focused on investigating the relationship between education and health suggests lack of education as a significant risk factor for poor health.

REGULATION OF HEALTH INFORMATION

The following examples illustrate policy mechanisms being used in the attempt to ensure that patients receive appropriate education.

National Introduction of Diabetes Teaching Programs in Germany

Although patient education has been widely accepted as an integral part of diabetes therapy for years, in many countries only a very limited number of persons with non-insulin-dependent diabetes mellitus (NIDDM) receive adequate structured education. In the United States a long struggle has taken place to arrange any reimbursement for provision of diabetes education as a professional service.

Beginning in 1991 nearly all German insurance funds covered physician fees for structured diabetes education programs, as well as reimbursement for the costs of teaching materials provided to patients. A prerequisite for this remuneration was completion of a specific postgraduate training course by both the physician and the office staff. Figure 11-1 shows the organization of the program's implementation. The training course for office-based physicians and their staffs followed the guidelines developed by the German Diabetes Association. It included microteaching techniques and preparation in basic methods of adult education. Although each team paid a significant fee for the seminar, by April 1995 more than 13,000 physicians and their staffs had participated in the training courses. Most teaching of patients is delivered by nonphysician providers; programs for patients are similar to those described in Chapter 7.[3]

Initial evaluation of this program showed that after provider participation the quality of diabetes care improved substantially: significant weight reduction occurred, relevant decrease of the prescription of oral antidiabetic agents was

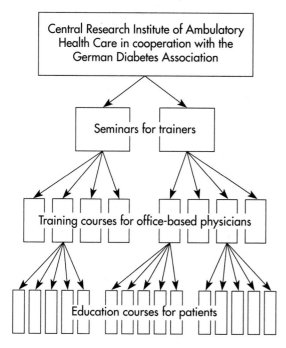

Central Research Institute of Ambulatory Health Care in cooperation with the German Diabetes Association

Seminars for trainers

Training courses for office-based physicians

Education courses for patients

Figure 11-1   Organization of nationwide implementation of structured treatment and education program for NIDDM patients in Germany. Central Institute is responsible for quality control and organization of trainer seminars for trainers (diabetologists and their diabetes educators) (1.5 days). (From Joergens V, Gruesser M: *Patient Educ Counsel* 26:195-202, 1995.)

achieved, and metabolic control improved significantly. Cost savings in the care of persons with diabetes are expected as a result of decrease in the rate of amputation, diabetic coma, and hospitalization. The number of patients participating in the program is to be monitored throughout Germany.[3]

Information About Advanced Directives

The Patient Self-Determination Act (PSDA), passed by the U.S. Congress in 1991, requires health care institutions that receive Medicare funds to inform patients at the time of admission about their rights and privileges in connection with life-support measures. Advance directives (ADs), such as living wills and durable powers of attorney for health care, are seen as ways for pa-

tients to provide direction to caregivers if the patient should not be able to speak for himself or herself. Under the PSDA provider organizations also are required to document whether patients have ADs, to implement policies to recognize ADs, and to educate their staff and communities about them.

The assumption underlying the PSDA is that persons will execute ADs if they are given sufficient information and encouragement. A growing body of research indicates that this assumption is simplistic. For example, persons older than 60 years are not executing ADs in significant numbers despite high levels of familiarity and understanding. Intervention studies have been shown to produce modest increases in use of ADs.[2] Yet the desired outcome from the AD movement is helping patients to knowledgeably make their own decisions about whether to have an AD and, if so, what to put in it.

Patients and families frequently need time to deal with losses and with conflicts among family members. Some believe that providers will abandon patients with ADs at some level. At the time of admission patients are often anxious, in pain, depressed, and cannot attend to information about ADs. In reality, many people need a teaching/counseling process to assist them with the decision about whether to develop an AD and what it will say. They need repeated explanations and discussions of options with a health care provider, as opposed to being informed by an admitting clerk that they can have an AD. It should be acknowledged that some patients defer action because their present perceived state of affairs does not urgently call for an AD or they are confident that they can rely on others and prefer the informality of decision making by family members. Indeed, intensive interventions, including repeated efforts to persuade patients to complete an AD, could be seen as coercive.

The box on p. 196 provides an example of a comprehension test on ADs, cardiopulmonary resuscitation (CPR), and artificial nutrition and hydration (ANH). An understanding of these issues if important to support end-of-life decision

■ PATIENT COMPREHENSION QUESTIONNAIRE

(a) Open-ended and
(b) Yes-or-No Questions

1. (a) What is an advance medical directive (often called a living will)?
   (b) Does an advance medical directive:
      Indicate a person's wishes about medical treatments?*
      Indicate the physician's opinions about medical treatments?

2. (a) When is the information a patient provides in the advance medical directive used?
   (b) Is the information a patient provides in the advance medical directive used when the patient:
      Enters the hospital for routine surgery?
      Comes for a routine check-up?
      Is unable to communicate?*
      Is unable to make decisions?*

3. (a) Why is the advance medical directive important?
   (b) Is the advance medical directive important because:
      It serves as a guide for family, friends, and physicians?*
      It helps with planning preventive health care measures?

4. (a) When is cardiopulmonary resuscitation (CPR) used?
   (b) Do physicians use CPR when:
      A patient has a stroke?
      A patient stops breathing?*
      A patient's heart stops beating?*
      A patient has dizziness?

5. (a) When physicians give CPR, what exactly do they do?
   (b) Does CPR involve:
      Giving the patient medications through an IV?

Pressing on the patient's chest?*
Bandaging the patient's chest?
Giving the patient artificial breathing?*
Taking x-rays of the patient's chest?
Giving the patient an electric shock?*
Measuring brain waves?
Inserting a heart catheter?

6. (a) What is artificial breathing?
   (b) Does artificial breathing involve:
      Providing oxygen through a face mask?
      Insertion of a tube into a windpipe?*
      Connecting the patient to a breathing machine?*
      Asking the patient to breathe rapidly?

7. (a) What is artificial feeding and fluids?
   (b) Is artificial feeding and fluids:
      A kind of antibiotic?
      A form of nourishment?*

8. (a) When do patients need to receive artificial feeding and fluids?
   (b) Do patients need to receive artificial feeding and fluids when:
      They are unable to eat or swallow enough food to stay alive?*
      They have a pain in their stomach?

9. (a) How are artificial feeding and fluids given to a patient?
   (b) Are artificial feeding and fluids given to patients:
      As a pill?
      Through a tube?*
   (c) Can artificial feeding and fluids be given to a patients through a tube that goes:
      Into a vein?*
      Into the liver?
      Into the lung?
      Through the skin to the stomach?*
      Through a catheter to the bladder?
      From the nose to the stomach?*

From Moore KA and others: *Arch Fam Med* 3:1057-1063, 1994.
*Indicates the correct response is yes.

making. Responses to open-ended questions were recorded verbatim.[5] What are the implicit learning objectives represented by this test? Is the questionnaire complete in testing the skills represented in the implicit objectives? What is the usefulness of such an instrument? Would you use it clinically?

Information About Prescription Drugs

Although information about prescription drugs has been regulated for a long time, recent trends reflect stronger efforts to ensure that patients receive relevant information. Two recent lines of regulation reflect this goal. The first is directed toward pharmacists, and the second is directed at the manufacturers of prescription drugs.

The Omnibus Reconciliation Act of 1990 (OBRA '90) contained several regulations regarding prescription drugs, including requiring pharmacists to offer counseling about these medications to patients whose care is funded by Medicaid. In fact, most states have adopted requirements for pharmacists to counsel all patients. In some instances written counseling is sufficient. The following information is to be included: route, dosage, duration, special directions and precautions, common severe side effects or adverse effects or interactions (including their avoidance and action required if they occur) techniques for self-monitoring drug therapy, storage, and action to be taken in the event of a missed dose.[4]

For many years the Food and Drug Administration (FDA) has regulated written information that comes with prescription drugs, known as patient package inserts (PPIs). As recently as the 1960s, physicians were viewed as the sole dispensers of such information. In 1980 the FDA proposed, on a pilot basis, a regulation that required mandatory patient information for 10 drugs or classes of drugs. Many physicians, pharmacists, and drug manufacturers opposed this program, contending that it would encourage self-diagnosis, produce adverse reactions in patients through suggestion, adversely affect liability of health care providers and manufacturers,

interfere with the physician-patient relationship, impose unnecessary burdens on manufacturers and pharmacists, and increase the costs of prescription drug products.[6]

The FDA suggested that PPIs could reduce inappropriate drug use and promote their optimal use. The proposed regulations requiring PPIs for most prescription drug products were revoked in 1982, with the expectation that the private sector would voluntarily distribute patient information. Such programs for distribution of drug information exist through physician organizations, the American Association of Retired Persons, and the United States Pharmacopeia.[6] In August of 1995 the FDA again proposed regulations for prescription drug labeling and medication guide requirements. A summary of those proposed regulations appears in the box on p. 198. The thrust of these regulations is to require standards for drug distribution and quality, to enhance patients' ability to understand the benefits and risks of treatment, and to use the drugs effectively. The voluntary program endorsed in the 1980s is judged to have made minimal progress in improving the distribution of drug information to patients. The information that actually reaches most patients is found to focus primarily on how to use the medication, with little precautionary or adverse drug information, and it varies highly in quality.[1]

This latest proposed ruling on the part of the FDA is still in process; time will tell whether the political climate in favor of wider access of patients to drug information will overcome the same objections raised a decade ago.

RELATIONSHIP BETWEEN EDUCATION AND HEALTH

Associations of higher socioeconomic status (SES) and better health have been reported for more than 150 years. Formal education is one component of SES, correlated with income and occupation, as well as with working and living conditions. The box on p. 199 lists possible mediational variables in this relationship. Low educational attain-

PROPOSED REGULATIONS FOR PRESCRIPTION DRUGS: DEPARTMENT OF HEALTH AND HUMAN SERVICES

Food and Drug Administration
21 CFR Parts 201, 208, 314, and 601
[Dockets No. 93N–0371]
RIN 0910–AA37

**Prescription drug product labeling;
medication guide requirements**

Agency: Food and Drug Administration, HHS.

Action: Proposed rule.

Summary: Inadequate access to appropriate patient information is a major cause of inappropriate use of prescription medications, resulting in serious personal injury and related costs to the health care system. The Food and Drug Administration (FDA) believes that it is essential that patients receive information accompanying dispensed prescription drugs. This information must be widely distributed and be of sufficient quality to promote the proper use of prescription drugs. Therefore, FDA is proposing performance standards that would define acceptable levels of information distribution and quality, and to assess supplied information according to these standards. Preliminary evidence suggests recent increases in the distribution of privately-produced patient medication information with dispensed prescriptions. Unfortunately, estimated distribution rates indicate that significant portions of patients do not receive information with their medications. FDA analyses also indicate that there is a high variability in the quality of this information. FDA believes that, with greater encouragement and clear objectives, the private sector will substantially improve the quality and distribution of patient information. Therefore, in concert with Healthy People 2000, FDA is proposing that private sector initiatives meet the goal of distributing useful patient information to 75 percent of individuals receiving new prescriptions by the year 2000 and 95 percent of individuals receiving new prescriptions by the year 2006. FDA is proposing two alternative approaches to help ensure that these goals (performance standards) are achieved. FDA would periodically evaluate and report on achievement of these goals. If the goals are not met in the specified timeframes, FDA would either (1) implement a mandatory comprehensive Medication Guide program, or (2) seek public comment on whether the comprehensive program should be implemented and what other steps should be taken to meet patient information goals. Regardless of the approach chosen, a mandatory Medication Guide program limited to instances where a product poses a serious and significant public health concern requiring immediate distribution of FDA-approved patient information would be implemented within 30 days of publication of a final rule based on this proposal. FDA believes that substantial health care cost savings can be realized by ensuring that consumers obtain the inherent benefits of proper use of prescription drugs, and by reducing the potential for harm caused by inappropriate drug use by the patient.

From Department of Health and Human Services: *Federal Register* 60:44182-44252, 1995.

ment is associated with high levels of infectious disease, many chronic noninfectious diseases, self-reported poor health, shorter survival when one is sick, and shorter life expectancy.[7] Those who have analyzed these relationships conclude that high educational attainments improves health directly through development of skills and information to help people deal with the stresses of life and indirectly through engendering a sense of personal control.[8]

Perhaps because the standard medical model does not incorporate these elements, they have been neglected. Related to the psychological and cognitive constructs listed in Box 11-3 is the serious impact of lack of functional literacy on the receipt of proper health care. The entire health care system assumes adequate literacy skills, for example, to read and understand labels on medication containers, appointment slips, informed consent documents, health education materials,

■ SOCIOECONOMIC STATUS AND HEALTH—POSSIBLE MEDIATIONAL VARIABLES BASED ON PERSONAL HEALTH BEHAVIORS AND PSYCHOLOGICAL AND COGNITIVE CONSTRUCTS

Personal health behaviors	Psychological and cognitive constructs
Diet and nutrition	Social support
Exercise	Anxiety
Smoking	Depression
Seat belt use	Health locus of control
Life stresses	Learned helplessness
Efficiency in use of medical services	Sense of coherence
Health insurance status	Self-efficacy
Use of preventive medical services	Optimism
Coping skills	Time preference
Problem-solving skills	Health knowledge

From Pincus T, Callahan LF: *J Clin Epidemiol* 47:355-361, 1994.

health insurance forms, and instructions pertaining to diagnostic tests. More specifically, those skills might include knowing how to take a medication four times a day, how to take a drug on an empty stomach, how many pills of a prescription should be taken, how many times a prescription can be refilled, or when the next appointment is scheduled. If patients cannot understand the forms, low literacy may also be an access barrier to receiving Medicaid assistance.[9]

This constellation of skills might be called functional health literacy—the ability to use reading, writing, and computational skills at a level adequate to meet the needs of everyday situations. Functional literacy varies by context and setting; the literacy skills of a patient might be adequate at home or work but marginal or inadequate in a health care setting. A study of two urban public hospitals found many patients (20% to 60%) to lack some of these skills.[9] In a Los Angeles public hospital, 11% of English-speaking and 33% of Spanish-speaking patients could not read well enough to understand preparation instructions—written at a fourth-grade level—for an upper gastrointestinal tract radiographic procedure. In an Atlanta public hospital, 43% of patients could not fully comprehend the "Rights and Responsibilities" section of the Medicaid application.

Patients are frequently discharged from a clinic and given only brief oral instructions, with health care providers assuming that they can read and understand important materials such as prescription bottles and appointment slips. This incorrect assumption certainly results in poorer health outcomes or adverse reactions among patients with low literacy skills. The problem is particularly acute among older adult patients. In the two public hospitals cited in the preceding paragraph, 48% to 81% of patients aged 60 years or older had inadequate functional health literacy.[9]

Thus adults with limited literacy face formidable problems in using the health care system. Even though appropriate availability of information and the opportunity to use it have increasingly been regulated, the needs of this group have not been seriously incorporated into mainstream health practice or the regulations governing it; nor have any measures been enforced. For example, the FDA's proposed rules for medication guide requirements do not address the extent of low literacy or illiteracy among the population.[1]

In our literacy-dependent society, lack of adequate patient education available to all the people we serve should be seen as a serious remediable deficit—a lack that stands in the way of achieving the health care outcomes and contributes to what many see as unjust differences among social classes.

SUMMARY

Slowly, but not very surely, patient education is moving from being perceived as a private matter managed by a patient's provider to being regulated by public policy. This chapter has provided several examples of the growing governmental regulation of this field, as well as highlighting an area in which well-designed and enforced regulation might serve to improve health care outcomes and ensure their more just distribution.

REFERENCES

1. Department of Health and Human Services, Food and Drug Administration: Prescription drug product labeling; medication guide requirements; proposed rule, 21 Code of Federal Regulations Part 201, *Federal Register* 60:44182-44252, 1995.

2. High DM: Advance directives and the elderly: a study of intervention strategies to increase use, *Gerontologist* 33:342-349, 1993.

3. Joergens, V, Gruesser M: Three years' experience after national introduction of teaching programs for type II diabetic patients in Germany: how to train general practitioners, *Patient Educ Counsel* 26:195-202, 1995.

4. Molzon JA: What kinds of patient counseling are required? *Am Pharm* NS32(3):50-57, 1992.

5. Moore KA and others: Elderly outpatients' understanding of a physician-initiated advance directive discussion, *Arch Fam Med* 3:1057-1063, 1994.

6. Nightingale SL: Written patient information on prescription drugs, *Int J Technol Assess Health Care* 11:399-409, 1995.

7. Pincus T, Callahan LF: Associations of low formal education level and poor health status: behavioral, in addition to demographic and medical explanations? *J Clin Epidemiol* 47:355-361, 1994.

8. Ross CE, Wu C: The links between education and health, *Am Sociol Rev* 60:719-745, 1995.

9. Williams MV and others: Inadequate functional health literacy among patients at two public hospitals, *JAMA* 274:1677-1682, 1995.

Postscript to Part II

Chapters 5 to 10 describe the best-developed areas of patient education practice, and Chapter 11 addresses the pressures in public policy to ensure that essential information reaches patients. The obvious question—How well are we doing in patient education?—is never asked. A review of these chapters elicits several observations.

1. In most instances, minority populations are heavily burdened by the diseases around which these educational programs have been organized. Yet we know very little about cultural models and educational approaches that are most effective with these populations.

2. Nearly all the indirect evidence available indicates that patient education is not accessible to significant portions of the population. Although the problem has been documented for a long time, persons with low or no literacy must be presumed to have very little access to the large number of printed materials used.

3. The needs patients have for education, which go well beyond the medical regimen, are focused on role changes associated with adapting to illness or maintaining good health. Of great interest is the emerging theme that for some disease entities for which patients are taught to access health care, lack of a common set of symptoms or varying interpretation of bodily sensations makes present education ineffective.

4. Each field of practice in patient education has developed with different strengths rather than according to some grand model. All deal with self-management. For example, cancer education focuses on self-assessment, especially breast self-examination, monitoring of symptoms, and pain management. Cardiac education focuses heavily on alteration of risk factors. Structures for quality management also differ. Diabetes education has opportunities both for accreditation of programs and certification of practitioners. In asthma and arthritis education, standardized, tested programs have been developed.

5. What patients need to learn has little to do with what is instructionally possible but rather with how the medical system is organized to deliver care. Almost no focus on longitudinal learning over a lifetime or over the course of self-management of a health care problem yet exists. Education is still not viewed as a long-term investment.

6. One widespread but untested assumption is that patient education does not have negative side effects. Conversely, there is almost no focus on the ethics of patient education, including when it is morally required, what conditions constitute manipulation, and other important questions.

7. Almost all policy documents focus on the right to information, completely ignoring the fact that education is necessary to use the information.

8. Most standards for patient education are process oriented, rather than outcome directed.

Although the accumulated meta-analyses of research show great promise for beneficial outcomes from patient education, only meager evidence exists for how it is carried out. A national survey of 6455 adults recently discharged from the medical or surgical units of 62 hospitals across the United States yielded the findings reported in Table 1. Patients are the best judges of the areas questioned: patient education and communication with providers, respect for patients' needs and preferences, provision of emotional and physical comfort, family involvement, and discharge preparation. Note that about 90% of patients said that medications, tests, and test results were explained in a way they could understand, but more than one fifth said that important side effects were not explained. More than 30% said that they were not told what foods they could or could not eat and that they were not informed of important side effects of their medications. Low income and poor health status showed the most pronounced association with patients' problem scores (see Table 1). Since this study was completed, the impact of managed care has probably changed hospital staffing conditions.

Although it is important, this kind of evaluation does not judge patients against a known standard of achievement. Such evaluation leaves unanswered the following questions: What performance level accomplished through patient education is good enough to optimally affect patient quality of life and health status? What portion of patients who do or do not receive education meet these standards? A badly needed next step in the development of patient education as a field of study and as a service is regular use of well-validated outcome measurement tools. These measured outcomes can then be compared against outcome standards and thus serve as a benchmark against the best that various delivery systems can accomplish.

Table 1   Frequency of problems reported by patients

DESCRIPTION OF PROBLEM EVENT	PATIENTS REPORTING PROBLEM (%)
Communication	
Not told about daily routine	44.9
Not told whom to ask for help, if needed	31.8
No doctor in charge of care or doctor in charge not available to answer questions	22.6
Doctor or nurse did not explain, before a test, how much pain or discomfort to expect	21.1
Not told before or shortly after admission things patient should have been told	10.3
Did not get understandable answers from nurses in response to important questions	7.2
Did not get understandable answers from doctors in response to important questions	6.4
Not given enough privacy while receiving important information about condition	4.5
Information about condition given in a way that upset patient	3.9
Financial information	
Not knowing how much would have to be paid worried patient	16.9
Needed help figuring out how to pay hospital bills and did not get it	11.4
Patients' needs and preferences	
Hospital staff did not go out of their way to meet patient's needs	19.9
Something was not done that patient thought should have been done	11.4
Not involved in decisions about care as much as patient wanted	10.2
Did not have enough say about medical treatment	10.0
Thought hospital staff put own needs first	9.9
Something done to patient in hospital that he or she thought should not have been done	9.7

From Picker-Commonwealth Survey of Patient-Centered Care; reprinted in Cleary PD and others: *Health Aff* 10:254-267, 1991.

Table 1   Frequency of problems reported by patients—cont'd

DESCRIPTION OF PROBLEM EVENT	PATIENTS REPORTING PROBLEM (%)
Doctors sometimes talked in front of patient as if he or she weren't there	9.3
Patient upset because examined or treated by someone who didn't explain what he or she was going to do	8.6
Nurses sometimes talked in front of patient as if he or she weren't there	7.0
Religious practices or preferences not respected	2.7
Not given enough privacy while being examined	2.4
Emotional support	
Did not have relationship of trust with any hospital staff other than doctor in charge of care	38.7
No one at hospital went out of way to make patient feel better	17.7
Difficult to find someone on staff to talk to about personal concerns	8.1
Did not have relationship of confidence or trust with doctor in charge of treatment at hospital	7.9
Physical comfort	
Nurses were overworked and too busy to take care of patient	28.4
Awakened for no reason by hospital staff	7.1
Needed, but did not get, help going to bathroom in time	6.6
Needed, but did not get, help bathing	6.4
On average, waited more than 15 minutes for help after pushing call button	4.9
Pain management	
Had moderate or severe pain that could have been eliminated by prompt attention by hospital staff	11.0
Pain experienced in hospital greater than patient told to expect	10.5
Waited, on average, more than 15 minutes for pain medicine	7.8
Received too little pain medicine	4.2
Education	
Important side effects of medicines not explained in a way patient could understand	23.6
Test results not explained in a way patient could understand	10.6
Why important tests were being done not explained in a way patient could understand	8.1
Purposes of medicines patient was getting in hospital not explained in a way patient could understand	8.0
Family participation	
Family or care partner not given all information needed to help patient recover at home	13.5
Family given too little information about care	8.8
Discharge preparation/continuity of care	
Not told which foods patient should or should not eat	36.5
Not told about important side effects of medicines	30.2

Continued.

Table 1   Frequency of problems reported by patients—cont'd

DESCRIPTION OF PROBLEM EVENT	PATIENTS REPORTING PROBLEM (%)
Discharge preparation/continuity of care—cont'd	
Not told what danger signals to watch for at home	26.5
Not told when patient could resume normal activities	24.2
Not told what activities patient should or should not do	18.6
Not told what to do to help recovery	16.7
Not told when patient could go back to work	16.2
No hospital staff tried to help patient with worries about returning home	8.6
Hospital did not assist patient prior to discharge in finding help needed after leaving the hospital	5.5
Purposes of discharge medicines not explained in a way patient could understand	4.6
Not told when and how to take medicines at home	2.9

Suggested Answers to Study Questions

CHAPTER 1 THE PRACTICE OF PATIENT EDUCATION: OVERVIEW

1. Answers will vary.
2. Parts of the teaching-learning process:
   a. The assessment of readiness for learning can use the mother's comments as the baby performs, including her comment about how frantic she gets when he cries.
   b. Learning goals are developed in response to the mother's comments, such as those about crying.
   c.-d. The teaching plan (intervention) follows the outline of the demonstration of the behavior, and the materials are the live baby and the interpersonal relationship between mother and provider, which, if formed as described, can be powerfully motivating.
   e. Evaluation is not as explicitly outlined as are other elements of the teaching process; however, one can presume that it would occur during a clinical interaction while stimulating and observing the baby's behavior. The mother's learning would be evaluated by her behavior with the baby and her responses to questions asked by the practitioner.

CHAPTER 2 MOTIVATION AND LEARNING

1. The implications are that all encounters with the health care system must advance the patient's understanding so that he or she can better manage his or her own health.
2. Evidence of wanting to learn is important for situations *a* and *b*.
   a. Your questions should determine the women's understanding and feelings about cancer, about preventive care in general, about manipulating their own breasts, and about the meaning of finding a lump. Some may have had instruction in the procedure and will be able to do some or all of it correctly.

   b. Some of your questions should enable you to discover the level of disability the boy is experiencing. Can he understand language and, if so, which words? How well can he grasp things and move his arms in a feeling motion? Other questions will deal with his independence and his caregiver's ability to cooperate in the training program. Does everyone in the family (including the boy) want the child to be independent? Is the caregiver patient yet precise enough to carry out a training program? Could she interpret the boy's behavior in terms of progress toward the goal?
3. You should not be surprised by these findings; they are what you would expect given an understanding of learning theory. Among the learning principles involved are that practice improves memory; direct experience of the skill helps the parent retain more learning than does an abstract review; and successful experience with feedback increases self-efficacy for that skill.
4. a. Establish baseline.
   b. Modeling.
   c. Setting up reinforcement; however, it would be useful to know if pennies for toys reinforce the child's behavior.
   d. Shaping.
   e. Contingent reinforcement.

CHAPTER 3 EDUCATIONAL OBJECTIVES AND INSTRUCTION

1. No, because the implicit (although never stated) objectives of discharge care involve observing the wound for evidence of complications, which requires being able to recognize such signs and symptoms.
2. The nurse can suggest that the mother place green peas, cereal bits, apple slices, and other similar foods on the baby's food tray to provide practice

of skills he or she needs to develop. Explanation of the organizing idea should also be given to the mother to show ways in which she can aid the baby's development. The U.S. Department of Agriculture has simple large-print booklets on this subject that can be read by mothers with limited literacy. The nurse can directly facilitate learning through modeling play and vocal games with the infant during visits and through his or her own expression of pleasure. All three of these strategies can be used. If this learning goal is needed by a number of mothers, consider developing a group teaching situation.

CHAPTER 4 EVALUATION AND RESEARCH IN PATIENT EDUCATION

1. To comprehend the means of attaining asepsis in giving an injection.
2. Transfer is involved every time the evaluation task is different from the learning tasks. Such is the case with all levels of the taxonomy with the possible exception of knowledge (cognitive). It is possible to index the degree of transfer of which the learner is capable by systematic testing of a wide variety of situations that require varying degrees of transfer (on a continuum from those tasks that are very much like the original learning task to those that are very little like it).
3. Factors and action:

Possible factors causing inattentiveness and rebelliousness	Nurse action
The complexity of the task the nurse was teaching might have been too great for the learner's ability, resulting in failure or even lack of willingness to begin learning.	Do a more careful analysis of prerequisite skills the learner possesses. If the goals are found to be too complex, break the skills into smaller units or teach the last part of the skill first (so that the learner experiences success).
The individual may be preoccupied with other life problems and therefore may not feel motivated to	Assess the accuracy of this hypothesis by talking with him and others who know him and by watching his behavior. It may be
develop this new behavior.	possible to create motivation by persuading him that learning the dressing skills can help him solve his other problem. Another alternative is to wait a few weeks and try again.
This may be the individual's usual response to many things.	Assess the validity of this statement. If true, it may be possible to do some teaching in spite of the inattentiveness and rebelliousness. The success of learning may alter these responses. Another alternative is teaching aimed first at altering these attitudes.

4. Analyzing patient's understanding:
   a. This person may not understand how blood sugar is measured—a certain amount per standard volume of blood. Investigate this.
   b. This is likely to be indicative of affective rather than cognitive learning. Because she is in the somewhat ambiguous situation of not being insulin-dependent, she is not motivated to move beyond the lower levels of the affective domain. It is also possible that she has not progressed beyond the denial or disbelief stage of psychosocial adaptation to illness.
   c. This comment may be evaluative of either cognitive objectives or affective objectives, or both. See if the rest of the conversation provides a more specific clue, and, if not, question the father yourself. The comment may mean that the man has not understood how diabetic patients accommodate such activities as hunting trips, or it may represent a seeking of verification from an experienced person that diabetic patients really can hunt and that his son can participate in such physically taxing activities.
5. The items test the objectives fairly well. It would seem unlikely that two providers would reach the same judgment inasmuch as the response, *correct,* is

not further refined. This tool was meant to be generic for use with many different medications. Providers would find it useful to define the correct responses about the drugs they are teaching most often.

6. Perhaps *believe* is a better term than *feel* because many of these items are cognitive. This content would be better suited to multiple-choice format. As it is, after the parent completed the tool, you know very little about why he agrees or disagrees or where misconceptions may lie.

CHAPTER 5 CANCER PATIENT EDUCATION

1. The critique should include (1) whether the questions test crucial elements, especially those that are commonly misunderstood by this population, (2) whether the reading level is so high that patients cannot understand the questions, (3) whether the score would represent true knowledge, and (4) whether the objective of increasing knowledge about screening will really contribute to any important clinical objective. My judgment is that the test is flawed on each of these criteria.

CHAPTER 7 DIABETES SELF-MANAGEMENT EDUCATION

1. Learning principles include the following:
   a. The assessment pinpointed changes that needed to be made from the perspectives of all stakeholders.
   b. People who would be delivering the program became committed to it by designing it.
   c. A teaching plan made expectations for the intervention clear and helped to ensure that appropriate materials would be available to carry it out.
   d. A cadre of nurses were certified (assured to have at least minimum skills) and could be ready resources to teach others on the units.
   e. Evaluation from several perspectives (outcomes, satisfaction) provided feedback for continuous improvement.

CHAPTER 8 EDUCATION FOR PREGNANCY AND PARENTING AND EDUCATION OF CHILDREN

1. Practice to overlearning; assessment and feedback from instructor and further instruction if necessary; speaking with parents who have used these skills successfully (modeling); and at least yearly re-education to maintain skills.

2. No, the concerns of the providers, particularly physicians, are not surprising because they frequently believe that "lay" people cannot handle technical health information. It will be necessary to develop at least one additional version of the VIP adapted to low reading level and to develop an audiotape or a videotape version for those who are illiterate.

3. Not really. One should be surprised by the ethical problem surrounding the intervention, which pays little attention to the values and informed choice of the mothers.

B Additional Study Questions and Suggested Answers

ADDITIONAL STUDY QUESTIONS

1. A radiology department found a problem of excessive repeat rates on some of its x-ray series, often because of poor bowel preparation. How would you justify development of a patient education program on preparation for these tests? What level of success could you promise?

2. One always has to be aware that messages in the environment or the content and behaviors one is teaching can be biased and not supportive of the patient's well-being. For example, an analysis of menstrual-product advertisements reveals the message that menstruation is a humiliating, shameful physiologic process that must be concealed and that the advertised products cleanse and deodorize.[5] Another example is the development of contraceptive technologies that make women more dependent on medical professionals for their administration and removal and frequently do not reflect women's reproductive needs or their experience in the use of various contraceptive methods.[9] In these situations, what is the patient educator's responsibility?

3. Patient package inserts (PPIs) are a prime educational tool for use of many drugs, including oral contraceptives. A study found that instructions in various brands of oral contraceptives were variable and confusing.[15] They differed in their recommendations of what to do after missing three or more pills and in what was considered the start day, including recommendations for using a backup method of contraception when first starting to use the pill. Should standards be set for these PPIs?

4. Compare the patient education standards for various disease entities contained in Appendix D. What conclusions can be drawn from the aggregate of this work?

5. Researchers in diabetes have found that self-care behaviors are often only weakly correlated with glycemic control.[8] What is the relevance of this finding for learning?

6. Studies show that feelings of control are important to psychosocial recovery from a cardiac event,[13] and that disease severity is not a reliable predictor of psychosocial recovery. This is also true for other illnesses such as cancer and rheumatoid arthritis. Perceptions of control are associated with increased adherence in persons with diabetes, patients undergoing cardiac rehabilitation, and individuals with hypertension. How can patient education be designed to develop perceived control by patients?

7. There are a number of theories of health behavior: health belief model, attribution theory, transtheoretic model of behavior change, and others. Faced with a patient education problem, how would you know which theories of behavior change to use?

8. Preparing patients to play a major role in choice of treatments is a goal of patient education. Some of the most structured work toward this goal has been done for persons choosing treatment for benign prostatic hypertrophy. The box on p. 209 contains symptom questions and value questions that reflect the patient's perspective and thus help him make a treatment decision.[1] Construct a similar set of symptom and value questions for helping patients with another disorder make a treatment decision.

9. Patients' knowledge of epilepsy has frequently been found to be inadequate, and because medication remains the most effective means to control seizure activity, medication knowledge is important.[6] Figure 1 shows a comparison of learning

SYMPTOM AND VALUE QUESTIONS

Symptom questions

Over the past month or so, how often have you:
1. Had a burning feeling when you urinate?
2. Had to push or strain to begin urination?
3. Had to urinate again shortly after you were finished urinating?
4. Found you stopped and started again several times when you urinated?
5. Dribbled urine after you thought you were finished urinating?

Ordered categorical responses: (1) not at all, (2) a few times, (3) fairly often, (4) usually, (5) always.

Value questions

1. Suppose your urinary symptoms stayed just the same as they are now for the rest of your life. How would you feel about that?
2. Suppose a treatment cured your urinary symptoms, but after the treatment any sexual climaxes would result in retrograde ejaculation. How would you feel about your situation?
3. Suppose a treatment cured your urinary symptoms, but you were not able to have sexual erections. How would you feel about your situation?
4. Suppose a treatment cured your urinary symptoms, but you occasionally dripped urine or wet your pants slightly. How would you feel about your situation?

Ordered categorical responses: (1) delighted, (2) pleased, (3) mostly satisfied, (4) mixed, (5) mostly dissatisfied, (6) unhappy, (7) terrible.

From Barry MJ and others: *Med Care* 33:771-782, 1995.

needs for persons with epilepsy, as rank-ordered by patients, nurses, and physicians. Were the differences among the three groups predictable? What lessons do these differences hold for teaching persons with epilepsy?

10. Fatigue is one of the most common complaints of newly delivered mothers. Fatigue affects the postpartum woman's quality of life and can interfere with her health and well-being and with development of the mother-infant relationship. The shortening of postpartum hospital stays seems to have increased both fatigue potential and difficulty for nurses to assess and assist in managing postpartum fatigue. A self-management guide[14] for patients with postpartum fatigue was developed by a process of:
   a. Content development by literature review to identify sources of fatigue and suggestions for its management
   b. Content validation by a panel of experts
   c. Pilot testing of the guide with patients.

   Develop a self-management guide with a group of patients. What potential negative side effects could be associated with such a guide, and how can you guard against them?

11. Families provide 60% to 80% of the total care received by impaired older adult relatives in such tasks as helping with eating, walking, dressing, taking medications, and managing chronic health problems such as incontinence. As the number of adults older than 85 years of age increases, the need for more physical care and assistance from family members will also increase. Where do families learn how to provide aid and physical care to their members? Because caregivers of stable or chronically impaired elders typically do not qualify for any Medicare-reimbursed nursing or other support services, they struggle with the responsibilities of caregiving without the benefit of any nursing assistance.

   Mahoney and Shippee-Rice[11] developed and piloted a training program for informal caregivers. The objectives are to help family caregivers achieve the following:
   a. Increase their knowledge of personal care techniques and needed adaptations
   b. Distinguish between normal changes associated with aging and pathologic processes
   c. Perform caregiving services in a more efficient manner
   d. Expand their range of caregiving skills
   e. Identify the meaning of the caregiver role to themselves and their care recipients
   f. Develop assertiveness techniques for use in the family system as well as in the formal caregiving system

   Using this model, design and pilot a program for informal caregivers in your neighborhood.

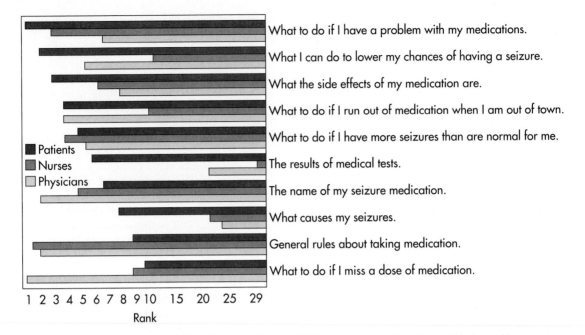

What to do if I have a problem with my medications.

What I can do to lower my chances of having a seizure.

What the side effects of my medication are.

What to do if I run out of medication when I am out of town.

What to do if I have more seizures than are normal for me.

The results of medical tests.

The name of my seizure medication.

What causes my seizures.

General rules about taking medication.

What to do if I miss a dose of medication.

■ Patients
■ Nurses
□ Physicians

1 2 3 4 5 6 7 8 9 10   15   20   25   29
Rank

Figure 1   Comparison of the rank order of the top 10 important items for patients with the rankings of nurse and physicians. (From Dilorio C, Faherty B, Manteuffel B: *Journal of Neuroscience Nurs* 25:22-29, 1993.)

12. Since 1981, the American Academy of Family Physicians Foundation has been developing a clearinghouse of evaluated patient education materials. The dilemma faced by busy clinicians is an overabundance of patient education materials, few of which have been appropriately evaluated. In 1989 a database describing such evaluated materials, including their cost and reading levels, became available and is now heavily used. The Materials Evaluation Questionnaire for health professionals and for patients is presented on pp. 211-213.[7] What suggestions would you make for its revision?

13. For a good example of identification of a patient education need and development of a program, read the article by Yetzer and others.[16] The parts of the teaching process are clearly labeled throughout the text. Based on what you know about patient education, what additional suggestions do you have for improving this program?

14. The patient questionnaire on p. 214 was used to assess the impact of a preoperative joint replacement patient education program.[10] The authors indicate that in an effort to intervene quickly with

pragmatic solutions, a dichotomous scale was chosen to focus on patients who had negative responses. Provide a critique of the tool.

15. Evaluate any teaching material for its suitability for persons with low literacy who have failing eyesight (remember that the final criterion of suitability is that persons of low literacy learn from it). Characteristics you might want to look for include the following[12]:

- Is the message behaviorally oriented and interactive?
- Is there use of stories and examples to describe difficult concepts?
- Does the material use language familiar to your patient population?
- Does it use short sentences of 12 to 15 words, alternating in length?
- Does it use techniques to draw attention to important ideas, such as arrows, underlining, bullets, bold face, and circles?
- Is there evidence that the material was pretested through focus groups, interviews, comprehension tests?

■ HEALTH PROMOTION PROJECT: MATERIALS EVALUATION QUESTIONNAIRE*

Directions: After reading over the material attached to this survey, please indicate your opinion by answering the questions below. If the question does not seem to apply, please circle NA. Comments are welcome. *Please* comment if you disagree or strongly disagree with any of the statements. Thank you.

Title:

Objective: In a few words, what do you think is the main purpose of this material?

It is designed to	Strongly disagree	Disagree		Agree	Strongly agree	
1. reinforce information.	1	2	3	4	5	NA
2. provide new information.	1	2	3	4	5	NA
3. stimulate behavior change.	1	2	3	4	5	NA

Appearance: Please rate the appearance of the material by answering each question below.

	Very low appeal	Low appeal		High appeal	Very high appeal	
4. At first glance it *attracted* my attention.	1	2	3	4	5	NA
5. It *held* my attention.	1	2	3	4	5	NA
6. Overall appearance	1	2	3	4	5	NA
7. Quality of illustrations	1	2	3	4	5	NA
8. Use of color	1	2	3	4	5	NA
9. Typeface (large enough, attractive, etc.)	1	2	3	4	5	NA
10. Highlighting of major concepts	1	2	3	4	5	NA

Comments _____

Content: Please rate the content of the material.

	Very poor	Poor		Good	Very good	
11. Up-to-date	1	2	3	4	5	NA
12. Scientifically accurate	1	2	3	4	5	NA
13. Adequate scope for objective(s)	1	2	3	4	5	NA
14. Overall organization	1	2	3	4	5	NA
15. Logical flow of ideas	1	2	3	4	5	NA
16. Needed background given to enable understanding	1	2	3	4	5	NA
17. Summary(ies) given when needed	1	2	3	4	5	NA
18. The management of fear content	1	2	3	4	5	NA
19. Fair presentation given (e.g., avoids sexism, ethnic bias, ageism, manufacturer bias, etc.)	1	2	3	4	5	NA
20. Does the bias interfere with the intent of the item?					Yes _____ (1) No _____ (2)	

Comments _____

From Gibson PA and others: *Bull Med Libr Assoc* 79:357-369, 1991.
*For use by health professionals.

Continued.

■ HEALTH PROMOTION PROJECT: MATERIALS EVALUATION QUESTIONNAIRE—cont'd

Usefulness: Please respond to the statements below by circling the best response.

	Strongly disagree	Disagree		Agree	Strongly agree	
21. It is useful for its intended audience.	1	2	3	4	5	NA
22. It is believable.	1	2	3	4	5	NA
23. The material is understandable.	1	2	3	4	5	NA
24. Requires little or no explanation.	1	2	3	4	5	NA

Comments _____

Overall: Please respond to the statements below.

	Strongly disagree	Disagree		Agree	Strongly agree	
25. Overall I would recommend that physicians use this material with patients.	1	2	3	4	5	NA
26. Overall this material meets its objectives.	1	2	3	4	5	NA

Remarks: _____

Placement: Please circle all that apply.

	Strongly disagree	Disagree		Agree	Strongly agree	
27. Should be placed in the physician's waiting room.	1	2	3	4	5	NA
28. Should be placed in the exam room.	1	2	3	4	5	NA
29. Should be stored for occasional use.	1	2	3	4	5	NA

30. Other suggested settings _____

Comments: _____

Please take a few seconds and complete the following:

Professional status:

		Number of years		
a. Resident	❑ PGY 1	❑ PGY 2		❑ PGY 3
b. Family physician faculty	❑ under 6	❑ 6-15	❑ 16-25	❑ 26 or over
c. Practicing physician	❑ under 6	❑ 6-15	❑ 16-25	❑ 26 or over
d. R.N.	❑ under 6	❑ 6-15	❑ 16-25	❑ 26 or over
e. Other (Specify) _____	❑ under 6	❑ 6-15	❑ 16-25	❑ 26 or over

Gender:

Age Range:

Male _____	(1)
Female _____	(2)
Under 25 _____	(1)
25-35 _____	(2)
36-45 _____	(3)
46-55 _____	(4)
56-65 _____	(5)
Over 65 _____	(6)

Name _____
            (Please print)

■ HEALTH PROMOTION PROJECT: MATERIALS EVALUATION QUESTIONNAIRE*

Directions: Please tell us what you think of the material attached to this form by answering all the questions below. For each question circle the number that best describes how you feel. If the question does not seem to apply to the material you are reviewing, please circle NA. If you wish to write comments, we would value your additional ideas.

Title: _____

Topic: _____

	Strongly disagree	Disagree		Agree	Strongly agree	
1. At first glance it *attracted* my attention.	1	2	3	4	5	NA
2. It *held* my attention.	1	2	3	4	5	NA
3. It is useful.	1	2	3	4	5	NA
4. I like the illustrations.	1	2	3	4	5	NA
5. I believe what it has to say.	1	2	3	4	5	NA
6. I would recommend it to a friend or relative to read.	1	2	3	4	5	NA
7. It is easy to understand.	1	2	3	4	5	NA
8. What is says is important.	1	2	3	4	5	NA
9. It reminds me of some things I need to think about.	1	2	3	4	5	NA
10. It gives me some new things to think about.	1	2	3	4	5	NA
11. It changes some of my thinking.	1	2	3	4	5	NA
12. It could change how I do things.	1	2	3	4	5	NA
13. Overall I recommend that doctors use this material with patients.	1	2	3	4	5	NA
14. Overall I am the right person to get this material from my doctor.	1	2	3	4	5	NA
15. Overall this material accomplishes its main purpose.	1	2	3	4	5	NA

Purpose: In just a few words, please write what you think is the main purpose of this material.

_____

_____

Comments: _____

_____

We would appreciate learning a little more about you.

( ) Male
( ) Female
Occupation _____
Years of school completed _____
Age range: ( ) Under 12
          ( ) 12-15
          ( ) 16-24
          ( ) 25-35
          ( ) 36-45
          ( ) 46-55
          ( ) 56-65
          ( ) Over 65

                    Thank you!

From Gibson PA and others: *Bull Med Libr Assoc* 79:357-369, 1991.
*For use by patients.

■ ASSESSMENT OF THE EDUCATION PROGRAM IN A JOINT REPLACEMENT CENTER
Patient Questionnaire

Letter

Dear

Our team is hopeful that your recent surgery is helping you to better enjoy life. To find out how you are doing since your joint replacement surgery, it is our hope that you will complete the enclosed questionnaire and return it to our office. We plan to write a research paper about the postoperative progress made by our patients. Your input would be greatly appreciated.

In gathering such information, we will be able to evaluate how our program can better serve patients before, during, and after their hospitalization. Emphasis will be on how you did once you were home. We also want to know your expectations of the surgical outcome. Did you do as well as you expected when you decided to have your operation?

We also would like to take this opportunity to say how much we enjoyed working with you and thank you in advance for helping us gather this information. We feel it will help others who are having this type of surgery know your feelings and suggestions for improvement of our program.

Sincerely,
Rhoda Lichenstein, CRNP
Case Manager

Questionnaire
Einstein/Moss Joint Replacement Center Patient Questionnaire

1. What was the date of your surgery? _____
2. Do you feel that the preoperative teaching you received helped you fully understand:

	Yes	No
Why you needed to have this operation	___	___
How the prosthesis looked and worked	___	___
What exercises you needed to do before your admission and when you were in the hospital	___	___
What our team expected you to report, i.e., drainage, redness and heat around incision, calf pain or swelling, etc.	___	___
Any additional comments you wish to make on this question?	___	___

_____

3. After your admission did you:

	Yes	No
Feel the medical staff was available for the care you required	___	___
Feel the nursing staff assisted you in your care	___	___

Comments please _____

_____

_____

4. Did the physical therapy department:

	Yes	No
See you on a daily basis	___	___
Help you understand the reasons behind the exercises you were doing	___	___
See that occupational therapy was part of your total program	___	___
Assign a reasonable length of time for each of your therapy sessions	___	___

From Lichtenstein R, Semaan S, Marmar EC: *Orthop Nurs* 12(6):17-25, 1993.

■ ASSESSMENT OF THE EDUCATION PROGRAM IN A JOINT REPLACEMENT CENTER
Patient Questionnaire—cont'd

	Yes	No
Too long?	____	____
Too short?	____	____
A bad time of the morning or afternoon	____	____
Too much time waiting while therapist was seeing other patients	____	____

Additional comments: Please indicate which hospital—AEMC, Willowcrest, or Moss—may have caused problems in your rehab. program.

_____

5. Upon discharge did the physical therapy and/or social services department:

	Yes	No
Arrange outpatient therapy appointments for you	____	____
See to it that you receive the necessary equipment you would need at home	____	____
Additional comments, please	____	____

_____

6. Did you have any problems at home that were not discussed with you by the hospital staff before your discharge that our team should know about?

7. Now that the surgery and recovery periods are over, do you feel that you are able to function as much as you anticipated prior to having this operation?

8. Do you have any suggestions that would help improve our present program?

- Is the material "friendly" for aging eyes, using 14- to 18-point type on nonshiny, cream-colored paper, with black letters, written at a very low reading level?

This is an example of 9-point type.

This is an example of 12-point type.

This is an example of 14-point type.

This is an example of 18-point type.

16. Butler and Beltran[3] describe adult persons with sickle cell anemia who were dissatisfied and angry with the treatment they received and were perceived by caregivers as exaggerating their pain, seeking drugs, and being noncompliant. Would you expect that an education/support group would be helpful in resolving these issues?

17. The quiz on p. 216 is given to elders in community settings to determine the adequacy of their knowledge about urinary incontinence.[2] Provide a critique of this tool for use in clinical practice.

18. Match the theory most identified with the following teaching approaches (theories may be used more than once).

◼ INCONTINENCE QUIZ

Statements for which:

Correct answer is "agree"

Most people who currently have involuntary urine loss live normal lives.

Many people with involuntary urine loss can be cured and almost everyone can experience significant improvement.

There are exercises that can help control urine if one leaks when they cough, sneeze, or laugh.

Involuntary loss of urine can be caused by several easily treatable medical conditions.

Women are more likely than men to develop urinary incontinence.

Many common over-the-counter medications can cause involuntary urine loss.

Correct answer is "disagree"

Once people start to lose control of their urine on a regular basis they usually can never regain complete control over it again.

The best treatment for involuntary urine loss is usually surgery.

Other than pads, diapers, and catheters, little can be done to treat or cure involuntary urine loss.

Most physicians ask their older patients whether they have bladder control problems.

Most people will involuntarily or accidentally lose control of their urine on a regular basis by the time they reach age 85.

Involuntary urine loss is caused by only one or two conditions.

Involuntary loss of urine, often called a leaky bladder or urinary incontinence, is one of the results of normal aging.

Most people with involuntary urine loss talk to their doctors about it.

From Branch LG and others: *J Am Geriatr Soc* 42:1257-1262, 1994.

Teaching approaches	Theories
___ 1. Emphasis on seriousness of consequences of not taking a health action	a. Self-efficacy theory
___ 2. Consciousness raising	b. Transtheoretic model of change
___ 3. Reinterpretation of physiologic signs and symptoms	c. Health belief model
___ 4. Relapse prevention	
___ 5. Modeling	
___ 6. Provision of cues to precipitate action	

Circle the correct answer

T F 7. A health care provider may be sued for a negative event resulting from the patient not understanding discharge instructions.

T F 8. Traditionally the goal of patient education has been compliance with the medical regimen.

REFERENCES

1. Barry MJ and others: Patient reactions to a program designed to facilitate patient participation in treatment decisions for benign prostatic hyperplasia, *Med Care* 33:771-782, 1995.
2. Branch LG and others: Urinary incontinence knowledge among community-dwelling people 65 years of age and older, *J Am Geriatr Soc* 42:1257-1262, 1994.
3. Butler DJ, Beltran LR: Functions of an adult sickle cell group: education, task orientation, and support, *Health Social Work* 18:49-56, 1993.
4. Clark NM, McLeroy KR: Creating capacity through health education: what we know and what we don't, *Health Educ Q* 22:273-289, 1995.
5. Coutts LB, Berg DH: The portrayal of the menstruating woman in menstrual product advertisements, *Health Care Women Int* 14:179-191, 1993.
6. Dilorio C, Faherty B, Manteuffel B: Learning needs of persons with epilepsy: a comparison of perceptions of persons with epilepsy, nurses and physicians, *J Neurosci Nurs* 25:22-29, 1993.
7. Gibson PA and others: A health/patient education database for family practice, *Bull Med Libr Assoc* 79:357-369, 1991.

8. Glasgow RE and others: Behavioral research on diabetes at the Oregon Research Institute, *Ann Behav Med* 17:32-40, 1995.

9. Hardon AP: The needs of women versus the interests of family planning personnel, policy-makers and researchers: conflicting views on safety and acceptability of contraceptives, *Soc Sci Med* 35:753-766, 1992.

10. Lichtenstein R, Semaan S, Marmar EC: Development and impact of a hospital-based perioperative patient education program in a joint replacement center, *Orthop Nurs* 12(6):17-25, 1993.

11. Mahoney DF, Shippee-Rice R: Training family caregivers of older adults: a program model for community nurses, *J Community Health Nurs* 11:71-78, 1994.

12. Meyer J, Rainey J: Writing health education material for low-literacy populations, *J Health Educ* 25:372-374, 1994.

13. Moser DK, Dracup K: Psychosocial recovery from a cardiac event: the influence of perceived control, *Heart Lung* 24:273-280, 1995.

14. Troy NW, Daigas-Pelish P: Development of a self-care guide for postpartum fatigue, *Appl Nurs Res* 8:92-101,1995.

15. Williams-Deane M, Potter LS: Current oral contraceptive use instructions: an analysis of patient package inserts, *Fam Plann Persp* 24:111-115, 1992.

16. Yetzer EA and others: Development of a patient education program for new amputees, *Rehabil Nurs* 19:355-358, 1994.

SUGGESTED ANSWERS TO STUDY QUESTIONS

1. You first need to consider who loses money if the tests have to be redone because payment does constitute a reinforcer. Are patients disgusted with having to come back several times? Are other services in the hospital affected? It is likely that a good patient-education program could improve bowel preparation, probably with increasing increments of improvements as the program and its delivery are refined.

2. Constantly be aware that such messages exist and that they serve interests other than those of your patient. Teaching of such messages can be considered unethical.

3. As a step toward improving women's ability to use the pill effectively, Family Health International believes that PPIs should provide standardized, simplified instructions on using oral contraceptives.[9]

4. These standards are just a beginning because they frequently do not include evidence that following them results in improved patient outcomes at a reasonable cost. Only one (enterostomal education) includes target patient outcomes.

5. This finding may say that no matter how much patients perform self-care behaviors as taught, their diabetes is not under control, which may mean that their medical treatments do not work very well. Under these circumstances, learning and doing self-care will not be reinforced because the patient continues to get worse. This finding may also reflect faulty self-reports on the patient's part.

6. Patient education can be designed to develop feelings of control by placing the patient in a major decision-making role in choice of treatment and by concentrating on development of self-efficacy for these behaviors.

7. The research base for these models has not made clear which components or critical mass of principles are needed to achieve change and which are more or less relevant to particular problems and populations of potential learners.[4] Your best bet is to use a theory that has been shown in studies to work with the problem you are facing.

8. Answers will vary.

9. The differences reflect expected perspectives of each of the groups and show especially that patients are interested in control of their symptoms, which should not be a surprise. The lesson to be learned is that patient education should clearly address the patient's concerns and not be constructed only from the providers' points of view. Unless this is done, patients lose interest in patient education, and satisfaction with their care frequently declines.

10.

Potential Negative Side Effects	Ways to Avoid
A serious complication that the patient does not recognize	Include those possibilities in the guide and note when to get help; have this advice validated by your panel of experts.
A feeling of lack of confidence if use of the guide does not ease the symptom	In the pilot test, verify that a wide range of users can understand and have the skills to use the guide effectively; include expected use of professional personnel if the symptoms do not abate.

11. Answers will vary.

12. Evidence about what a wide variety of patients learn from the materials.

13. It would have been helpful to obtain need-to-know behaviors from persons at various stages of recovering from amputation and to focus on development of a sense of self-efficacy in dealing with the various aspects of life with an amputation. Some of the objectives should be more focused on the actual behavior needed. For example, instead of stating that the patient should look for any red, discolored, or open areas daily, it would have been better to see if the patient could identify such areas on real amputations or at least in pictures. The use of a support group is excellent; what objectives should be accomplished through it? Would it be useful to put this process on a critical pathway to help identify benchmarks for patient progress in reaching the outcomes? It would also be helpful to have evaluation tools such as anchored scales. Although this program is a good start, persons with amputations no doubt need ongoing patient education services until they have reached optimal rehabilitation.

14. It is important that the questions are not focused on outcomes from patient education (except indirectly in Question 2); indeed, clear outcome objectives were not found in the article. Most of the questions are focused on patient satisfaction with process. This questionnaire clearly does not measure the impact of the perioperative joint replacement patient education program. "Yes-no" answers lead to socially desirable answers. Scoring on a nondichotomous scale could still have served to alert providers to patients with problems or dissatisfaction.

15. Answers will vary.

16. Perhaps. These patients were described as having disabling pain (and depended on medication to control it), depression, defenses for coping with developmental delays caused by the disease, death anxiety, and disability.[3] The education/social support group can, however, help them gain self-efficacy with a sense of control over their options, as well as the knowledge and skill base undergirding it. The support group can provide opportunities for modeling those who are coping successfully with this disease and for the emotional support of peers, which can help to ease conflicts between patients and providers.

17. Incontinence Quiz
    a. The agree/degree response provides very limited information about what people know and is easily influenced by guessing.
    b. Develop for yourself a content grid of what people who have incontinence want to know and want to be able to do and what you think they should know and be able to do. What is missing from this test? (In other words, compare the test against a set of learning objectives.) Questions 7 through 9 are not central to my sense of what is important, whereas more detail about what patients know relative to the other questions would be important.
    c. An important question should be: How much knowledge is enough? What is the outcome behavior desired? Enough to get people to treatment if they are incontinent? Without clarity about outcome and formal studies that show that particular test scores predict the outcome, it is very difficult to use the tool clinically.

18. (1) c, (2) b, (3) a, (4) b, (5) a, (6) c, (7) T, (8) T

C Meta-analyses and Other Research Reviews

A number of articles summarize research on patient education. Many of these have been cited throughout the text. In the field of research summarization a series of techniques, called *meta-analysis,* is now being used. These techniques select studies and extract findings by means of a rigorous procedure. The findings are summarized across studies statistically. The goal of the procedure is to decrease the subjectivity that can be involved in traditional methods of summarization by narrative or by counting studies in which the experimental treatment does or does not show a positive effect. Increasing numbers of reviews available for patient education use meta-analysis.

Anderson KO, Masur FT III: Psychological preparation for invasive medical and dental procedures, *J Behav Med* 6:1-40, 1983.

Psychologic preparation for invasive medical and dental procedures has been based on the rationale that high levels of preprocedural fear are detrimental to patients' later adaptation. However, what constitutes an adaptive level of preprocedural concern has yet to be established. Outcome studies have employed informative, psychotherapeutic, modeling, behavioral, cognitive-behavioral, and hypnotic techniques. The research, although frequently flawed, suggests that each of these approaches can be effective.

Bates TA, Broome M: Preparation of children for hospitalization and surgery: a review of the literature, *J Pediatr Nurs* 1:230-239, 1986.

The three most commonly reported hospital and surgery preparation methods for children are hospital tours, play therapy, and filmed modeling. The research on preparation reveals that younger children tend to benefit from programs using play therapy, dolls, and puppets, whereas older children will benefit from verbal explanations, diagrams, and audiovisual aids. The school-aged child can be prepared several days in advance, but preschool children benefit from preparation closer to the actual event. For children with previous hospital experience, information formats with built-in coping procedures will be more beneficial in decreasing anxiety. Health care providers should allow children and parents the freedom to verbalize fears, anxieties, and questions.

Bernard-Bonnin AC and others: Self-management teaching programs and morbidity of pediatric asthma: a meta-analysis, *J Allergy Clin Immunol* 95:34-41, 1995.

This meta-analysis, which summarizes 11 studies published between 1970 and 1991, found that self-management teaching programs do not seem to reduce morbidity.

Broom ME, Lillis PP, Smith MC: Pain interventions with children: a meta-analysis of research, *Nurs Res* 38:154-158, 1989.

A combination of cognitive and affective pain management interventions was reported in more than 40% of the studies, and 70% of interventions were introduced immediately before the painful event. The pain management programs resulted in at least a 30% reduction in children's distress responses.

Brown SA: Studies of educational interventions and outcomes in diabetic adults: a meta-analysis revisited, *Patient Educ Counsel* 16:189-215, 1990.

This study expanded a 1988 summary of research on effectiveness of diabetes education. Results indicate that patients who receive diabetes patient education experience improved knowledge, self-care behaviors, metabolic outcomes, and psychologic outcomes.

Brown SA: Meta-analysis of diabetes patient education research: variations in intervention effects across studies, *Res Nurs Health* 15:409-419, 1992.

Reanalysis of 73 studies from previously reported meta-analyses of diabetes patient education literature found that patient education appeared to be more effective in younger patients. For all patients, glycosylated hemoglobin levels improved between 1 and 6 months postintervention but decreased to 1-month levels after 6 months. Length of the educational intervention did not appear to influence outcomes.

Devine EC, Cook TD: A meta-analytic analysis of effects of psychoeducational interventions on length of post-surgical hospital stay, *Nurs Res* 32:267-274, 1983.

Forty-nine studies of the relationships between brief psychoeducational interventions and the length of post-surgical hospitalization were reviewed. The interventions were often multidimensional and included providing the patient with information about procedures, pain, and sensations to expect; skills training or teaching the patient exercises to promote recovery by preventing complications or reducing anxiety; and psychosocial support by a health care provider who prepared interactions to reduce the patient's anxiety or enhance his or her ability to cope with hospitalization. Results showed that interventions reduced hospital stay by about 1¼ days and had an effect size of 0.38 standard deviation units (up to 0.3 standard deviation is small, 0.3-0.5 is moderately large, and over 0.5 is large.)

Devine ED, Cook TD: Clinical and cost-saving effects of psychoeducational interventions with surgical patients: a meta-analysis, *Res Nurs Health* 9:89-105, 1986.

A meta-analysis of 102 studies was conducted to examine how psychoeducational interventions influenced recovery, pain, psychologic well-being, and satisfaction with care among hospitalized adult surgery patients. Statistically reliable and positive effects were reported on each of these four classes of outcome. The average duration of treatments included in the meta-analysis was 42 minutes. The average effect size across all measures of recovery was 0.50, which means that these interventions reliably facilitate the recovery of surgical patients.

Devine EC: Effects of psychoeducational care for adult surgical patients: a meta-analysis of 191 studies, *Patient Educ Counsel* 19:129-142, 1992.

This is a quantitative review of 191 studies, issued between 1963 and 1989, of the effects of psychoeducational care on adult surgical patients. Statistically reliable, small-to-moderate sized beneficial effects were found on recovery, postoperative pain, and psychologic distress.

Glanz K: Compliance with dietary regimens: its magnitude, measurement and determinants, *Prev Med* 9:787-804, 1980.

Studies of patient compliance with dietary regimens for cardiovascular disease risk reduction, weight reduction, renal disease, diabetes, and other conditions were reviewed. Patient noncompliance with dietary regimens was found to be at least as frequent as noncompliance with medication regimens. Health professionals might increase their effectiveness by recognizing that nonhealth motivations may lead individuals to take appropriate actions and that social and familial influences may affect patients' willingness, desire, and ability to adhere to diets.

Glanz K: Nutrition education for risk-factor reduction and patient education: a review, *Prev Med* 14:721-725, 1985.

Studies of adult nutrition education and counseling for weight reduction, diabetes, cancer, low-fat diets, sodium-restricted diets, and renal diets were also reviewed. These studies draw on a variety of theories from communications, anthropology, education, sociology, and psychology, although before the last 15 to 20 years nutrition education was usually thought of as informational or persuasive. A wide gap exists between the development of behavioral science strategies for nutrition education and the testing of these strategies in practice. On the basis of this review, several basic educational principles for patient nutrition education should be considered in the design of all educational efforts: tailoring of both dietary regimens and educational strategies, use of social support within and outside of the health care setting, provision of skills training in addition to information, effective patient-provider communication, and attention to follow-up, monitoring, and reinforcement.

Glanz K: Patient and public education for cholesterol reduction: a review of strategies and issues, *Patient Educ Counsel* 12:235-257, 1988.

Current knowledge regarding patient and public education for cholesterol reduction lags behind the epidemiologic and clinical evidence that forms the basis for controlling blood cholesterol levels.

Greenland P, Chu JS: Efficacy of cardiac rehabilitation services with emphasis on patients after myocardial infarction, *Ann Intern Med* 109:650-663, 1988.

Cardiac rehabilitation programs commonly offer education about the heart, causes of myocardial infarction, cardiac risk factors, and other general teaching designed to reassure patients with cardiac disease by making them more knowledgeable about their heart conditions. The evidence that teaching or counseling, or both, are helpful in cardiac programs after infarction is not conclusive.

Hansel NK: Review of oral hygiene patient education, *Patient Educ Counsel* 5:89-93, 1983.

Most attempts to improve oral hygiene practices have relied heavily on instructional approaches of the lecture-demonstration type or on such strategies combined with practice sessions in brushing and flossing. Frequently, behavior change may persist for only a short time after the preventive program ends.

Hathaway D: Effect of preoperative instruction on postoperative outcomes: a meta-analysis, *Nurs Res* 35:269-275, 1986.

A meta-analysis was performed on 68 studies of traditional preoperative instruction, using both physiologic and psychologic dependent variables. An average effect size of 0.44 was found. This result was not dissimilar to the findings of other analyses on these kinds of preoperative interventions.

Hirano PC, Laurent DD, Lorig K: Arthritis patient education studies, 1987-1991: a review of the literature, *Patient Educ Counsel* 24:9-54, 1994.

Clinical studies have shown that medical care, including the use of medications, can offer a 20% to 50% improvement in reported arthritis symptoms. Data from patient education studies suggest that a further improvement of 15% to 30% is attainable through patient education interventions.

Hunsberger M, Love B, Byrne C: A review of current approaches used to help children and parents cope with health care procedures, *Matern Child Nurs J* 13:145-165, 1984.

Programs that prepare children for hospitalization are designed to inform the child about what will happen and to familiarize the child with the hospital environment. Even though the reason that information is beneficial is unclear, benefits have been demonstrated. Information about health care procedures was provided through modeling, procedural and sensory information, and stress-point nursing. The research findings tended to oppose the notions that young children should not receive information, that all children benefit equally from the same type and timing of preparation, that a child who has had a previous experience requires less preparation, and that a one-time preadmission program provides adequate preparation. Techniques that assist the child in gaining a sense of control suggest that children can benefit from being helped to gain a sense of mastery over a stressful event. Progressive muscle relaxation and desensitization have been shown to reduce anxiety and discomfort during health care procedures.

Janz NK, Becker MH, Hartman PE: Contingency contracting to enhance patient compliance: a review, *Patient Educ Counsel* 5:165-178, 1983.

The contingency contract is a specific negotiated agreement that provides for the delivery of positive consequences or reinforcers contingent on desirable behavior. It has its theoretic roots in operant conditioning. The 15 studies reviewed demonstrated at least short-term positive effects from contingency contracting across a variety of medical conditions and health-related behaviors. Most of the studies were conducted with motivated volunteers rather than with random samples of some defined population.

Janz NK and others: Interventions to enhance breast self-examination: a review, *Pub Health Rev* 17:89-169, 1989/90.

Intensive interventions result in better outcomes. The provisions of information seem sufficient to obtain breast self-examination (BSE) initiation but not necessarily adequate to maintain practice or to establish proficiency. The addition of skills training and corrective feedback leads to significantly improved BSE proficiency. Prompts and reminder aids seem also to contribute to long-term frequency.

Jones LC: A meta-analytic study of the effects of childbirth education on the parent-infant relationship, *Health Care Women Int* 7:357-370, 1986.

Twenty-seven studies of the effect of childbirth education on knowledge, behavior, or attitude in the parent-infant relationship (completed from 1960-

1981) were analyzed. Average effect size was 0.38 (equivalent to a correlation of 0.20) even though the major focus of these childbirth classes was on helping women cope with labor and delivery with few medications and minimum pain. Compared with parents who did not take childbirth education, parents participating in it were more attentive and responsive to their infants, were more satisfied with the behavior of the infants, reported fewer feeding problems, had more positive feelings and attitudes toward their infants, and spent more time playing with and cuddling their infants. Few negative effects of childbirth education were found. Larger effect sizes were obtained for middle-income parents (0.40) as compared with parents of low income (0.16). Flaws in the research included the researchers' acknowledging allegiance to childbirth education, conducting the research while knowledgeable of the composition of the groups or while teaching the classes, or using instruments that could be easily controlled by the investigator.

Kirscht JP: Preventive health behavior: a review of research and issues, *Health Psychol* 2:277-301, 1983.

Preventive behavior is any behavior that people engage in spontaneously or can be induced to perform with the intention of alleviating the impact of potential risks and hazards in their environment. Sociocultural perspectives and cognitive and behavioral models were used to explain the behavior, with each point of view having its own intervention strategies.

Kottke TE and others: Attributes of successful smoking cessation interventions in medical practice: a meta-analysis of 39 controlled trials, *JAMA* 259:2883-2889, 1988.

Group and individual sessions combined were better than either alone. Success was the product of personalized smoking cessation advice and assistance repeated in different forms by several sources over the longest feasible period. It is reinforcement—the number of contacts and the number of people making them—that produces results. Withdrawing reinforcement contributes to relapse.

Levy SR, Iverson BK, Walberg HJ: Adolescent pregnancy programs and educational interventions: a research synthesis and review, *J Soc Health* 3:99-103, 1983.

Research from 1970-1980 contained in studies of educational programs designed for the adolescent par-

ent in diverse settings such as schools, communities, hospitals, and clinics was synthesized. Examples of topics emphasized in these various settings include family life, parenting, birth defects, nutrition, and prenatal care. The mean overall effect size was 0.35 standard deviation units. (An effect size contrasts the average performance of a treatment group with that of another treatment or control group.) The programs being evaluated were not being compared with true control groups, which receive no treatment. They were being compared with different groups of clients who receive some services similar to those of the target program; therefore the effect size can be considered both statistically significant and an advantageous result of educational programs. Interestingly, the effect size for reducing or delaying repeat pregnancies was only 0.177.

Lindeman CA: Patient education, *Rev Nurs Res* 6:29-60, 1988.

Patient-education influences learning, with the greatest impact on knowledge and skills. Most teaching strategies, such as booklet, programmed instruction, modeling, and lecture-discussion, are effective. Group teaching is as effective as individual teaching. The organizational structure of the hospital is less important than the value the staff and administration attaches to patient-teaching. The effectiveness of patient education as a nursing intervention is clearly established.

Lipsey MW, Wilson DB: The efficacy of psychological, educational and behavioral treatment; confirmation from meta-analysis, *Am Psychol* 48:1181-1209, 1993.

This study examined large bodies of meta-analyses of treatment research, many focused on mental health but including some on patient education. It is most useful as a reference work.

Lorig K, Konkol L, Gonzalez V: Arthritis patient education: a review of the literature, *Patient Educ Counsel* 10:207-252, 1987.

Patient education can influence a variety of arthritis-related behaviors, such as exercise, relaxation, and joint protection. With patient education, 61% of health status measures of pain, disability, count of painful joints, depression, and quality of life demonstrated improvement. The effect of arthritis patient education is potentially similar to that of other standard arthritis treatment, such as nonsteroid anti-inflammatory drugs (NSAIDs).

Mazzuca SA: Does patient education in chronic disease have therapeutic value? *J Chron Dis* 35:521-529, 1982.

From a pool of 320 articles on patient education, 30 were found that documented controlled experiments in chronic disease. These experiments had dependent variables that included (1) compliance with a therapeutic regimen, (2) physiologic progress of patients, or (3) long-range health outcomes. Diseases in the sample included hypertension (10), other heart disease (5), asthma and obesity (3 each), and others.

A summary of all experimental effects shows that patient education was most successful in altering compliance (average improvement = 0.67 standard deviation over control) but was also statistically significant in improving physiologic progress (0.49 standard deviation) and health outcomes (0.20 standard deviation).

Studies were divided according to those in which (1) the emphasis was didactic, having a standard presentation to all subjects, with information transfer accomplished by numerous vehicles, or (2) the emphasis was behavioral, focusing on the patient's own regimen and daily routine as the content of instruction, with attempts made to affect the patient's home or work environment in ways that promoted effective self-management, use of social support, medication monitoring, and telephone follow-up.

Behaviorally oriented programs were found to be consistently more successful in improving the clinical course of chronic disease.

McCain NL, Lynn MR: Meta-analysis of a narrative review: studies evaluating patient teaching, *West J Nurs Res* 12:347-358, 1990.

This meta-analysis summarized studies previously summarized in narrative reviews and found a clear benefit of patient teaching. The score of the average individual in the experimental group exceeded that of 69% of the individuals in the control group.

Meyer TJ, Mark MM: Effects of psychosocial interventions with adult cancer patients: a meta-analysis of randomized experiments, *Health Psychol* 14:101-108, 1995.

This study summarizes results of 45 studies of psychosocial interventions intended to improve the qual-

ity of life of adult cancer patients. The analysis found an effect size of 0.24 for emotional adjustment, 0.19 for functional adjustment, and 0.26 for treatment and disease-related symptoms. These are moderate effect sizes.

Mullen PD: Health promotion and patient education benefits for employees, *Annu Rev Public Health* 9:305-332, 1988.

For reducing risk of disease and promoting well-being, group programs at the worksite or those contracted by the employer in the community can be moderately effective in changing behavior for some groups of employees. For increasing competence in self-care of minor complaints, several rigorous studies suggest that providing materials and support to guide and encourage self-care for common complaints can safely reduce outpatient visits. Education is an important component of programs to substitute home care for hospital and outpatient care. Currently, however, a patient cannot rely on usual providers of medical care to offer adequate education.

Mullen PD, Green LW, Persinger GS: Clinical trials of patient-education for chronic conditions: a comparative meta-analysis of intervention types, *Prev Med* 14:753-781, 1985.

The findings of 70 published evaluations of education programs for people with long-term health problems and regimens that include drugs were synthesized. The overall effect size was 0.37, indicating a substantially decreased number of drug errors. Effect size for decreased drug errors for one-to-one counseling was 0.43; for group education, 0.34; for written or other audiovisual materials except patient package inserts (PPIs), 0.43; for PPIs, 0.01 (almost no effect on increasing patients' knowledge); for counseling or group plus materials, 0.44; for labels, special containers, or memory aids, 0.42; for behavior modification and self-administration, 0.50. The higher the educational quality of an intervention in terms of relevance, individualization, feedback, reinforcement, and so on, the larger the effect size value for decreased drug errors.

Mullen PD, Mains DA, Velez R: A meta-analysis of controlled trials of cardiac education, *Patient Educ Counsel* 9:143-162, 1992.

Twenty-eight controlled studies of cardiac patient education programs showed an average effect size of 0.51 for blood pressure and 0.24 for mortality.

Mullen PD, Ramirez G, Groff JY: A meta-analysis of randomized trials of prenatal smoking cessation interventions, *Am J Obstet Gynecol* 171:1328-1334, 1994.

Most of the programs included individual counseling sessions of no more than 10 minutes; all used material specifically directed to pregnancy rather than to a general audience. More intensive interventions with multiple contacts, multiple formats, and some form of follow-up reaped a larger effect.

Mullen PD and others: Efficacy of psychoeducational interventions on pain, depression, and disability in people with arthritis: a meta-analysis, *J Rheumatol* (suppl 15)14:33-39, 1987.

Summary of 15 studies of the effects of psychoeducational interventions in individuals with arthritis showed moderate effect sizes of 0.2 for pain, 0.27 for depression, and 0.13 for disability.

Mumford E, Schlesinger HJ, Glass GV: The effects of psychological intervention on recovery from surgery and heart attacks: an analysis of the literature, *Am J Public Health* 72:141-151, 1982.

Thirty-four controlled experimental studies were reviewed. On the average, surgical or coronary patients, who were provided information or emotional support to help them master the medical crisis, did better than patients who received only ordinary care. The effect size was 0.50 standard deviation, consistent across studies. A combination of both approaches seems clearly superior to either alone.

A review of 13 studies that used hospital days after surgery or after heart attack as outcome indicators showed that, on the average, psychologic intervention reduced hospitalization approximately 2 days below the control group's average of 9.92 days.

Most of the interventions were modest, and in most studies they were not matched in any way to the needs or coping styles of particular patients. Beyond the intrinsic value of offering humane and considerate care, the evidence shows that psychologic care can be cost-effective.

Nunes EV, Frank KA, Kornfeld DS: Psychologic treatment for the type A behavior pattern and for coronary heart disease: a meta-analysis of the literature, *Psychosom Med* 48:159-173, 1987.

The type A behavior pattern (TABP) is a recognized risk factor for coronary heart disease; yet treatments aimed at its modification are not widely used. Eighteen controlled studies of the psychologic treatment of TABP found an effect size of 0.61. Treatment modalities include education about coronary heart disease, education about TABP, relaxation training, cognitive therapy, imaging, behavior modification, emotional support, and psychodynamic interpretation. A combination of treatment techniques is most effective.

Padgett D and others: Meta-analysis of the effects of educational and psychosocial interventions on management of diabetes mellitus, *J Clin Epidemiol* 41:1007-1030, 1988.

Diet instruction showed an effect size of 0.68, and social learning and behavior modification interventions, an effect size of 0.57. The weakest effect size was for relaxation training (0.30). Positive effects decreased but were retained at 6- and 12-month follow-up, with the exception of weight loss.

Posavac EJ: Evaluation of patient-education programs: a meta-analysis, *Eval Health Prof* 3:47-62, 1980.

A literature search identified 23 evaluations of patient-education programs that used a randomly selected experimental or quasi-experimental design. The mean effect size was 0.74; for measures of compliance, it was 1.08, and for anxiety, 0.60.

Posavac EJ and others: Increasing compliance to medical treatment regimens: a meta-analysis of program evaluation, *Eval Health Prof* 8:7-22, 1985.

A total of 58 studies evaluating the effectiveness of programs to increase compliance with medical treatment regimens were quantitatively integrated to assess their impact on the behavior of clients. Mean effect size was 0.47. The advantage of the program groups dropped as the amount of life-style changes required by the treatment regimen increased. The most successful interventions involved improving the facility providing care and helping patients to incorporate the treatment regimen into their daily routine. One program using several interventions had the largest impact, and two based on the behavioral principle of rewarding successive approximations of outpatient compliant behavior were very strong as well.

Reading AE: The short-term effects of psychological preparation for surgery, *Soc Sci Med* 13A:641-654, 1979.

Accumulating evidence exists on the short-term effects of psychologic preparation for surgery; however, the way in which these effects are produced is not clear. Worry, information, and coping models have been used. It seems likely that the effects of psychologic preparation will vary according to the nature of the situation as well as the personality of the patient.

Suls J, Wan CK: Effects of sensory and procedural information on coping with stressful medical procedures and pain: a meta-analysis, *J Consult Clin Psychol* 57:372-379, 1989.

Combined sensory-procedural preparation yielded the strongest and most consistent benefits in terms of reducing negative affect, pain reports, and other-rated distress. Procedural details provide a map of specific events, whereas sensory information facilitates their interpretation as nonthreatening.

Theis SL, Johnson JH: Strategies for teaching patients: a meta-analysis, *Clin Nurse Spec* 9:100-120, 1995.

This meta-analysis synthesized the body of research examining teaching strategies used in patient education—a total of 72 studies. The mean effect size was a moderate 0.41, indicating that 66% of subjects receiving planned teaching had better outcomes than did control group subjects receiving routine care. Structure yielded the highest effect size, with reinforcement, independent study, and use of multiple strategies also above the study mean.

Thompson RH: Where we stand: twenty years of research on pediatric hospitalization and health care, *Child Health Care* 14:200-210, 1986.

More than 300 research reports appearing since 1965 were summarized. This literature encompassed children's responses to hospitalization and health care, the effects of separation and parental rooming-in, parental responses to hospitalization, the hospital environment, play, and preparation for hospitalization.

Turley MA: A meta-analysis of informing mothers concerning the sensory and perceptual capabilities of their infants: the effects on maternal-infant interaction, *Matern Child Nurs J* 14:183-197, 1985.

Twenty research studies conducted between 1970 and 1981 were analyzed. These studies investigated the effects of providing information to mothers concerning the sensory and perceptual capabilities of their newborns and the effects this treatment had on maternal-infant interaction. The overall effect size in terms of maternal-infant interaction was significantly increased by the intervention. The fourth week after discharge was shown to be the most effective time to present the information.

Vallejo BC: Is structured presurgical education more effective than nonstructured education? *Patient Educ Counsel* 9:283-290, 1987.

None of the literature synthesis techniques showed that structured presurgical education was more effective than unstructured education in promoting compliance with the postsurgical therapeutic regimen.

D Patient Education: Rights, Standards, Guidelines, Accreditation, and Organizational Statements

A PATIENT'S BILL OF RIGHTS

Introduction

Effective health care requires collaboration between patients and physicians and other health care professionals. Open and honest communication, respect for personal and professional values, and sensitivity to differences are integral to optimal patient care. As the setting for the provision of health services, hospitals must provide a foundation for understanding and respecting the rights and responsibilities of patients, their families, physicians, and other caregivers. Hospitals must ensure a health care ethic that respects the role of patients in decision making about treatment choices and other aspects of their care. Hospitals must be sensitive to cultural, racial, linguistic, religious, age, gender, and other differences as well as the needs of persons with disabilities.

The American Hospital Association presents *A Patient's Bill of Rights* with the expectation that it will contribute to more effective patient care and be supported by the hospital on behalf of the institution, its medical staff, employees, and patients. The American Hospital Association encourages health care institutions to tailor this bill of rights to their patient community by translating and/or simplifying the language of this bill of rights as may be necessary to ensure that patients and their families understand their rights and responsibilities.

Bill of Rights*

1. The patient has the right to considerate and respectful care.
2. The patient has the right to and is encouraged to obtain from physicians and other direct caregivers relevant, current, and understandable information concerning diagnosis, treatment, and prognosis.

Except in emergencies when the patient lacks decision-making capacity and the need for treatment is urgent, the patient is entitled to the opportunity to discuss and request information related to the specific procedures and/or treatments, the risks involved, the possible length of recuperation, and the medically reasonable alternatives and their accompanying risks and benefits.

Patients have the right to know the identity of physicians, nurses, and others involved in their care, as well as when those involved are students, residents, or other trainees. The patient also has the right to know the immediate and long-term financial implications of treatment choices, insofar as they are known.

3. The patient has the right to make decisions about the plan of care prior to and during the course of treatment and to refuse a recommended treatment or plan of care to the extent permitted by law and hospital policy and to be informed of the medical consequences of this action. In case of such refusal, the patient is entitled to other appropriate care and services that the hospital provides or transfer to another hospital. The hospital should notify patients of any policy that might affect patient choice within the institution.

4. The patient has the right to have an advance directive (such as a living will, health care proxy, or durable power of attorney for health care) concerning treatment or designating a surrogate decision maker with the expectation that the hospi-

tal will honor the intent of that directive to the extent permitted by law and hospital policy.

Health care institutions must advise patients of their rights under state law and hospital policy to make informed medical choices, ask if the patient has an advance directive, and include that information in patient records. The patient has the right to timely information about hospital policy that may limit its ability to implement fully a legally valid advance directive.

5. The patient has the right to every consideration of privacy. Case discussion, consultation, examination, and treatment should be conducted so as to protect each patient's privacy.

6. The patient has the right to expect that all communications and records pertaining to his/her care will be treated as confidential by the hospital, except in cases such as suspected abuse and public health hazards when reporting is permitted or required by law. The patient has the right to expect that the hospital will emphasize the confidentiality of this information when it releases it to any other parties entitled to review information in these records.

7. The patient has the right to review the records pertaining to his/her medical care and to have the information explained or interpreted as necessary, except when restricted by law.

8. The patient has the right to expect that, within its capacity and policies, a hospital will make reasonable response to the request of a patient for appropriate and medically indicated care and services. The hospital must provide evaluation, service, and/or referral as indicated by the urgency of the case. When medically appropriate and legally permissible, or when a patient has so requested, a patient may be transferred to another facility. The institution to which the patient is to be transferred must first have accepted the patient for transfer. The patient must also have the benefit of complete information and explanation concerning the need for, risks, benefits, and alternatives to such a transfer.

9. The patient has the right to ask and be informed of the existence of business relationships among the hospital, educational institutions, other health care providers, or payers that may influence the patient's treatment and care.

10. The patient has the right to consent to or decline to participate in proposed research studies or hu-

man experimentation affecting care and treatment or requiring direct patient involvement, and to have those studies fully explained prior to consent. A patient who declines to participate in research or experimentation is entitled to the most effective care that the hospital can otherwise provide.

11. The patient has the right to expect reasonable continuity of care when appropriate and to be informed by physicians and other caregivers of available and realistic patient care options when hospital care is no longer appropriate.

12. The patient has the right to be informed of hospital policies and practices that relate to patient care, treatment, and responsibilities. The patient has the right to be informed of available resources for resolving disputes, grievances, and conflicts, such as ethics committees, patient representatives, or other mechanisms available in the institution. The patient has the right to be informed of the hospital's charges for services and available payment methods.

The collaborative nature of health care requires that patients, or their families/surrogates, participate in their care. The effectiveness of care and patient satisfaction with the course of treatment depend, in part, on the patient fulfilling certain responsibilities. Patients are responsible for providing information about past illnesses, hospitalizations, medications, and other matters related to health status. To participate effectively in decision making, patients must be encouraged to take responsibility for requesting additional information or clarification about their health status or treatment when they do not fully understand information and instructions. Patients are also responsible for ensuring that the health care institution has a copy of their written advance directive if they have one. Patients are responsible for informing their physicians and other caregivers if they anticipate problems in following prescribed treatment.

Patients should also be aware of the hospital's obligation to be reasonably efficient and equitable in providing care to other patients and the community. The hospital's rules and regulations are designed to help the hospital meet this obligation. Patients and their families are responsible for making reasonable accommodations to the needs of the hospital, other patients, medical staff, and hospital employees. Patients are responsible for providing necessary information for insurance claims and for working with the hospital to make payment arrangements, when necessary.

A person's health depends on much more than health care services. Patients are responsible for recognizing the impact of their life-style on their personal health.

Conclusion

Hospitals have many functions to perform, including the enhancement of health status, health promotion, and the prevention and treatment of injury and disease; the immediate and ongoing care and rehabilitation of patients; the education of health professionals, patients, and the community; and research. All these activities must be conducted with an overriding concern for the values and dignity of patients.

NATIONAL STANDARDS FOR DIABETES SELF-MANAGEMENT EDUCATION PROGRAMS*

In 1993, the National Diabetes Advisory Board charged The American Diabetes Association to coordinate a task force of representatives of diabetes and other organizations to review, and revise if indicated, the National Standards for Diabetes Patient Education Programs. The task force consisted of representatives from the following organizations: the American Association of Diabetes Educators, the American Diabetes Association, the American Dietetic Association, the Centers for Disease Control and Prevention, the Department of Defense, the Department of Veterans Affairs, the Diabetes Research and Training Centers, the Indian Health Service, and the Juvenile Diabetes Foundation. The task force decided to revise the standards to reflect recent research and current health care trends. Thus, the standards were revised and are now termed the National Standards for Diabetes Self-Management Education Programs. These revised standards have been endorsed by the organizations involved in their development.

Introduction

Diabetes mellitus is a chronic metabolic disorder. Individuals affected by diabetes must learn self-management skills and make lifestyle changes to effectively manage diabetes and to avoid or delay the complications associated with this disorder. For these reasons, self-management education is the cornerstone of treat-

*From Task Force to Revise the National Standards: *Diabetes Educ* 21(3):189-193, 1995. Approved August 1994. For a technical review on this subject, see *Diabetes Care* 21:18, 1995.

ment for all people with diabetes. These National Standards, which were developed in collaboration with diabetes organizations, will provide guidance for the establishment and maintenance of quality diabetes self-management education programs.

The term "patient education" traditionally has been used to describe the process of teaching people with chronic diseases, such as diabetes, to take care of their disorders. However, over time, this designation has changed to "self-management training" and "self-management education" as well as patient education. This article will use the term self-management education to refer to the process of teaching individuals to manage their diabetes.

These standards provide:
1. Diabetes educators with the means to:
   - develop quality self-management education programs.
   - assess the quality of their education programs.
   - identify areas in their programs where changes and improvements are needed.
2. People with diabetes with the means to:
   - assess the quality of the diabetes-related services they receive.
   - gain an understanding of the skills needed for self-management.
3. Referral sources, insurers, employers, government agencies, and the general public with:
   - a description of quality self-management education services for people with diabetes.
   - an awareness of the importance of comprehensive self-management education to enable people with diabetes to effectively manage this disorder.

Quality diabetes self-management education programs can be measured in terms of structure, process, and outcomes. Each of these program components include one or more elements with specific standards. The broad outline of these standards is as follows:

Structure
- Organization
- Needs assessment
- Program management
- Program staff
- Curriculum
- Participant access

Process
- Assessment
- Plan and implementation
- Follow-up

Outcomes
- Program outcome evaluation
- Participant outcome evaluation

Structure

The structure necessary to provide quality diabetes self-management education consists of the human and material resources and the management systems needed to achieve program and participant goals. Such structure includes the support and commitment of the organization that is sponsoring the program, the program administration and management systems, the qualifications and diversity of the personnel involved in the program, the curriculum and instructional methods and materials, and the accessibility of the program.

Organization. The sponsoring organization must provide the support and structure within which the program functions. Organizational commitment to self-management education, including operational support, adequate space, personnel, budget, and materials, must be clearly evident. Because multiple health care professionals from a variety of disciplines are involved in diabetes care, clear lines of authority and efficient communication systems should be established.

Standard 1. The sponsoring organization shall have a written policy that affirms education as an integral component of diabetes care.

Standard 2. The sponsoring organization shall identify and provide the educational resources required to achieve its educational objectives in terms of its target population. These resources include adequate space, personnel, budget, and instructional materials.

Standard 3. The organizational relationships, lines of authority, staffing, job descriptions, and operational policies shall be clearly defined and documented.

Needs assessment. A successful program is based on the needs of the population that the program is intended to serve. Because diabetes populations vary, each organization should assess its service area and match resources to the needs of the defined target population. Needs assessments should guide program planning and management. Periodic reassessment should be done to allow the program to adapt to changing needs.

Standard 4. The service area shall be assessed to define the target population and determine appro-

priate allocation of personnel and resources to serve the educational needs of the target population.

Program management. Effective management is essential to implement and maintain a successful program and to ensure that resources are adequate for the defined tasks. To ensure that management policies and program design reflect broad perspectives relevant to diabetes, the organization should designate a standing advisory committee that includes health care professionals and people with diabetes to assist staff with program planning and review. Involvement and support from the medical community are also necessary. At times, resources outside the sponsoring institution may be required to enable individuals affected by diabetes to maximize their health outcomes.

Standard 5. A standing advisory committee consisting of a physician, nurse educator, dietitian, an individual with behavioral science expertise, a consumer, and a community representative, at a minimum, shall be established to oversee the program.

Standard 6. The advisory committee shall participate in the annual planning process, including determination of target audience, program objectives, participant access mechanisms, instructional methods, resource requirements (including space, personnel, budget, and materials), participant follow-up mechanisms, and program evaluation.

Standard 7. Professional program staff shall have sufficient time and resources for lesson planning, instruction, documentation, evaluation, and follow-up.

Standard 8. Community resources shall be assessed periodically.

Program staff. Qualified personnel are essential to the success of a diabetes self-management education program. The sponsoring organization should identify the program personnel, which must include a program coordinator who has overall responsibility for the program. Because diabetes is a chronic disorder requiring lifestyle changes, instructors need to be skilled and experienced health care professionals with recent education in diabetes, educational principles, and behavior change strategies.

Standard 9. A coordinator shall be designated who is responsible for program planning, implementation, and evaluation.

Standard 10. Health care professionals with recent didactic and experimental preparation in diabetes clinical and educational issues shall serve as the program instructors. The staff will include at least a nurse educator and a dietitian who collaborate routinely. Certification as a diabetes educator by the National Certification Board of Diabetes Educators is recommended.

Standard 11. Professional program staff shall obtain education about diabetes, educational principles, and behavior change strategies on a continuing basis.

Curriculum. A quality diabetes self-management education program should provide comprehensive instruction in the content areas relevant to the target population and to the participants being served. The curriculum, instructional methods, and materials should be appropriate for the specified target population, considering type and duration of diabetes, age, cultural influences, and individual learning abilities.

Standard 12. Based on the needs of the target population, the program shall be capable of offering instruction in the following content areas:

a. Diabetes overview
b. Stress and psychosocial adjustment
c. Family involvement and social support
d. Nutrition
e. Exercise and activity
f. Medications
g. Monitoring and use of results
h. Relationships among nutrition, exercise, medication, and blood glucose levels
i. Prevention, detection, and treatment of acute complications
j. Prevention, detection, and treatment of chronic complications
k. Foot, skin, and dental care
l. Behavior change strategies, goal setting, risk factor reduction, and problem solving
m. Benefits, risks, and management options for improving glucose control
n. Preconception care, pregnancy, and gestational diabetes
o. Use of health care systems and community resources

Standard 13. The program shall use instructional methods and materials that are appropriate for the target population and the participants being served.

Participant access. Quality programs must be readily accessible to those in need of education. The sponsoring organization should facilitate access to self-management education in the target population identified in the needs assessment. Access is promoted by a commitment to routinely inform referral sources and the target population of the availability and benefits of the program.

Standard 14. A system shall be in place to inform the target population and potential referral sources of the availability and benefits of the program.

Standard 15. The program shall be conveniently and regularly available.

Standard 16. The program shall be responsive to requests for information and to referrals from consumers, health care professionals, and health care agencies.

Process

Process refers to the methods or means by which resources are used to attain stated goals. The process of providing diabetes self-management education involves the integration of an individual assessment, goal setting, education plan development, implementation, evaluation, and follow-up. Each component requires documentation that can be evaluated.

Assessment. Because individuals are unique, their educational needs will vary with age, disease processes, culture, and lifestyles. Effective instruction can only be accomplished by a collaborative effort between educators and participants to identify individualized educational needs.

Standard 17. An individualized assessment shall be developed and updated in collaboration with each participant. The assessment will include relevant medical history, present health status, health service or resource utilization, risk factors, diabetes knowledge and skills, cultural influences, health beliefs and attitudes, health behaviors and goals, support systems, barriers to learning, and socioeconomic factors.

Plan and implementation. For the educational experience to meet the participant's needs, an individual assessment should be used to develop the education plan. All information about the educational experience should be documented in the participant's permanent medical or education record. Because different health care professionals may be involved in the provision of the educational experience, effective communication and coordination are essential.

Standard 18. An individualized education plan, based on the assessment, shall be developed in collaboration with each participant.

Standard 19. The participant's educational experience, including assessment, intervention, evaluation, and follow-up, shall be documented in a permanent medical or education record. There will be documentation of collaboration and coordination among program staff and other providers.

Follow-up. Because diabetes is a chronic disorder requiring a lifetime of self-management, follow-up services will be needed. Participants' lifestyles, knowledge, skills, attitudes, and disease characteristics change over time, so that ongoing education is necessary and appropriate. Programs should be able to offer periodic reassessment and education as part of comprehensive services.

Standard 20. The program shall offer appropriate and timely educational interventions based on periodic reassessments of health status, knowledge, skills, attitudes, goals, and self-care behaviors.

Outcomes

Outcomes are the desired results for the program and participants. For programs, the desired results include achievement of stated objectives, reaching the defined target population, and helping participants improve their health outcomes. For participants, outcomes include the knowledge and skills necessary for self-management, desired self-management behaviors, and improved health outcomes. Assessing outcomes and using the assessments in regular program evaluation and subsequent planning are essential to maintain quality programs.

Program outcome evaluation. The advisory committee should periodically review the program to ascertain that the program continues to meet the National Standards for Diabetes Self-Management Education Programs. The results of this review should be documented and used in subsequent program planning and modification.

Standard 21. The advisory committee shall review program performance annually, including all components of the annual program plan and curriculum, and use the information in subsequent planning and program modification.

Participant Outcome Evaluation

Participants' outcomes, such as success in incorporating self-management into their lifestyles, should be periodically reviewed. The specific outcomes evaluated will vary with the program, but the program's effectiveness in helping participants improve their health outcomes should be documented and used for future program planning and modification.

Standard 22. The advisory committee shall annually review and evaluate predetermined outcomes for program participants.

SCOPE OF PRACTICE FOR DIABETES EDUCATORS*

Purpose

The American Association of Diabetes Educators developed this Scope of Practice to delineate: (1) selected beliefs and definitions related to the practice of diabetes education, and (2) the dimensions of this practice in relation to other components of care for persons with diabetes, their families, and appropriate support systems. This Scope of Practice describes the present practice of diabetes education by multidisciplinary health care professionals.

Beliefs and definitions

Living well with diabetes requires a positive psychosocial adaptation to, and the effective self-management of, the disease. To achieve effective self-management of diabetes mellitus, a patient must learn the body of knowledge, attitudes, and self-management skills related to the control of this chronic disease. *Diabetes education* is defined as the teaching and the learning of this body of knowledge and skills, with the ultimate goal being to promote the behavior changes necessary for optimal health outcomes, psychosocial adaptation, and quality of life. This planned educational experience is most effectively provided by qualified diabetes educators. Diabetes education is considered a therapeutic modality, and it is integral to the care of these patients.

A *diabetes educator* is defined as a health care professional who has mastered the core of knowledge and skill in the biological and social sciences, communication and counseling, and education, and who has experience in the care of patients with diabetes. The role of the diabetes educator can be assumed by various health care professionals, including but not limited to: registered

---

*From American Association of Diabetes Educators: *Diabetes Educ* 18:52-56, 1992.

dietitians, registered nurses, physicians, pharmacists, social workers, podiatrists, and exercise physiologists. A goal for all diabetes educators should be to meet the academic, professional, and experiential requirements to become a certified diabetes educator (CDE).

Dimensions of practice

The role of the diabetes educator is multidimensional, with boundaries for accountability that interface with other members of the health care team. This role involves the education of patients, their families, and appropriate support systems, as well as other health care professionals who do not specialize in diabetes management, and the public. While a multidisciplinary team approach is the preferred delivery system for diabetes education, this specialty practice can occur successfully in a wide variety of settings and formats.

The primary area of responsibility for diabetes educators is the education of patients, their families, and appropriate support systems about diabetes self-management and related issues. The content of this educational experience should include, but not be limited to, the following topics:

- Pathophysiology of diabetes mellitus
- Nutrition management and diet
- Pharmacologic interventions
- Exercise and activity
- Self-monitoring for glycemic control
- Prevention and management of acute and chronic complications
- Psychosocial adjustment
- Problem-solving skills
- Stress management
- Use of the health care delivery system

The diabetes educator should present the necessary information, using established principles of teaching-learning theory and life-style counseling. The instruction is individualized for persons of all ages, incorporating their cultural preferences, health beliefs, and preferred learning styles, when feasible. The diabetes educator should perform the following:

- Assessment of educational needs
- Planning of the teaching-learning process
- Implementation of the educational plan
- Documentation of the process
- Evaluation based on outcome criteria

The Scope of Practice of a diabetes educator *should intersect* with the practice of other members of the health care team. The diabetes educator should appreciate the impact of acute or chronic problems on patients' health behaviors and on the teaching-learning process. Such appreciation is essential for the development of a comprehensive plan for continuing education and cost-effective, managed care.

Members of the various health care professions who practice diabetes education bring their particular focus to the educational process. This phenomenon widens or narrows the Scope of Practice for individual educators, as is appropriate within the boundaries of each health profession, which may be regulated by national or state agencies or accrediting bodies. Other roles for the diabetes educator may involve consultation with other health care providers or agencies and research in diabetes management and education.

Diabetes education occurs in a variety of settings, depending on the needs of the patient, the practice of the educator, and the local environment. Inpatient and outpatient settings, as well as home settings, are used effectively for both individual and group education. Diabetes education should be a planned, individualized, and evaluated activity wherever it occurs.

Summary

This Scope of Practice incorporates definitions of *diabetes educator* and *diabetes education,* while providing statements of beliefs regarding the educational process inherent in this practice. The scope of practice of a diabetes educator has changing dimensions because of the multidisciplinary nature of the health care professionals who provide it. The primary role of a diabetes educator is to provide an educational experience for patients, their families, and appropriate support systems to learn the effective management of diabetes. Thus, the Scope of Practice delineates the multifaceted role and responsibilities of the health care professional who engages in this teaching-learning process. This Scope of Practice does not constitute an exhaustive description of diabetes education as a specialty practice because there are various interpretations of the role of the diabetes educator in a health care team.

STANDARDS OF PRACTICE FOR DIABETES EDUCATORS*

Purpose

This document has been developed by the American Association of Diabetes Educators to: (1) provide

---

*From American Association of Diabetes Educators: *Diabetes Educ* 18:52-56, 1992.

standards for a nationally acceptable level of practice for diabetes educators; and (2) assure quality in the professional practice of diabetes education. The individual diabetes educator is responsible for adhering to these Standards.

The Standards of Practice will provide:
1. Diabetes educators with
   - direction to assess and improve the quality of their practice
   - a framework within which to practice
2. Patients with
   - a means of assessing the quality of diabetes education services provided
   - a basis for forming expectations of the diabetes education experience
3. Health care professionals who do not specialize in diabetes management with a means of
   - understanding the role of the diabetes educator
   - assessing the quality of diabetes education services provided
   - understanding diabetes education as an integral component of diabetes patient care
4. Insurers, government agencies, industry, and the general public with
   - a description of the specialized educational services provided by a diabetes educator
   - information about the benefits of diabetes education in developing self-management skills
   - an awareness of the importance of diabetes education in improving the quality of life for persons with diabetes

Standards of education

Standard I assessment. The diabetes educator should conduct a thorough, individualized needs assessment with the participation of the patient, family, or support systems, when appropriate, prior to the development of the education plan and intervention.

Practice guidelines

The needs assessment should include information from the patient on the following:
1. Health history
2. Medical history
3. Previous use of medication
4. Diet history
5. Current mental health status
6. Use of health care delivery systems
7. Life-style practices such as occupation, vocation, education, financial status, social, cultural, and religious practices
8. Physical and psychological factors including age, mobility, visual acuity, hearing, manual dexterity, alertness, attention span, and ability to concentrate
9. Barriers to learning such as education, literacy levels, perceived learning needs, motivation to learn, and attitudes
10. Family and social supports
11. Previous diabetes education, actual knowledge, and skills

Standard II use of resources. The diabetes educator should strive to create an educational setting conducive to learning, with adequate resources to facilitate the learning process.

Practice guidelines

Appropriate resources for effective teaching should include:
1. A teaching environment that
   a) provides privacy, safety, and accessibility
   b) includes ample teaching and storage space, adequate furniture, lighting, and ventilation
2. A variety of teaching materials and audiovisual teaching aids to meet the individual patient's needs
3. Adequate staffing for the needs of the patient population

Standard III planning. The written educational plan should be developed from information obtained from the needs assessment and based on the components of the educational process: assessment, planning, implementation, and evaluation. The plan is coordinated among diabetes health team members, including the patient with diabetes, family, and support system.

Practice guidelines

The written educational plan should include the following:
1. Goals of the educational intervention
2. Measurable, behaviorally stated learner objectives
3. Content outline
4. Instructional methods, including discussion, demonstration, role playing, simulations
5. Learner outcomes based on the evaluation process

Standard IV implementation. The diabetes educator should provide individualized education based on a progression from basic survival skills to advanced information for daily self-management.

Practice guidelines

Considerations in developing the individualized education plan should include:

1. The need for diabetes education to be lifelong because of the chronicity of the condition
2. The need for a dynamic education plan that will reflect the inevitable changes in life-style
3. Survival skills that include safe practices of medication administration, meal planning, self-monitoring for glycemic control, and recognition of when to access professional assistance for emergencies
4. Advanced information for daily self-management practices that may include prevention and management of chronic complications, problem-solving skills, exercise, psychosocial adjustment, stress management, and travel situations

Standard V documentation. The diabetes educator should completely and accurately document the educational experience.

Practice guidelines

Accurate documentation:

1. Establishes a record to substantiate the provision of education
2. Contributes information for retrospective, concurrent, and prospective reviews
3. Provides data for scientific and economic analysis
4. Serves as a resource for continuity of care
5. Aids in planning subsequent diabetes education

Standard VI evaluation and outcome. The diabetes educator should participate in at least an annual review of the quality and outcome of the education process.

Practice guidelines

Evaluation of the diabetes education process should:

1. Occur periodically and as part of a comprehensive quality assurance program
2. Be consistent with the National Standards for Diabetes Patient Education Programs as established by the National Diabetes Advisory Board
3. Determine the impact of education on patients, institutions, and the community
4. Use outcome measures such as:
   a) cost-effectiveness
   b) changes in use of health care delivery systems (e.g., emergency room visits, hospital length of stay)
   c) changes in knowledge and attitudes
   d) changes in physiological measures (e.g., glycosylated hemoglobin values, weight)

Standards of professional practice

Standard VII multidisciplinary collaboration. The diabetes educator should collaborate with the multidisciplinary team of health care professionals and integrate their knowledge and skills to provide a comprehensive educational experience.

Practice guidelines

The multidisciplinary education team should:

1. Include, but not be limited to, the registered nurse, registered dietitian, physician, pharmacist, social worker, psychologist, exercise physiologist, and podiatrist
2. Observe professional practice boundaries in light of each member's discipline
3. Have a responsibility to:
   a) share with team members information from individual patient assessments
   b) prioritize learning needs
   c) make education relevant to medical management
   d) promote delivery of consistent information from various team members to patients
   e) hold patient management conferences on a regular basis
   f) provide referrals for appropriate follow-up

Standard VIII professional development. The diabetes educator should assume responsibility for professional development and pursue continuing education to acquire current knowledge and skills.

Practice guidelines

The diabetes educator should:

1. Incorporate into practice the generally accepted new techniques and knowledge acquired through continuing education
2. Deliver education based on a continuous process of review and evaluation of scientific theory, clinical and educational research
3. Pursue professional education based on progression from basic through advanced curriculum
4. Strive to meet the academic, professional, and experiential requirements to become a certified diabetes educator (CDE)

Standard IX professional accountability. The diabetes educator should accept responsibility for self-assessment of performance and peer review to assure the delivery of high quality diabetes education.

Practice guidelines

The diabetes educator should:

1. Participate in an annual systematic review and evaluation of practice

2. Incorporate into practice the appropriate changes based on the results of self-evaluation, peer review, and patients' evaluations

Standard X ethics. The diabetes educator should respect and uphold the basic human rights of all persons.

Practice guidelines

The diabetes educator should:

1. Maintain confidentiality of appropriate information, and allow freedom of expression, decision making, and action
2. Demonstrate concern for personal dignity
3. Consider that a person with diabetes balances many daily tasks for management which may require a gradual incorporation into life-style
4. Appreciate the impact of diabetes management on daily living so that reasonable expectations are established with the patient
5. Display honesty, warmth, and openness to reinforce positive behavior change.

Bibliography

American Diabetes Association. Standards of medical care for patients with diabetes mellitus. Diabetes Care 1991; 14(suppl 2):10-13

American Nurses' Association and Association of Rehabilitation Nurses. Standards of rehabilitative nursing practice. Kansas City, Mo: American Nurses' Association, 1986.

Bartlett E. At last a definition of patient education [Editorial]. Patient Educ Couns 1985;7:323-24.

Beebe CA. Self-monitoring of blood glucose: an adjunct to dietary and insulin management of the patient with diabetes. J Am Diet Assoc 1987;87:61-65.

Brookfield SD. Understanding and facilitating adult learning. San Francisco: Jossey-Bass, 1986.

Dunst C, Trivette C, Deal A. Enabling and empowering families: principles and guidelines for practice. Cambridge, Mass: Brookline Books, 1988.

Green LW, Kreuter MW. Health promotion planning: an educational and environmental approach. 2d ed. Mountain View, Calif: Mayfield Publishing Co, 1991.

Guthrie DW, ed. Diabetes education: a core curriculum for health professionals. Chicago: American Association of Diabetes Educators, 1988.

National Coalition for Recognition of Diabetes Patient Education Programs. Self-study and application handbook. Rockville, Md: NACOR, 1986.

Powers MA, ed. Nutrition guide for professionals: diabetes education and meal planning. Alexandria, Va/Chicago: American Diabetes Association/American Dietetic Association, 1987.

Redman BK. The process of patient education. 6th ed. St. Louis: CV Mosby, 1988.

Van Hoozer HL. The teaching process: theory and practice in nursing. East Norwalk, Conn: Appleton and Lange, 1987.

ARTHRITIS AND MUSCULOSKELETAL PATIENT EDUCATION STANDARDS*

I. Introduction

Background. Patient education is a powerful strategy intervention that can improve the lives of persons with rheumatic disease. Most forms of arthritis are chronic in nature and extend over many years. Therefore, along with the routine, ongoing education given by caregivers during individual clinical contacts, the patient needs a formal body of knowledge and skills in order to manage the disease on a day-to-day basis. Effective, efficient management of chronic disease is possible only when patients are knowledgeable participants in decisions about their care and are able to follow through on these decisions.

Patient education is considered an integral part of the treatment of the more than 100 forms of rheumatic disease. More than 75 education programs, reported in the literature, have shown beneficial effects on various aspects of health status, such as functional ability, psychological state, and pain. Furthermore, considerable effort has been made to develop and/or test instruments to evaluate important health outcomes of rheumatic disease care.

This document addresses suggested standards for formal rheumatic disease patient education programs. The purposes of the standards are to: (1) assure the quality of patient education programs, (2) promote the easy access to education for the patient with rheumatic disease, and (3) secure documentation of outcomes of patient education that can be used to improve care.

Definitions. The following terms are defined for use in this document.

1. **Patient Education.** Patient education is planned, organized learning experiences designed to facilitate voluntary adoption of behaviors or beliefs conducive to health. It is a set of planned educational activities that are separate from clinical patient care. The activities of a patient education program must be designed to attain goals the patient has participated in formulating. The primary focus of these activities includes acquisition of information, skills, beliefs

---

*From Burchhardt CS: *Arthritis Care Res* 7:1-4, 1994.

and attitudes which impact on health status, quality of life, and possibly health care utilization.

2. **Program.** A program consists of three parts:
   a. Specific objectives oriented to each individual or group
   b. Content tailored to meet these objectives
   c. Education processes which deliver the content in a manner which enables the patient to achieve the objectives

   A program can be delivered in a variety of ways and in different settings dependent upon the needs of patients and the availability of resources.

3. **Standards.** Standards are written statements that describe the expectations of the quality of a given education program.

4. **Review Criteria.** Review criteria are measurable methods of determining whether the standards have been met.

5. **Provider.** The provider may be an individual practitioner, an organization or an institution. In all cases the provider is responsible for upholding the standards.

6. **Approved Program.** An approved program is one that has been found to meet the rheumatic disease patient education standards as determined by the designated authority.

II. Needs assessment standards

Standard. The numbers and needs of persons with rheumatic disease vary. Therefore, patient education programs must begin with an assessment of the needs of the target population. This includes the patient and his/her family members and significant care providers.

The provider of the patient education program will conduct an educational needs assessment of the target patient population. This assessment will include, but not be limited to, problems caused by the rheumatic disease, skills needed to manage the disease, and current level of knowledge and skills. Preferred language of instruction and reading level will also be assessed, if applicable. Additional need assessments, as appropriate, may be conducted with health care providers, administrators, or family members and significant others.

Review criterion

1. The provider will document how the needs assessment was conducted and the findings of the needs assessment.

III. Planning/management standards

Standard. Planning is a comprehensive process that should involve health professionals and educators as well as persons with rheumatic diseases and members of their families.

In addition, it entails good communication and clearly delineated responsibilities and functions. Communication must occur among program personnel, health care givers, community health agencies, patients, and their family members. A program coordinator with ultimate responsibility and authority for the quality and operation of the program should be designated. The program should be readily accessible to all patients for whom it has been designed.

Review criteria

1. Provider will document the participation of a rheumatologist, one or more other health professionals and patients in the selection or planning of a program.
2. Each provider will designate one person as coordinator. At a minimum, this person will be responsible for coordinating and documenting patient education activities and is responsible for the quality and operation of the program.
3. Information about patient participation in educational programs shall be documented.
4. Information about each patient's participation shall be retained in a patient's record or similar file for at least 5 years. This record will be available for the patient's personal or other consented use.

IV. Curriculum standards

Standard. The program curriculum organizes the content and documents the educational process. It is also expected that the educational program will be reasonably supported by professional consensus and the research literature on arthritis patient education.

The provider periodically assesses the availability of community resources for their potential contribution to rheumatic disease education. In addition, programs should be updated in a timely manner.

Review criteria

1. The program shall have written patient outcome objectives which reflect the findings of the needs assessment(s) and the patients' goals.
2. The program shall offer information and skills in the content areas determined by the needs assessment and patients' goals. These will be doc-

umented by a written curriculum plan which includes content outlines, instructional methods, and instructional materials.

3. Documentation is available to show that curriculum and instructional materials are appropriate for the specified target audience.
4. The curriculum is reviewed and updated as necessary or at least every 5 years.
5. The provider shows evidence of an initial assessment of community resources and repeats the assessment at least every 2 years. The assessment includes the name, address, telephone number and a brief statement of what the particular resource offers.

V. Instructor standards

Qualified personnel are essential to the success of a rheumatic disease education program. Instructors should have recent training and experience in both rheumatic disease and educational principles, including teaching approaches specific to the target audience (e.g., children, adults, geriatric, culturally diverse population, etc.).

Review criteria (instructor-led patient education)

1. Instructors are health professionals or lay persons with special education and/or training and experience appropriate to the instructional needs of the program.
2. Documentation of rheumatic disease related training and/or experience is provided.
3. Personnel are expected to participate in continuing education in their areas of expertise on a regular basis.
4. Evidence is provided of regular meetings between instructors and program coordinator.

Review criteria (mediated patient education)

1. Some educational programs such as those utilizing interactive computers, interactive video, or packages utilizing written, audio tape, and/or video components do not require an instructor. When such programs are used, a person knowledgeable in program content and rheumatology care must be readily available to answer questions or assist with problems. Access may be in person or by telephone. Resource persons for mediated programs must meet the same criteria as outlined in section V, 1-4.

VI. Evaluation standards

Standard. In order for a program to meet the standards of this document, it must demonstrate its effectiveness in maintaining or improving health status (i.e., pain, functional ability, psychological state, social functioning, and/or quality of life). For example, decreased pain, depression, disability, fatigue, and improvement of quality of life can be determined by assessing the patient with a standardized measurement tool. Maintenance and/or improvement may be shown in terms of group or individual change (e.g., a third of a standard deviation) or other definitions that can be justified by the provider. In addition, satisfaction data from patients and family members must be collected and reviewed annually.

Review criteria. For new, not previously approved, programs.

1. Effectiveness is documented by scores on standard validated instruments.
2. Providers do not need to present new evaluation data when using already approved programs.
3. Any provider who chooses to use an approved program which has been demonstrated to meet the criteria in section VI,1 for patients who differ in some major way from the patient groups for which the program was designed, must show evidence that the program is effective for this new patient group.

VII. Documentation standards

Standard. Documented program planning and evaluation serves as the basis for future program development and modification. All aspects of the program shall be recorded by the program coordinator or other designated person.

Review criteria

1. Documentation shall include:
   a. How needs assessment(s) were conducted
   b. Results of needs assessment
   c. Curriculum
   d. Instructors/resource persons—qualifications, training, retraining, supervision, evaluation by participants
   e. Program outcome evaluation for new program
   f. Number of participants entering the program
   g. Number of participants completing the program

h. Satisfaction data from patients and family members

i. Any other documentation required by this document

2. The provider shall conduct and record a yearly internal review of the program documentation.

NATIONAL GUIDELINES FOR ENTEROSTOMAL PATIENT EDUCATION*

Prepared by the Standards Development Committee of the United Ostomy Association with the Assistance of Prospect Associates (See acknowledgments for complete list of contributors and affiliations.)

Background on the National Guidelines for Enterostomal Patient Education

In October 1988, the National Digestive Diseases Advisory Board (NDDAB) sponsored a conference where patients and health care professionals developed recommendations to improve enterostomal patient education. These recommendations may be used as a model for improving patient education on other digestive diseases. Following the conference, a task group, which included an enterostomal nurse, a gastroenterologist, and a patient, met to develop an action plan and identify the lead organizations responsible for implementing the conference recommendations. One recommendation was to develop national standards for enterostomal patient education as a tool for planning, implementing, and evaluating quality of care. The task group identified the United Ostomy Association (UOA) as the appropriate lead organization for coordinating the development of these standards. The UOA invited other relevant professional and voluntary organizations to participate. This document is a result of their efforts. A list of the individuals and organizations that contributed to this document is provided. At its May 1993 meeting, the Board reviewed and endorsed the original document with the provision that they be called "guidelines," not standards, consistent with current terminology used by the medical community (e.g., practice care guidelines).

Introduction

The following guidelines for enterostomal patient education have been formulated to assist the educator in providing the self-care skills and psychosocial support needed by patients to successfully manage their stomas. Studies have suggested that ostomy patient education reduces the patient's hospital length of stay, postoperative complications, need for additional surgery, and hospital readmissions. Additionally, teaching self-management techniques may improve the patient's compliance with treatment and reduce excessive use of medications and supplies.

The term "educator," as used in this document, includes various members of the multidisciplinary health care team who play important roles in caring for the ostomy patient. The educator may be a surgeon (e.g., general, colorectal, urologic, pediatric), a gastroenterologist, a nurse, a psychosocial health care professional, a registered dietitian, or a trained volunteer from a lay organization (e.g., UOA, ACS, CCFA). Each area of information should be administered by the appropriate educator (i.e., a surgeon should discuss surgical procedures, a registered dietitian should provide diet counseling, etc.) Many resources are available to assist the educator in meeting these guidelines and achieving optimal patient outcomes. A list of individuals and organizations that may serve as important resources is provided.

The term "patient," as used in this document, is defined as the enterostomal patient (temporary or permanent) as well as spouse, parent, guardian, or other home care provider. The patient encompasses all age groups from neonates to the elderly. Age, stage of developmental maturation, or disability of the patient may influence expected outcomes. Therefore, the educator will need to adapt his or her approach to accommodate such differences. Also in this context, the term "self-care," as used in this document, may refer when applicable to care or assisted care by a home care provider.

These guidelines are designed to ensure continuing patient education from diagnosis through rehabilitation. The guidelines are divided into three segments: preoperative, postoperative, and long-term rehabilitation. Guidelines, rationale, outcome criteria, and interventions have been identified for each segment. Ideally, the enterostomal patient's education begins in the preoperative period and continues throughout the hospital stay and after discharge. However, in emergency situations, the patient may be unable to receive information before an operation. In these cases, it is appropriate that the education process begin after the operation for the patient, and before the operation for the person giving permission for surgery.

---

*From Standards Development Committee of the United Ostomy Association: *Dis Colon Rectum* 37:559-563, 1994.

The long-term outcome of an ostomy operation is highly dependent on patient education. Educators provide patient education to potentially reduce the length of hospital stay for the patient, to avoid stoma-related postoperative complications, and to reduce fears, depression, and negative feelings associated with having an ostomy. The UOA Ostomate Bill of Rights states that the ostomy patient has the right to have access to and obtain systematic teaching from knowledgeable individuals.

These guidelines are directed to educators responsible for delivering enterostomal patient education and may improve patient awareness and knowledge concerning life with an ostomy.

National Guidelines for Enterostomal Patient Education

Preoperative period
Guidelines

Patient education begins during the preoperative period. At this stage, the educator(s) will:

Review changes in anatomy and physiology as it relates to the planned surgery.

Define the structure, care, and function of an ostomy, including related equipment and supplies.

Explain the anticipated surgical procedure, indications, alternative procedures, reason for stoma site selection, anticipated postoperative course, expectations for self-care, potential complications, and follow-up care.

Describe the relationship between the planned procedure and the disease process, including the potential effects on prognosis and future interventions.

Explain the physiological and psychological changes that may be associated with the ostomy, including potential effects on body image, self-esteem, sexuality, social function, nutrition, employment or schooling, and growth and development where applicable.

Inform the patient of the existence of community resources and support systems.

Rationale

Providing the patient with adequate and accurate information during the preoperative period should facilitate self-care in the rehabilitative process and should reduce postoperative apprehension and complications related to ostomy care and function.

Outcome criteria

The patient will:

Describe the stoma and its function including related equipment and supplies.

List community resources for equipment, supplies, and emotional support.

Describe the anticipated surgical procedure, changes in anatomy and physiology, indications, alternative procedures, reason for stoma site selection, anticipated postoperative course, expectations for self-care, potential complications, and follow-up care.

Describe the disease process, including prognosis, potential future therapies, and expected outcomes.

Discuss the potential impact of the stoma on body image, self-esteem, sexuality, social function, and employment or schooling as applicable.

Describe dietary modifications to prevent/manage diarrhea, constipation, bloating, stoma obstruction, food blockage, malnutrition, flatulence, dehydration, urinary tract infection, and urinary calculus formation.

Explain potential effects of the stoma on growth and development, as appropriate.

Interventions

Suggested interventions include:

Provision of educational materials (see resource section).

Nutrition counseling.

Enterostomal consultation.

Educator/patient conferences including lay visitor.

Social services consultation.

Postoperative period
Guidelines

To facilitate the patient's recovery and return to self-care, the educator will:

Provide strategies for attaining an appropriate level of self-care.

Clarify the patient's understanding of the changes in anatomy and physiology, structure, care, and function of the ostomy, including related equipment and supplies.

Reinforce the patient's knowledge of the surgical procedure and its implications.

Clarify the relationship between the surgical procedure and the disease process, including the prognosis.

Discuss the impact of the stoma on body image, self-esteem, sexuality, employment, and social function.

Provide strategies for the prevention and management of stoma-related complications.

Instruct the patient regarding the continued need for adequate nutritional and fluid intake, including individual requirements and those related to the specific surgery.

Inform the patient of the existence of community resources and support systems.

Instruct the patient regarding sources of obtaining and receiving reimbursement for equipment.

Rationale

Providing postoperative education and psychosocial support should lead to improved patient function and facilitate recovery.

Outcome criteria

The patient will:

Demonstrate an appropriate level of self-care.

Describe the prevention and management of potential complications resulting from ostomy surgery.

Demonstrate an understanding of types of equipment needed in ostomy management and reasons for use.

Explain ostomy management within activities of daily living, work, play, and sexual life.

Communicate concerns and potential problems related to altered body image and function.

Describe dietary means to prevent/manage diarrhea, constipation, bloating, stoma obstruction, food blockage, malnutrition, flatulence, dehydration, urinary tract infection, and urinary calculus formation.

Identify sources of equipment and resources for reimbursement.

Demonstrate an appropriate understanding of stoma-related complications.

List community resources for mutual aid and support, rehabilitation, and education.

Interventions

Suggested interventions include:

Provision of educational materials (see resource section).

Educator/patient conferences, including lay visitor.

Nutrition counseling.

Enterostomal consultation.

Social services consultation.

Long-term rehabilitation period

Guidelines

To prepare the patient for the long-term rehabilitation period, the educator will:

Explain long-term nutritional, social, pharmacologic, and other therapeutic needs.

Assist the patient in achieving optimal physiologic and psychosocial status and level of activity.

Define long-term follow-up approaches including monitoring for potential complications and ongoing education to facilitate self-care.

Explain the difference between the effects of the disease process and the effects of the ostomy on long-term rehabilitation.

Rationale

Optimal understanding, acceptance, and management of the ostomy and possible ongoing disease process should minimize complications and maximize the patient's quality of life. Educational activities should prepare the patient for the long-term rehabilitation period. The patient must be prepared for possible adjustments in areas of medications, equipment, diet, fluid intake, routines of daily living, and self-care expectations.

Outcome criteria

The patient will:

Manage care of the stoma and appropriately select and utilize equipment and supplies.

Identify and describe prevention, detection, and management strategies related to potential complications, adaptive and environmental changes, and the disease process, within the limits of the patient's level of education and understanding.

Use professional, community, family, and personal resources to maximize level of functioning and, when applicable, to optimize growth and development.

Interventions

Suggested interventions include:

Referral to appropriate support group(s).

Provision of educational materials (see resource section).

Nutrition counseling.

Enterostomal consultation.

Educator/patient conferences, including lay visitor.

Social services consultation.

An appropriate, individualized follow-up protocol.

Resources

Numerous professional and voluntary organizations provide relevant materials and information on ostomy patient education that assist educators in implementing these standards. Health care professionals located within local communities are also excellent resources. These include: surgeons, (e.g., general, colorectal, urologic, pediatric), gastroenterologists, enterostomal therapy nurses, registered dietitians, pharmacists, gastrointestinal nurses and associates, social workers, trained lay visitors, and psychotherapists. In addition, manufacturers and suppliers of ostomy equipment and pharmaceuticals produce patient education materials.

The following organizations provide a variety of useful information related to ostomy patient education and may have local chapters, support services, or representatives in the educator's community.

American Cancer Society, Ostomy Rehabilitation Program, 1599 Clifton Road, N.E., Atlanta, Georgia 30329. 1-800-227-2345.

American Dietetic Association, 216 West Jackson Boulevard, Suite 800, Chicago, Illinois 60606-6995. (312) 899-0040.

American Society of Colon and Rectal Surgeons, 800 East N.W. Highway, Suite 1080, Palatine, Illinois 60067. (708) 359-9184.

American Urological Association Allied, Inc., 11512 Allecingie Parkway, Richmond, Virginia 23235. (804) 379-1306.

Association of Rehabilitation Nurses, 5700 Old Orchard Road, First Floor, Skokie, Illinois 60077. (708) 966-3433.

Crohn's & Colitis Foundation of America, Inc. (formerly National Foundation for Ileitis and Colitis), 444 Park Avenue, S., 11th floor, New York, New York 10016-7374. 1-800-343-3637.

International Association for Enterostomal Therapy, 27241 LaPaz Road, Laguna Niguel, California 92656. (714) 476-0268.

National Digestive Diseases Information Clearinghouse, Box NDDIC, 9000 Rockville Pike, Bethesda, Maryland 20892. (301) 468-6344.

Society of Gastroenterology Nurses and Associates, 1070 Sibley Tower, Rochester, New York 14604. (716) 546-7241. 1-800-245-SGNA.

United Ostomy Association, Inc., 36 Executive Park, Suite 120, Irvine, California 92714-6744. (714) 660-8624. 1-800-826-0826.

Acknowledgments

Coordinated for the United Ostomy Association (UOA) by Marilyn A. Mau, Past President
STANDARDS DEVELOPMENT STEERING COMMITTEE
CHAIR: James Fleshman, M.D.
Washington University School of Medicine, St. Louis, MO
Chair, UOA Medical Advisory Committee

INVITED TO PARTICIPATE
American Cancer Society (ACS)
American College of Physicians (ACP)
American Dietetic Association (ADA)
American Gastroenterological Association (AGA)
American Nephrology Nurses Association (ANNA)
American Nurses' Association (ANA)
American Society of Colon and Rectal Surgeons (ASCRS)
American Society of Gastroenterology Endoscopy (ASGE)
American Urological Association Allied, Inc. (AUAA)
Association of Rehabilitation Nurses (ARN)
Crohn's and Colitis Foundation of America (CCFA)
Digestive Disease National Coalition (DDNC)
National Digestive Diseases Information Clearinghouse (NDDIC)
North American Society for Pediatric Gastroenterology (NASPG)
Society of Gastroenterology Nurses and Associates (SGNA)
Wound, Ostomy and Continence Nurses Society (WOCN)

CONTRIBUTORS TO THE STANDARDS
Linda K. Aukett,* UOA
Rebecca Bonsaint, ASGE
Cheryl Corbin, M.S., R.D., ADA
Frederick Daum, M.D., NASPG
Judy Ebbert, ACP
Linda Farah, ANNA
John Farrar, M.D., DDNC
Jim Fleshman,* M.D., UOA and ASCRS
Linda Gabrielson,* M.S., R.D., ADA
Michael Gray, Ph.D., AUAA
Cecilia Grindel,* Ph.D., R.N., ANA
TennieBee Hall,* UOA, CCFA, past member of the NDDAB
Marsha Hardick, R.N., CGC and SGNA
John Latimer,* M.D., NASPG
Malcolm Malooh, M.S., R.N., R.N.C.
Marilyn A. Mau,* Past President, UOA
Kenneth Mirkin,* M.D., AGA
Nancy J. Reilly, R.N., M.S.N., C.U.R.N., AUAA
Dale Singer,† Prospect Associates

---

*Represents members of the Steering Committee.
†This document was prepared with the assistance of Prospect Associates under a contract with the United Ostomy Association.

Beth Stevenson, M.P.H., ACS
Kristy Wright, R.N., B.S.N., C.E.T.N., WOCN

References

Bartlett EE. How can patient education contribute to improved health care under prospective pricing? Health Policy 1986;6:283-94.

Karam JA, Sundre SM, Smith GA. Cost/benefit analysis of patient education. Hosp Health Serv Adm 1986;31:82-90.

Kreps GL, Ruben BD, Baker MW, Rosenthal SR. Survey of public health knowledge about digestive health and diseases: implications for health education. Public Health Rep 1987;102:270-7.

Ostomate bill of rights. United Ostomy Association. Irvine, California, 1977.

IAET Standards Committee. Outcome standards for the ostomy client. J Enterostomal Ther 1983;10:128-31.

Stanton M. Patient education-implications for nursing. Todays OR Nurse 1987;9:16-20.

Wainwright P. Information and the surgical patient. Nurs Times 1982;78:1480-2.

Williams D. Preoperative patient education: in the home or in the hospital? Orthop Nurs 1986;5:37-41.

Ziemer MM. Effects of information on postsurgical patient coping. Nurs Res 1983;32:282-7.

SELECTIONS FROM JCAHO 1995 ACCREDITATION MANUAL FOR HOSPITALS
Education Standards*

Preamble

The **goal** of educating the patient and/or, when appropriate, family† is to improve patient health outcomes by promoting recovery, speeding return to function, promoting healthy behavior, and appropriately involving patients in his or her care and care decisions. Education should

- facilitate the patient's and/or, when appropriate, family's understanding of the patient's health status, health care options, and consequences of options selected;
- encourage patient and/or family participation in decision making about health care options;

- increase the patient's and/or, when appropriate, family's potential to follow the therapeutic health care plan;
- maximize patient and/or family care skills;
- increase the patient's and/or, when appropriate, family's ability to cope with the patient's health status/prognosis/outcome;
- enhance the patient's and/or, when appropriate, family's role in continuing care; and
- promote a healthy patient life-style.

The "Education" standards address the need for a systematic approach to education throughout the organization. However, the standards do not require any specific structure for providing education, such as an education department,‡ a patient education committee, or the employment of an educator. The standards allow the organization to focus on its current processes and how these processes are implemented in relation to the patient's care plan, the level of care, the setting in which teaching occurs, and continuity of care.

The performance-improvement framework in the "Improving Organizational Performance" chapter of this *Manual* is used to design, measure, assess, and improve the organization's performance of the education function.

The terms used in this chapter are defined as they are used in the context of the patient-focused function and may not reflect common dictionary usage.

PF.1

The patient and/or his or her family are provided with appropriate education and training to increase their knowledge of the patient's illness and treatment needs and to learn skills and behaviors that promote recovery and improve function.

PF.2

The patient and/or, when appropriate, his or her family receive education specific to the patient's assessed needs, abilities, and readiness, as appropriate to the patient's length of stay.

---

*From the Joint Commission on Accreditation of Health Care Organizations: *Accreditation manual for hospitals,* vol 1, *Standards,* Chicago, 1994, The Commission.

†**Family** refers to the person(s) who plays a significant role in the patient's life. This includes an individual(s) who may or may not be legally related to the patient.

‡A **department** is defined in this *Manual* as any structural unit of the health care organization, whether it is called a department, a service, a unit, or something similar.

PF.2.I. The patient and/or, when appropriate, his or her family have their learning needs, abilities, and readiness to learn assessed.

PF.2.1.1   When indicated, the assessment includes cultural and religious practices, emotional barriers, desire and motivation to learn, physical and/or cognitive limitations, and language barriers.

PF.2.2. The patient and/or, when appropriate, his or her family are provided with the knowledge and/or skills required to meet the patient's ongoing health care needs. Such instruction is presented in ways understandable to the patient and/or his or her family and includes, but is not limited to,

PF.2.2.1   the safe and effective use of medication, when applicable, in accordance with legal requirements and patient needs;

PF.2.2.2   the safe and effective use of medical equipment, when applicable;

PF.2.2.3   instruction on potential drug-food interactions and counseling on nutrition intervention and/or modified diets, as appropriate;

PF.2.2.4   instruction in rehabilitation techniques to facilitate adaptation to and/or functional independence in the environment, if needed;

PF2.2.5   access to available community resources, if needed;

PF.2.2.6   when and how to obtain further treatment, if needed; and

PF.2.2.7   the patient's and/or, when appropriate, family's responsibilities in the patient's care.

PF.3

Any discharge instructions given to the patient and/or, when appropriate, his or her family are provided to the organization or individual responsible for the patient's continuing care.

PF.4

The organization plans and supports the provision and coordination of patient and/or, when appropriate, family education activities and resources.

PF.4.I. The organization identifies and provides the educational resources required to achieve its educational objectives.

PF.4.2. The patient and/or, when appropriate, family educational process is interdisciplinary, as appropriate to the care plan.

Scoring Guidelines*

Preamble

The goal of educating the patient and/or, when appropriate, family† is to improve patient health outcomes by promoting recovery, speeding return to function, promoting healthy behavior, and appropriately involving the patient in his or her care decisions. Education should

- facilitate the patient's and/or, when appropriate, family's understanding of the patient's health status, health care options, and consequences of options selected;
- encourage patient and/or, when appropriate, family participation in the decision-making process about health care options;
- increase the patient's and/or, when appropriate, family's potential to follow the therapeutic health care plan;
- maximize patient and/or, when appropriate, family care skills;
- increase the patient's and/or, when appropriate, family's ability to cope with the patient's health status/prognosis/outcome;
- enhance the patient's and/or, when appropriate, family's role in continuing care; and
- promote a healthy patient lifestyle.

The "Education" standards address the need for a systematic approach to education throughout the organization. However, they do not require any specific structure for providing education, such as an education department,‡ a patient education committee, or the employment of an educator. The standards allow the organization to focus on its current processes and how these processes are implemented in relation to

---

*From the Joint Commission on Accreditation of Health Care Organizations: *Accreditation manual for hospitals,* vol 2, *Scoring guidelines,* Chicago, 1995, The Commission.

†**Family** refers to the person(s) who play a significant role in the patient's life. This includes an individual(s) who may or may not be legally related to the patient.

‡A **department** is defined in this *Manual* as any structural unit of the health care organization, whether it is called a department, a service, a unit, or something similar.

the patient's care plan, level of care, setting in which teaching occurs, and continuity of care.

The performance-improvement framework in the "Improving Organizational Performance" chapter of this *Manual* is used to design, measure, assess, and improve the organization's performance of the education function.

The terms used in this chapter are defined as they are used in the context of the patient-focused function and may not reflect common dictionary usage.

Practical application

The flowchart for the education function (Figure 1) illustrates the three areas of impact on the patient: the organization's focus on education; the direct impact of education on the patient and family; and the evaluation of the program for patient and family education relative to goal achievement (assessed as part of the pediatric intensive care unit's [PICU] ongoing measurement, assessment, and improvement of quality patient care outcomes).

1. A 4-year-old girl and her family receives education throughout her stay in the hospital. This example limits its focus to her care in the PICU. The goals established for the patient and family education program for the PICU include (1) decreasing fear of equipment used, and (2) promoting family involvement in the patient's care. In service of these two goals, while the child was comatose, the PICU staff continuously provided what they call "casual education." Casual education includes assessing the parents' level of knowledge about intensive care unit equipment, explaining what is being used on their child, and why it is needed for her care. More formal information is available through the use of booklets prepared by PICU staff in collaboration with staff in the pediatric unit. The allocation of resources to support the provision of the program is included in the PICU's budget planning processes each year and analyzed on an ongoing basis by comparing identified needs to available resources.

2. The areas of the program that directly impact the child include talking to her while care is being administered because the staff recognizes that many coma patients do hear and are able to understand. After becoming alert and able to visually recognize her parents and objects, she is taught to use hand signals and a "Needs Cartoon Chart." At this point, the parents are also instructed in the chart's

use, and they take turns working with their child using the chart each time they stay with her in the PICU.

3. Finally, as mentioned above and as part of the PICU's ongoing measurement and assessment of the care provided to patients in the unit, the effectiveness of the educational program(s) provided is also assessed.

Standard

PF.1 The patient and/or, when appropriate, his or her family are provided with appropriate education and training to increase knowlege of the patient's illness and treatment needs and to learn skills and behaviors that promote recovery and improve function.

Intent of PF.1

Educating the patient and/or, when appropriate, his or her family is integral to providing patient care. A positive outcome of a patient's care is often dependent on (1) the instructions given to a patient and/or, when appropriate, family before care or treatment (such as before diagnostic testing or surgery); (2) the patient's and/or his or her family's activities subsequent to the patient's discharge from the health care organization; and (3) information given about the patient's health maintenance. The organization provides a framework to assist the patient and/or his or her family in gaining the knowledge and skills to meet the patient's ongoing health care needs.

Example of implementation—PF.1

An organization could prioritize specific diseases for education interventions, such as heart disease, cancer, diabetes, hypertension, and other leading causes of death where lifestyle impacts the disease process.

Scoring for PF.1

This standard is not scored.

Standards

PF.2. The patient and/or, when appropriate, his or her family receive education specific to the patient's assessed needs, abilities, and readiness, as appropriate to the patient's length of stay.

PF.2.1. The patient and/or, when appropriate, his or her family have their learning needs, abilities, and readiness to learn assessed.

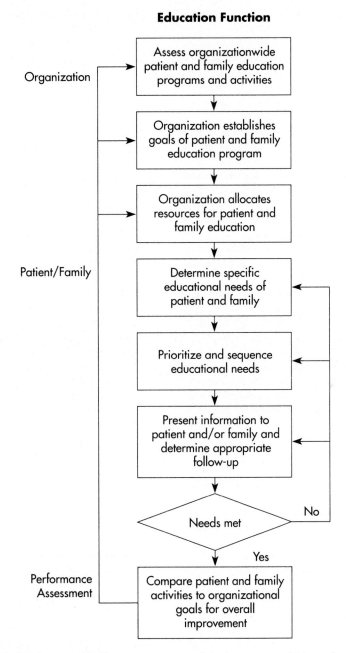

Figure 1   This flowchart graphically represents most of the important activities and processes, particularly the risk points, in the education function.

PF.2.1.1. When indicated, the assessment includes cultural and religious practices, emotional barriers, desire and motivation to learn, physical and/or cognitive limitations, and language barriers.

PF.2.2. The patient and/or, when appropriate, his or her family are provided with the specific knowledge and/or skills required to meet the patient's ongoing health care needs. Such instruction is presented in ways understandable to the patient and/or his or her family and includes, but is not limited to,

PF.2.2.1. The safe and effective use of medication in accordance with legal requirements and patient needs, when applicable;

PF.2.2.2. The safe and effective use of medical equipment, when applicable;

PF.2.2.3. Instruction on potential drug-food interactions and counseling on nutrition intervention and/or modified diets, as appropriate;

PF.2.2.4. Instruction in rehabilitation techniques to facilitate adaptation to and/or functional independence in the environment, if needed;

PF.2.2.5. Access to available community resources, if needed;

PF.2.2.6. When and how to obtain further treatment, if needed; and

Intent of PF.2 through PF.2.2.6

The process for identifying the patient's learning needs addresses the patient's anticipated length of stay, appropriate use of applicable organization and community resources, and the patient's and family's ability to comprehend and implement the education provided.

Patient learning needs, when indicated, are identified and prioritized, as are the learning needs of the family who participate in the patient's care. However, not all patients need education concerning their care plan. The patient's and/or, when appropriate, family's ability to learn is also assessed, thereby enabling the provider to impart pertinent information to the patient and/or, when appropriate, family in a manner that is as understandable as possible.

When assessing the learning needs, abilities, and readiness to learn of the patient and/or, when appropriate, family, staff considers, when indicated, such variables as the patient's and/or, when appropriate, family's beliefs, values, literacy, and language. Staff should be open and flexible when teaching the individual(s). These variables can influence the patient's and/or, when appropriate, family's choice to follow or not to follow instructions.

Examples of Implementation—PF.2 through PF.2.2.6

1. The quality of life for a patient with chronic obstructive pulmonary disease could be improved by educating him or her about treatment modalities that can be carried out in the home.

2. A family coping with an illness that is particularly traumatic because of its duration, severity, or effect on the patient's physical or psychological development could benefit from having a list of appropriate community organizations providing support programs. Some examples of such patient education resources include support groups, courses, self-help groups, transportation to get health care, and community clinics for follow-up care.

3. An organization could increase a patient's and his or her family's understanding of and compliance with treatment procedures if it considers the significance of cultural influences on the patient's recovery and health maintenance. For instance, in male-dominant cultures, the family's male figurehead must fully understand and respect a female patient's recovery requirements to ensure compliance with treatment procedures and thus promote a favorable outcome.

4. For neonatal intensive care, parents learn—before the infant's discharge—the special procedures they must perform. Parental participation is encouraged to facilitate baby-parent bonding and family adjustment as well as continuity of care following discharge.

5. Rehabilitation patients are instructed in using adaptive bathroom equipment so they can function independently.

6. For hospitals providing maternity services, pregnant women are provided with information regarding the management of breastfeeding, instructed in proper breastfeeding technique and proper nutrition while lactating, and re-evaluated prior to discharge. Breastfeeding mothers are provided with breastfeeding educational information and breastfeeding community contact names and telephone numbers for postdischarge assistance with any feeding concern(s).

Examples of evidence of performance—PF.2 through PF.2.2.6

- Organizationwide policies and procedures defining responsibilities for patient and/or, when appropriate, family
- Progress notes

- Flowsheets
- Referral and consultation notes
- Interviews with clinical staff

Scoring for PF.2

Score 1. The organization educates patients and/or, when appropriate, his or her families using an approach defined by the leaders of the medical staff, nursing staff, and other professional disciplines, as appropriate.

And

91% to 100% of medical records reviewed indicate that the patients' learning needs pertaining to the care of the patient are assessed, identified, and addressed.

Score 2. The organization educates patients and/or, when appropriate, his or her families using an approach defined by the leaders of the medical staff, nursing staff, and other professional disciplines, as appropriate.

And

76% to 90% of medical records reviewed indicate that the patient's learning needs pertaining to the care of the patient are assessed, identified, and addressed.

Score 3. The organization does not have a defined approach for patient education.

Or

51% to 75% of medical records reviewed indicate that the patients' learning needs pertaining to the care of the patient are assessed, identified, and addressed.

Score 4. 26% to 50% of medical records reviewed indicate that the patients' learning needs pertaining to the care of the patient are assessed, identified, and addressed.

Score 5. Fewer than 26% of medical records reviewed indicate that the patients' learning needs pertaining to the care of the patient are asssessed, identified, and addressed.

Scoring for PF.2.1

Score 1. 91% to 100% of medical records reviewed indicate that patient and/or, when appropriate, family learning needs are assessed. At a minimum, this evidence of assessment includes tasks the patient can or cannot accomplish as related to his or her current health problem.

Score 2. 76% to 90% of medical records reviewed indicate that patient and/or, when appropriate, family learning needs are assessed. At a minimum, this evidence of assessment includes tasks the patient can or cannot accomplish as related to his or her current health problem.

Score 3. 51% to 75% of medical records reviewed indicate that patient and/or, when appropriate, family learning needs are assessed. At a minimum, this evidence of assessment includes tasks the patient can or cannot accomplish as related to his or her current health problem.

Score 4. 26% to 50% of medical records reviewed indicate that patient and/or, when appropriate, family learning needs are assessed. At a minimum, this evidence of assessment includes tasks the patient can or cannot accomplish as related to his or her current health problem.

Score 5. Fewer than 26% of medical records reviewed indicate that patient and/or, when appropriate, family learning needs are assessed. At a minimum, this evidence of assessment includes tasks the patient can or cannot accomplish as related to his or her current health problem.

Scoring for PF.2.1.1

Score 1. 91% to 100% of medical records reviewed indicate that the assessment considers cultural values and religious beliefs, emotional barriers, desire and motivation to learn, physical and/or cognitive limitations, and language barriers, as indicated.

Score 2. 76% to 90% of medical records reviewed indicate that the assessment considers cultural values and religious beliefs, emotional barriers, desire and motivation to learn, physical and/or cognitive limitations, and language barriers, as indicated.

Score 3. 51% to 75% of medical records reviewed indicate that the assessment considers cultural values and religious beliefs, emotional barriers, desire and motivation to learn, physical and/or cognitive limitations, and language barriers, as indicated.

Score 4. 26% to 50% of medical records reviewed indicate that the assessment considers cultural values and religious beliefs, emotional barriers, desire and motivation to learn, physical and/or cognitive limitations, and language barriers, as indicated.

Score 5. Fewer than 26% of medical records reviewed indicate that the assessment considers cultural values and religious beliefs, emotional barriers, desire and motivation to learn, physical and/or cognitive limitations, and language barriers, as indicated.

Scoring for PF.2.2

This standard is not scored.

Scoring for PF.2.2.1

Score 1. The education in the safe and effective use of medication is guided by policies and procedures, the development of which involves all appropriate disciplines.

And

The policies and procedures guiding patient and/or, when appropriate, family education in the safe and effective use of medication are implemented.

And

91% to 100% of medical records reviewed indicate that the patient's and/or, when appropriate, family's specific learning needs concerning the safe use of medication are identified and addressed, when such instruction is necessary.

Score 2. The education in the safe and effective use of medication is guided by policies and procedures; however, the development of the policies and procedures does not involve all appropriate disciplines.

And

The policies and procedures guiding patient and/or, when appropriate, family education in the safe and effective use of medication are implemented.

And

76% to 90% of medical records reviewed indicate that the patient's and/or, when appropriate, family's specific learning needs concerning the safe use of medication are identified and addressed, when such instruction is necessary.

Score 3. The education in the safe and effective use of medication is guided by policies and procedures; however, the development of the policies and procedures does not involve the appropriate disciplines.

Or

The policies and procedures guiding patient and/or, when appropriate, family education in the safe and effective use of medication are not implemented.

Or

51% to 75% of medical records reviewed indicate that the patient's and/or, when appropriate, family's specific learning needs concerning the safe use of medication are identified and addressed, when such instruction is necessary.

Score 4. 26% to 50% of medical records reviewed indicate that the patient's and/or, when appropriate, family's specific learning needs concerning the safe use of medication are identified and addressed, when such instruction is necessary.

Score 5. Fewer than 26% of medical records reviewed indicate that the patient's and/or, when

appropriate, family's specific learning needs concerning the safe use of medication are identified and addressed, when such instruction is necessary.

Scoring for PF.2.2.2

Score 1. The education in the safe and effective use of medical equipment is guided by policies and procedures, the development of which involves all appropriate disciplines.

And

The policies and procedures guiding patient and/or, when appropriate, family education in the safe and effective use of medical equipment are implemented.

And

91% to 100% of medical records reviewed indicate that the patient's and/or, when appropriate, family's specific learning needs concerning the safe use of medical equipment are identified and addressed, when such instruction is necessary.

Score 2. The education in the safe and effective use of medical equipment is guided by policies and procedures; however, the development of the policies and procedures does not involve all appropriate disciplines.

And

The policies and procedures guiding patient and/or, when appropriate, family education in the safe and effective use of medical equipment are implemented.

And

76% to 90% of medical records reviewed indicate that the patient's and/or, when appropriate, family's specific learning needs concerning the safe use of medical equipment are identified and addressed, when such instruction is necessary.

Score 3. The education in the safe and effective use of medical equipment is guided by policies and procedures; however, the development of the policies and procedures does not involve all appropriate disciplines.

Or

The policies and procedures guiding patient education in the safe and effective use of medical equipment are not implemented.

Or

51% to 75% of medical records reviewed indicate that the patient's and/or, when appropriate, family's specific learning needs concerning the safe use of medical equipment are identified and addressed, when such instruction is necessary.

Score 4. 26% to 50% of medical records reviewed indicate that the patient's and/or, when appropriate, family's specific learning needs concerning the safe use of medical equipment are identified and addressed, when such instruction is necessary.

Score 5. Fewer than 26% of medical records reviewed indicate that the patient's and/or, when appropriate, family's specific learning needs concerning the safe use of medical equipment are identified and addressed, when such instruction is necessary.

Scoring for PF.2.2.3

Score 1. Dietary and nutritional instruction is guided by policies and procedures, the development of which involves all appropriate disciplines.

And

The policies and procedures guiding patient and/or, when appropriate, family education in dietary and nutritional instruction are implemented.

And

91% to 100% of medical records reviewed indicate that the patient's and/or, when appropriate, family's specific learning needs concerning diet and nutrition are identified and addressed, when such instruction is necessary.

Score 2. Dietary and nutritional instruction is guided by policies and procedures; however, the development of the policies and procedures does not involve all appropriate disciplines.

And

The policies and procedures guiding patient and/or, when appropriate, family education in dietary and nutritional instruction are implemented.

And

76% to 90% of medical records reviewed indicate that the patient's and/or, when appropriate, family's specific learning needs concerning diet and nutrition are identified and addressed, when such instruction is necessary.

Score 3. Dietary and nutritional instruction is guided by policies and procedures; however, the development of the policies and procedures does not involve all appropriate disciplines.

Or

The policies and procedures guiding patient and/or, when appropriate, family education in dietary and nutritional instruction are not implemented.

Or

51% to 75% of medical records reviewed indicate that the patient's and/or, when appropriate, family's specific learning needs concerning diet and nutrition are identified and addressed, when such instruction is necessary.

Score 4. 26% to 50% of medical records reviewed indicate that the patient's and/or, when appropriate, family's specific learning needs concerning diet and nutrition are identified and addressed, when such instruction is necessary.

Score 5. Fewer than 26% of medical records reviewed indicate that the patient's and/or, when appropriate, family's specific learning needs concerning diet and nutrition are identified and addressed, when such instruction is necessary.

Scoring for PF.2.2.4

Score 1. Rehabilitation instruction is guided by policies and procedures, the development of which involves the appropriate disciplines.

And

The policies and procedures guiding patient and/or, when appropriate, family education in rehabilitation instruction are implemented.

And

91% to 100% of medical records reviewed indicate that the patient's and/or, when appropriate, family's specific learning needs concerning rehabilitation are identified and addressed, when such instruction is necessary.

Score 2. Rehabilitation instruction is guided by policies and procedures; however, the development of the policies and procedures does not involve all appropriate disciplines.

And

The policies and procedures guiding patient and/or, when appropriate, family education in rehabilitation instruction are implemented.

And

76% to 90% of medical records reviewed indicate that the patient's and/or, when appropriate, family's specific learning needs concerning rehabilitation are identified and addressed, when such instruction is necessary.

Score 3. Rehabilitation instruction is guided by policies and procedures; however, the development of the policies and procedures does not involve all appropriate disciplines.

Or

The policies and procedures guiding patient and/or, when appropriate, family education in rehabilitation instruction are not implemented.

Or

51% to 75% of medical records reviewed indicate that the patient's and/or, when appropriate, family's specific learning needs concerning rehabilitation are identified and addressed, when such instruction is necessary.

Score 4. 26% to 50% of medical records reviewed indicate that the patient's and/or, when appropriate, family's specific learning needs concerning rehabilitation are identified and addressed, when such instruction is necessary.

Score 5. Fewer than 26% of medical records reviewed indicate that the patient's and/or, when appropriate, family's specific learning needs concerning rehabilitation are identified and addressed, when such instruction is necessary.

Scoring for PF.2.2.5

Score 1. The provision of information about other patient educational resources is guided by policies and procedures, the development of which involves the appropriate disciplines.

And

The policies and procedures guiding patient and/or, when appropriate, family education in the provision of information about other educational resources are implemented.

And

91% to 100% of medical records reviewed indicate that the patient's and/or, when appropriate, family's specific needs concerning referral services are identified and addressed, when such instruction is necessary.

Score 2. The provision of information about other patient educational resources is guided by policies and procedures; however, the development of the policies and procedures does not involve all appropriate disciplines.

And

The policies and procedures guiding patient and/or, when appropriate, family education in the provision of information about other educational resources are implemented.

And

76% to 90% of medical records reviewed indicate that the patient's and/or, when appropriate, family's specific needs concerning referral services are identified and addressed, when such instruction is necessary.

Score 3. The provision of information about other patient education resources is guided by policies and procedures; however, the development of the policies and procedures does not involve all appropriate disciplines.

Or

The policies and procedures guiding patient education in the provision of information about other patient education resources are not implemented.

Or

51% to 75% of medical records reviewed indicate that the patient's and/or, when appropriate, family's specific needs concerning referral services are identified and addressed, when such instruction is necessary.

Score 4. 26% to 50% of medical records reviewed indicate that the patient's and/or, when appropriate, family's specific needs concerning referral services are identified and addressed, when such instruction is necessary.

Score 5. Fewer than 26% of medical records reviewed indicate that the patient's and/or, when appropriate, family's specific needs concerning referral services are identified and addressed, when such instruction is necessary.

Scoring for PF.2.2.6

Score 1. Patient instruction in any follow-up care is guided by policies and procedures, the development of which involves the appropriate disciplines.

And

The policies and procedures guiding patient and/or, when appropriate, family education in patient instruction in follow-up care are implemented.

And

91% to 100% of medical records reviewed indicate that the patient and/or, when appropriate, family are instructed as to any follow-up care needed and how to obtain that care, when such instruction is necessary.

Score 2. Patient instruction in any follow-up care is guided by policies and procedures; however, the development of the policies and procedures does not involve all appropriate disciplines.

And

The policies and procedures guiding patient and/or, when appropriate, family instruction in follow-up care are implemented.

And

76% to 90% of medical records reviewed indicate that the patient and/or, when appropriate, family are instructed as to any follow-up care needed and how to obtain that care, when such instruction is necessary.

Score 3. Patient instruction in any follow-up care is guided by policies and procedures; however, the development of the policies and procedures does not involve all appropriate disciplines.

Or

The policies and procedures guiding patient and/or, when appropriate, family education in patient instruction in follow-up care are not implemented.

Or

51% to 75% of medical records reviewed indicate that the patient and/or, when appropriate, family are instructed as to any follow-up care needed and how to obtain that care, when such instruction is necessary.

Score 4. 26% to 50% of medical records reviewed indicate that the patient and/or, when appropriate, family are instructed as to any follow-up care needed and how to obtain that care, when such instruction is necessary.

Score 5. Fewer than 26% of medical records reviewed indicate that the patient and/or, when appropriate, family are instructed as to any follow-up care needed and how to obtain that care, when such instruction is necessary.

Standard

PF.2.2.7. The patient and/or, when appropriate, his or her family are provided with the specific knowledge and/or skills required to meet the patient's ongoing health care needs. Such instruction is presented in ways understandable to the patient and/or his or her family and includes, but is not limited to, the patient's and family's responsibilities in the patient's care.

Intent of PF.2.2.7

Health care organizations are entitled to reasonable and responsible behavior, considering the nature of the illness, on the part of the patient and his or her family. The organization identifies the responsibilities of patients and their families and then educates them accordingly. Such responsibilities may include, but need not be limited to, the following:

- **Provision of information.** The patient and/or, when appropriate, family are responsible for providing to the best of their knowledge, accurate and complete information about present complaints, past illnesses, hospitalizations, medications, and other matters relating to the patient's health. The patient and/or, when appropriate, family are re-

sponsible for reporting unexpected changes in the patient's condition to the responsible practitioner and whether the patient clearly comprehends a contemplated course of action and what is expected of him or her.

- **Compliance with instruction.** The patient and/or, when appropriate, family is responsible for following the treatment plan developed with the practitioner. The patient should express any concerns regarding his or her ability to comply with a proposed course of treatment, and every effort should be made to adapt the treatment plan to the patient's specific needs and limitations. Where such adaptation to the treatment plan is not clinically indicated, the patient and/or, when appropriate, family are responsible for understanding the consequences of the treatment alternatives and of noncompliance with the proposed course of treatment.

- **Refusal of treatment.** The patient and/or, when appropriate, family is responsible for the outcomes if the patient and/or, when appropriate, family refuses treatment or does not follow the practitioner's instructions.

- **Rules and regulations.** The patient and/or, when appropriate, family are responsible for following the health care organization's rules and regulations affecting patient care and conduct.

- **Respect and consideration.** The patient and/or, when appropriate, family is responsible for being considerate of the rights of other patients and organization personnel and for assisting in the control of noise, smoking, and distractions. The patient and/or, when appropriate, family is responsible for being respectful of the property of other persons and of the health care organization.

Example of implementation—PF.2.2.7

1. Early in the admission process, an adolescent admitted for conduct disorder is oriented to the treatment process and treatment team guiding his/her treatment plan. The patient's age is considered to determine whether the parent(s) or guardian(s) should be involved in the treatment plan. In the orientation, the patient and, if appropriate, the parent(s) or guardian(s) learn about schedules and treatment modalities as well as activities in which the patient is expected to participate.

   Behavioral expectations are also spelled out. The adolescent is informed about his or her rights and warned that aggressive, assaultive, or destructive behavior will result in a reduction of his or her privileges. If the adolescent was voluntarily admitted and he or she refuses treatment, then he or she may be discharged. If the adolescent was involuntarily admitted and he or she refuses treatment, then state law and organization policy guide the organization. If the patient is considered a threat to others, then he or she may be treated as an involuntary admission.

2. Education of patients and families regarding their responsibilities can take many forms. Pre-admission information mailed to the patient or presented at an earlier visit outlines the patient's rights and responsibilities. Criteria for admission to a specialized care unit, such as a comprehensive physical rehabilitation program, might include a set of patient responsibilities that is provided during the pre-entry phase. During admission, the patient could be provided with a verbal explanation or a booklet; or the responsibilities could be posted in a patient area available to all and the patient informed about their location.

3. The organization may not agree with a patient's choice of treatments and does not agree with the patient's wish to transfer to another organization to receive the treatment. The organization, however, has a procedure to inform the patient and his or her family that they can assume the responsibility to make arrangements for such transfers.

Examples of evidence of performance—PF.2.2.7
- Medical record entries
- Posted signs
- Policies and procedures
- Statement on patient rights and responsibilities
- Written information given to patients and families

Scoring for PF.2.2.7

Score 1. The organization has identified the patient's and family's responsibilities.

And

The organization has a mechanism in place designed to educate patients and families about their responsibilities.

Score 2. Note: *Although the surveyor will score this standard at an organization's actual level of performance, the impact of the score will be no greater*

than a Score 2. See the "Explanatory Notes" in the Introduction of this Manual.

Score 5. The organization has not identified the patient's and family's responsibilities.

Or

The organization does not have a mechanism in place designed to educate patients and families about their responsibilities.

Standard

PF.3. Any discharge instructions given to the patient and/or, when appropriate, his or her family are provided to the organization or individual responsible for the patient's continuing care.

Intent of PF.3

Patient and/or, when appropriate, family education, discharge planning, and continuity of care are interrelated. Discharge planning helps the patient and his or her family develop and implement a feasible postdischarge plan of care. Discharge planning involves teaching the patient and/or, when appropriate, the family about care after discharge, understanding treatment, making life-style changes, and managing continuing care, whether it is carried out at home (for example, by the patient and/or, when appropriate, the family, with home health care services) or by discharge to another care facility. The discharge instructions are communicated to anyone responsible for the patient's health care needs. For example, a copy of the discharge summary and instructions, if pertinent, are forwarded to the patient's primary care provider.

Example of implementation—PF.3

1. Patients returning home to manage their own care may have been taught procedures foreign to their understanding before hospitalization (for instance, wound care following an extensive incision and drainage procedure, colostomy care, insulin administration, self-catheterization). Besides learning how to perform procedures, patients are also taught to look for signs and symptoms of complications. A copy of the discharge summary and instructions, if pertinent, are forwarded to the patient's primary care practitioner. A primary care practitioner may be an attending physician in the community where the patient resides following treatment at an out-of-town tertiary care center, a home health agency, a rehabilitation center, or a skilled nursing facility.

2. Patients and their family members need to continue portions of the rehabilitation treatment plan upon leaving the acute phase of their biopsychosocial treatment program. Education is provided throughout the acute phase of treatment, immediately before discharge, and clarification is available by telephone after discharge.

Scoring for PF.3

Score 1. 91% to 100% of medical records reviewed indicate that any discharge instructions given to the patient and/or, when appropriate, his or her family were provided to the organization or individual responsible for the patient's continuing care.

Score 2. 76% to 90% of medical records reviewed indicate that any discharge instructions given to the patient and/or, when appropriate, his or her family were provided to the organization or individual responsible for the patient's continuing care.

Score 3. 51% to 75% of medical records reviewed indicate that any discharge instructions given to the patient and/or, when appropriate, his or her family were provided to the organization or individual responsible for the patient's continuing care.

Score 4. 26% to 50% of medical records reviewed indicate that any discharge instructions given to the patient and/or, when appropriate, his or her family were provided to the organization or individual responsible for the patient's continuing care.

Score 5. Fewer than 26% of medical records reviewed indicate that any discharge instructions given to the patient and/or, when appropriate, his or her family were provided to the organization or individual responsible for the patient's continuing care.

Standard

PF.4. The organization plans and supports the provision and coordination of patient and/or, when appropriate, family education activities and resources.

Intent of PF.4

Within the context of its mission and scope, the health care organization plans and provides for patient education to promote and maintain health. The multiplicity of settings and types of patients requiring patient education are considered (for example, patient education in outpatient and inpatient settings, patient teaching for different sociocultural backgrounds, patient education across lifespan, and education about appropriate community resources to support needed life-style changes). Patient education can contribute to other activities and outcomes, such as risk management, obtaining informed consent, and patient satisfaction.

To implement the goals and processes of patient and/or, when appropriate, family education, health care organizations should

- establish an environment that fosters patient and/or, when appropriate, family questioning, learning, and participating in care and in health care decision making;
- assure that staff who provide patient and/or, when appropriate, family education are competent to do so;
- establish mechanisms designed to identify and respond to patient and/or, when appropriate, family learning needs, requests, abilities, and resources, including the identification of community resources;
- ensure that educational resources are appropriate, available, effective, and efficacious, and are delivered in a continuous, safe, timely, efficient, caring, and respectful manner;
- provide education in a manner understandable to the patient and/or, when appropriate, the family, that is, with respect to cultural and religious variables, language, age, abilities, resources, and hearing and/or speaking impairments; and
- assess and improve educational systems and outcomes as part of the organization's performance improvement process.

Example of implementation—PF.4

When defining educational requirements in response to health care needs and patient characteristics, the organization considers what will be taught (methods and resources used), who will teach (discipline roles), where teaching will be conducted (inpatient or ambulatory), and when teaching will occur (preadmission, during hospitalization, or postcare).

Examples of evidence of performance—PF.4

- Long- and short-range plans
- Budgets
- Interviews
- Meeting minutes
- Policies and procedures
- Reports to committees and/or the governing body
- Staff development documentation

Scoring for PF.4

Score 1. Evidence indicates that the organization plans and supports the provision of patient and/or, when appropriate, family education.

Score 3. Note: *Although the surveyor will score this standard at an organization's actual level of performance, the impact of the score will be no greater than a Score 3.*

Score 5. Evidence indicates that the organization does not plan and support the provision of patient and/or, when appropriate, family education.

Standard

PF.4.1. The organization identifies and provides the educational resources required to achieve its educational objectives.

Intent of PF.4.1

Educational resources are selected based on the patient's and family's learning needs. Such resources may include, but are not limited to, teaching by appropriate member(s) of the health care team; types of material (for example, pamphlets, videotapes); teaching methods; teaching by community resource, if needed; and patient referrals to programs that can meet special needs as required. The organization provides these resources as part of its commitment to patient and/or, when appropriate, family education. Educational material and resources are available, as required, in modalities that accommodate persons with disabilities (for example, braille, tape recording, large print). Medical record documentation of the verbal information method used satisfies the intent of the standard.

Example of implementation—PF.4.1

Implementation may consist of formal teaching plans or informal teaching opportunities for many of the patient and family education activities. Health care professionals determine how to best meet the patient's and/or, when appropriate, family's specific learning needs. Examples of educational formats include
- nutrition class for diabetics;
- information on community resource availability and access;
- closed-circuit television system within the organization;
- multimedia library consisting of books, tapes, and videos;
- development of a patient and/or, when appropriate, family education materials database;

- group presentations; and
- one-on-one presentations.

Scoring for PF.4.1

Score 1. Evidence indicates that appropriate educational resources are available and allocated. Priorities are established according to need.

Score 3. Evidence indicates that appropriate educational resources are available and allocated; however, priorities are not established according to need.

Score 5. There is no evidence that educational resources are available and allocated.

Standard

PF.4.2. The patient and/or, when appropriate, family educational process is interdisciplinary, as appropriate to the care plan.

Intent of PF.4.2

Understanding other health care professionals' contributions to patient education increases its effectiveness and facilitates collaboration among the health care team. Collaboration ensures that the patient and/or, when appropriate, the family receive consistent education about health care and maintenance. However, this collaborative effort does not preclude the physician educating the patient in his or her office or in the organization. This standard recognizes that patient and/or, when appropriate, family education may be provided by a single discipline (for example, only the physician, only the nurse) or may be multidisciplinary (for example, the physician, nurse, physical therapist). When it is the latter, the education is coordinated among the various involved disciplines (it should be interdisciplinary).

Example of implementation—PF.4.2

Patient education is enhanced for the newly diagnosed diabetic when a multidisciplinary approach is used. Professionals involved in the coordinated effort may include a physician, nurse, pharmacist, and dietician, for example. This teaching function is carried out in accordance with an organizational mechanism addressing patient and family education.

Examples of evidence of performance—PF.4.2
- Organizational policy
- Departmental policy
- Meeting minutes

- Medical records (for example, progress notes, discharge plans, patient care plans)

Scoring for PF.4.2

Score 1. The organization's patient and/or, when appropriate, family education process is interdisciplinary, as required by the severity of illness, patient needs, and patient problems.

And

A written mechanism describes the organization's interdisciplinary process for patient and/or, when appropriate, family education.

And

91% to 100% of medical records reviewed indicate an interdisciplinary process for patient and/or, when appropriate, family education.

Score 2. The organization's patient and/or, when appropriate, family education process is interdisciplinary, as required by the severity of illness, patient needs, and patient problems.

And

A written mechanism describes the organization's interdisciplinary process for patient and/or, when appropriate, family education.

And

76% to 90% of medical records reviewed indicate an interdisciplinary process for patient and/or, when appropriate, family education.

Score 3. The organization's patient and/or, when appropriate, family education process is interdisciplinary, as required by the severity of illness, patient needs, and patient problems.

And

A written mechanism describes the organization's interdisciplinary process for patient and/or, when appropriate, family education.

And

51% to 75% of medical records reviewed indicate an interdisciplinary process for patient and/or, when appropriate, family education.

Score 4. The organization's patient and/or, when appropriate, family education process is inter-

disciplinary, as required by the severity of illness, patient needs, and patient problems.

And

A written mechanism describes the organization's interdisciplinary process for patient and/or, when appropriate, family education.

And

26% to 50% of medical records reviewed indicate an interdisciplinary process for patient and/or, when appropriate, family education.

Score 5. There is no written mechanism that describes the organization's interdisciplinary process for patient and/or, when appropriate, family education.

Or

Fewer than 26% of medical records reviewed indicate an interdisciplinary process for patient and/or, when appropriate, family education.

Suggested readings and other resources

Barry K: Patient self-medication: An innovative approach to medication teaching. *J Nurs Care Qual* 8(1):75-82, 1993.

Uses a case study to examine the concept of a unit-based self-medication program. Discusses problems prior to the development of the program, which methods best improve patient knowledge, the phases involved in developing a self-medication program, implementing the program, and some of the issues that arise with patients on the program.

Gilmour DM: Navigating the teaching-learning process. Education standards for reaching quality improvement destination. *J Nurs Care Qual* 8(1):67-74, 1993.

Case study. Explains the process the Department of Education and Nursing Research at the Medical Center of Delaware in Wilmington underwent in switching from a quality assurance mode to a quality improvement plan.

Whitman NI, et al: *Teaching in Nursing Practice:* A Professional Model, 2nd ed. Norwalk, CT: Appleton & Lange, 1992.

Provides a comprehensive approach to the process of health education. Divides text into four units that focus on the development and implementation of an educational program, the learning environment, the learner, and teaching strategies. Intended to aid in assessing, planning, implementing, and evaluating teaching. Includes examples of educational activities.

Patient/Family Education
Standard I
Oncology nurse
The oncology nurse at both the generalist and advanced practice levels is responsible for patient/family education related to cancer.

Standard II
Resources
Adequate resources to achieve the objectives of patient/family education related to cancer care are available and appropriate.

Standard III
Curriculum
Knowledge, skills, and attitudes related to the management of human responses to cancer are reflected in the educational activity for the patient/family experiencing cancer.

Standard IV
Teaching–learning process
Teaching-learning theories are applied to the development, implementation, and evaluation of learning experiences related to cancer care.

Standard V
Learner: the patient family
The patient/family apply knowledge, skills, and attitudes to management of actual or potential human responses to the cancer experience.

Public Education
Standard I
Oncology nurse
The oncology nurse provides formal and informal cancer-related public education commensurate with personal education and experience.

Standard II
Resources
Adequate resources for public education related to cancer prevention, detection, treatment, and care are current and appropriate to achieve education objectives.

Standard III
Curriculum
Knowledge, skills, and attitudes related to the physical and psychosocial aspects of cancer prevention, early detection, treatment, and care are included in public education activities.

Standard IV
Teaching–learning process
Teaching-learning theories are applied to the development, implementation, and evaluation of learning experiences related to cancer education for the public.

Standard V
Learner: the public
Personal behaviors and public policy related to cancer prevention, detection, treatment, rehabilitation, and supportive care are influenced by formal and informal cancer public education.

From Oncology Nursing Society: *Standards of oncology education: patient/family and public nursing,* Pittsburgh, 1995, The Society.

E Resources for Patient Education

Finding, developing, and evaluating teaching materials are recurring responsibilities in patient education. This appendix provides additional resources for these functions.

GUIDELINES FOR DESIGNING AND EVALUATING PRINTED EDUCATION MATERIALS

Printed education materials (PEMs) are among the most economical and frequently used methods for educating individuals about health matters. Bernier and Yasko[1] have developed the model for evaluating printed materials that is shown on pp. 258-260. In their article they describe testing the model, including development of a self-report questionnaire. Clearly, congruence between desired outcomes as specified by PEM developers and the actual learning achieved by the target population represents the ultimate measure of the PEM quality, although it appears that little evaluation of actual learning outcomes is carried out by developers of PEMs. It is important to note that Bernier and Yasko make the assumption that the process and criteria used in creating PEMs and contained in their model influence the quality of the product and subsequent learning outcomes. The model, which was created by harvesting criteria from existing literature and the practice of educators, has been validated by expert opinion.

As noted in Chapter 3, development of educational materials involves a predesign phase of needs assessment and a design phase of decisions about educational objectives, content, structure, and format. After initial development of the product, evaluation of actual learning that it creates in target patients should be used to revise and refine it. Then the PEM is distributed and tested more broadly on much larger populations.

READING LEVEL, WORD FAMILIARITY, AND SIMPLIFIED INSTRUCTIONS

The single most commonly used quantitative method for evaluating patient education materials is probably the readability formula. Several chapters in this book provide information about how readability indices are computed and interpreted, as well as their limitations (at least when used alone) in evaluating patient education materials. This appendix provides several analyses of the readability of a variety of patient education materials. Because the formulas used to determine readability may not take into account the unfamiliarity of medical words, examples from published studies of the understandability of medical words to specific population are noted.

The evidence on readability of pediatric patient education materials verifies the difficulty in obtaining materials appropriate for the broad range of populations that health care professionals serve. The inability to read and understand written information can interfere with a parent's ability to follow a treatment regimen. Table 1 indicates the grade level at which many materials for parents are written—as based on the FOG index. Table 2, on the other hand, demonstrates the variability of grade level obtained by means of three different readability formulas, therefore reinforcing the usefulness of multiple formulas in analyzing a particular piece of patient education material. Table 3, an analysis of teaching materials from the American Cancer Society and the National Cancer Institute, provides additional evidence about the high reading-level bias in available materials.

Possible word substitutions for complex medical terms are shown in Table 4 (p. 269), and examples of original and simplified text appear in the box on p. 273. The commonly occurring health-related words in the box on pp. 271-272, which is based on an anal-

---

■ A MODEL FOR DESIGNING AND EVALUATING PRINTED EDUCATION MATERIALS (PEMs)

I Pre-design phase: assessment

A. An educational need/problem/issue exists and it is clearly identified

B. Target populations (PEMs recipients) are clearly identified

C. A review of the literature (ROL) about the topic is conducted:
   1. periodicals and texts are reviewed
   2. existing PEMs in the topic area are reviewed

D. Deficits in existing PEMs are identified in the ROL

E. Needs assessment and informational data about the topic are obtained from:
   1. former patients and their families, or previously affected groups and communities
   2. current patients and their families, or currently affected groups and communities
   3. health professionals involved in the care of persons, groups, or communities for whom the PEM is intended
   4. experts from other disciplines relating to the topic

F. The purpose of the PEM is established and it relates to the assessment data

G. The learning objectives are designated and they relate to the assessment data

H. Minimum levels of performance, knowledge, or behavioral change to be achieved by the target group are decided upon by the PEM developers

I. The question of how the developer(s) will determine whether the PEM has fulfilled its purpose and achieved the desired learning outcome is decided

J. The budget for the project is developed

K. Person(s) distributing the PEM to target groups(s) are knowledgeable about the content or will have access to experts who can answer questions of the target group

II Design phase: writing of the first draft

Educational content

A. The purpose of the PEM is made clear to the target group(s)

B. The learning objectives of the PEM relate to the intended outcome of the PEM

C. Only the most essential information about the topic is presented using no more than 3-4 main points (e.g., what, when, where, how)

D. Supplemental information is separated from the main points and is provided as appendices or in a special section of the PEM

E. Content is verified as accurate and current by persons with experience in the topic area:
   1. former patients and their families, groups and communities
   2. current patients and their families, groups and communities
   3. experts in the health professions
   4. experts in other professions and disciplines

Structure and format: text

F. Readability tests (grade level) specific for the intended target group(s) are conducted throughout the development of the PEM (computer software available for determining readability levels; SMOG and Frye formulas for manual calculation)

G. Specialized vocabulary lists are developed and placed at the front of the PEM for easy reader access

From Bernier MJ, Yasko J: *Patient Educ Counsel* 18:253-263, 1991.

A Model for Designing and Evaluating Printed Education Materials (PEMs)— cont'd

Structure and format: illustrations

H. Drawings and illustrations to convey content and improve understanding are discussed and drafted

I. Drawings and illustrations present only essential content relevant to the educational purpose

J. Drawings and illustrations are recognizable to target group(s) with or without explanatory text

K. Each drawing conveys a single idea or concept

L. The lines of the drawings are heavy enough to be seen by the target group(s)

Structure and format: organization

M. The information considered most important by target group(s) is presented first

N. Topic headings and advance organizers are used

O. One idea per paragraph is presented

P. The first sentence of each paragraph is a topic sentence

Q. Short, simple sentences are used to convey one idea at a time

R. Ideas are expressed using one and two syllable words instead of three (or more) syllable words as much as possible

S. Necessary health terms are defined

T. The active voice is used (e.g., "Many persons with colostomies find it helpful to be a member of an Ostomy Support Group" instead of "Many persons with colostomies have found that they benefited from an Ostomy Support Group.")

U. The second person, YOU, is used instead of the third person

V. Consideration is given to eye span or characters per line for easy reading. Use no more than 60-70 characters for ideal eye span

W. Both upper and lower case letters are used for ease of reading

X. The leading (space between each line of type), type style, and font (print size) are selected for ease of reading (1-2 point leading, serif type style, and 12 point print size are easy to read)

Y. Color is used as a cueing agent to highlight material and promote learning; use sensitivity in selecting color in keeping with subject and mood of topic

Z. The size of the PEM is one that is easily handled by the target group(s). Size 8.5 in vertical by 5.5 in horizontal is easy to handle

AA. The title of the PEM is short and conveys the meaning of the material

BB. The cover of the PEM is attractive and eye catching

III Pilot phase

A. A draft of the PEM is pilot tested with the following groups:
   1. former patients and their families or previously affected groups and communities
   2. current patients and their families or currently affected groups and communities
   3. health professionals involved in the care of persons, groups, or communities for whom the PEM is intended
   4. experts from other disciplines who have knowledge about the PEM content

B. Pilot subjects are instructed on their role and they understand what they are being asked to do

C. The purpose of the PEM is clear to pilot subjects

D. The intended outcome of the PEM is clear to the pilot subjects

E. Feedback (verbal or written) about the PEM is received from pilot subjects

F. Feedback from pilot subjects is used to revise and improve the PEM

G. A revised draft of the PEM is distributed to a second group of pilot subjects for further feedback and evaluation

Continued.

■ A MODEL FOR DESIGNING AND EVALUATING PRINTED EDUCATION MATERIALS (PEMs)—
cont'd

IV Distribution and implementation

A. A means of making the PEM available and accessible to the target group(s) is established

B. Direction (instruction and education) is provided to persons, groups, or communities distributing the PEM to target populations

V Evaluation of intended outcome of the PEM

A. The procedures for evaluation considered during the Pre-Design phase are carried out

B. Procedures for evaluation are consistent with desired learning outcomes

C. Findings of the evaluation are shared with the developers of the PEM

D. If results of evaluation suggest that the intended outcome has not been achieved, the PEM is revised by the developer

E. News ideas, questions, and topics emerging from the evaluation of the PEM are noted and shared with persons qualified and interested in the topic area

---

ysis of articles in *Family Health,* a health education magazine, provide information about the grade levels at which these words are comprehensible. The list would be helpful in choosing terms to use in patient education materials targeted at populations at particular reading levels.

Table 5 (p. 270) presents original and simplified sets of instructions for emergency department patients.

Meade and Howser [7] offer examples for revision of informed-consent documents, which are consistently written at a college level. Obviously, the intent of informed-consent documents is subverted if patients cannot read and understand conditions to which they are asked to consent.

Text continued on p. 273.

Table 1 Reading levels of pediatric patient education materials: A guide for parents

TITLE	FOG INDEX GRADE LEVEL
American Academy of Pediatrics	
The Injury Prevention Program (TIPP) Pamphlets	
Safe Driving . . . A Parental Responsibility: HE0038	12
The Child as Passenger on an Adult's Bicycle: HE0037	10
Safe Bicycling Starts Early: HE0036	11
Choosing the Right Size Bicycle for Your Child: HE0035	10
Safe Swimming for Your Young Child: HE0034	11
Protect Your Home Against Fire . . . Planning Saves Lives: HE0039	10
Protect Your Child . . . Prevent Poisoning: HE0033	12
Baby Sitting Reminders: HE0031	10
Infant Furniture: Cribs: HE0030	7
Framingham Safety Survey From Ten to Twelve Years: HE0067-B	6
Framingham Safety Survey From Six to Nine Years: HE0067-A	7
Framingham Safety Survey From One to Five Years (Part 2): HE0022-C	7
Framingham Safety Survey From One to Five Years (Part 1): HE0022-B	9
Framingham Safety Survey the First Year of Life: HE0022-A	7
Safety for Your Child 10 Years: HE0064-D	8
Safety for Your Child 8 Years: HE0062-C	7
Safety for Your Child 6 Years: HE0064-B	6
Early Childhood Years Birth to Six Months: HE0021-A	8
Early Childhood Years Seven to Twelve Months: HE0021-B	8
Early Childhood Years One to Two Years: HE0021-C	9
Early Childhood Years Two to Four Years: HE0021-D	10
Safety for Your Child 5 Years: HE0064-A	7
Safety Tips for Home Playground Equipment . . . : HE0032	9
Guidelines for Parents	
Child Sexual Abuse: What It Is and How to Prevent It: HE0029	10
Hepatitis B: HE0120	13
Other Pamphlets	
Newborns: Care of the Uncircumcised Penis: HE0023R (Rev 2/92)	12
Child Care: What's Best for Your Family: HE0028 (Rev 2/92)	10
Television and the Family: HE0015A	13
Guidelines For Your Family's Health Insurance: HE0077	12
Sex Education: A Bibliography of Educational Materials for Children, Adolescents, and Their Families: HE0024A (Rev 11/90)	17
A Guide to Children's Dental Health: HE0085	10
Sports and Your Child: HE0058 (Rev 2/92)	11
Deciding to Wait: Guidelines for Teens: HE0125	8
Guidelines for Teens: Acne Treatment and Control: HE0087	9
Marijuana: Your Child and Drugs: HE0052	13
Better Health Through Fitness: HE0090	12
Smoking: Straight Talk for Teens: HE0088	10
Tobacco Use: A Message to Parents and Teens: HE0065	9
Choking Prevention and First Aid for Infants and Children: HE0066	8

From Davis TC and others: *Pediatrics* 93:460-468, 1994.
DTP, Diphtheria-tetanus-pertussis; *WIC*, The Special Supplemental Food Program for Women, Infants, and Children.

Continued.

Table 1   Reading levels of pediatric patient education materials: A guide for parents—cont'd

TITLE	FOG INDEX GRADE LEVEL
Other Pamphlets—cont'd	
Important Information for Teens Who Get Headaches: HE0107	14
Surviving: Coping with Adolescent Depression and Suicide: HE0046	11
Teens Who Drink and Drive: Reducing the Death Toll: HE0026	16
Cocaine: Your Child and Drugs: HE0056	11
Alcohol: Your Child and Drugs: HE0059	10
Making the Right Choice: Facts Young People Need to Know About Avoiding Pregnancy: HE0055	11
Hepatitis B: HE0118	12
Healthy Start Food to Grow On Program	
Produced as a cooperative effort by:	
The American Academy of Pediatrics (AAP)	
The American Dietetic Association (ADA)	
The Food Marketing Institute (FMI)	
Feeding Kids Right Isn't Always Easy	9
Tips for Preventing Food Hassles: HE0097	
Growing Up Healthy: Fat, Cholesterol and More: HE0096	9
Right from the Start:	8
ABC's of Good Nutrition for Young Children: HE0095	
What's to Eat? Healthy Foods for Hungry Children: HE0094	10
Patient Medication Instructions	
Codeine: PM1005	12
Diphenhydramine: PM1004	10
Acetaminophen: PM1006	10
Pseudoephedrine: PM1018	11
Posters	
Choking/CPR: HE0008 (Rev 1/89)	8
Cards	
Child Vaccination Record Card	12
Parenting Books	
Caring for Your Baby and Young Child: Birth to Age 5. New York: Bantam Books; 1991	12
Caring for Your Adolescent: Ages 12 to 21. New York: Bantam Books; October 1991	15
Magazines	
Healthy Kids Birth-3, Spring/Summer 1992	12
Healthy Kids 4-10, Spring/Summer 1993	10
Centers for Disease Control and Prevention	
Immunization Pamphlets	
Before It's Too Late Vaccinate: Diphtheria, Tetanus, and Pertussis: HE0054	11
Before It's Too Late Vaccinate: Ten Questions and Answers About How to Help Protect Your Child From Getting Deadly Diseases: HE0109	10
Diphtheria, Tetanus, and Pertussis: What You Need to Know: HE0113 (Rev 2/92)	10
Measles, Mumps, and Rubella: What You Need to Know: HE0114	12
Polio: What You Need to Know: HE0115	10

Table 1   Reading levels of pediatric patient education materials: A guide for parents—cont'd

TITLE	FOG INDEX GRADE LEVEL
Other sources	
Caddo-Shreveport Health Unit	
Pamphlet	
Important Information About Polio and Oral Polio Vaccine (Rev 3/83)	14
American Dietetic Association	
Pediatric diets	
Guidelines for Daily Food Intake	13
Citizens for Public Action on Blood Pressure and Cholesterol, Inc.	
Pamphlet	
Cholesterol and Kids: A Parent's Guide—1991. Bethesda, MD	13
Fisher-Price Family Alert Program	
Pamphlet	
Information for Parents About Choking Risks Involving Little People and Other Small Objects	15
Louisiana Drug and Poison Information Center	
US Consumer Product Safety Commission Poison Lookout Checklist (Rheumatology)	11
Louisiana State University Medical Center Pediatric Clinic	
Pediatric endocrinology and diabetes education	
Information about Diabetes for School Personnel	13
Forms	
Vaccine Administration Record (DTP 10/15/91)	17
Influenza Vaccine Consent Form	13
After-care Instructions	10
Leaflets	
Feeding Guide	8
When Your Child Has Asthma	12
House Dust	10
Home Instructions Chicken Pox	10
Sick Day	14
Instructions for Home Under 10	9
Pediatrics Endocrinology and Diabetes Education	13
Instructions for Home Age 10+	9
Louisiana Office of Public Health	
Nutrition section	
Feeding Children One to Two Years	8
Feeding Children Three to Five Years	8
Participating in the WIC Program, Special Food for Special People	9
Scriptographic booklets	
About Hepatitis B (No. 37762F-7-92)	7
Your Child's Hearing, A Guide for Parents (No. 11809)	10
Shots for Tots (No. 11551AF-6-92)	10
When Your Child is Ill (No. 11502)	9
About Childhood Communicable Diseases (No. 37200)	10
About Pregnancy and Drugs (No. 37309C-6-92)	9
Parents and Stress (No. 37663B-6-92)	8

Continued.

Table 1 Reading levels of pediatric patient education materials: A guide for parents—cont'd

TITLE	FOG INDEX GRADE LEVEL
Other sources—cont'd	
March of Dimes	
Pamphlets	
3 Words About Drinking While Pregnant: Don't Do It!	8
Double Trouble Drugs, Alcohol, Tobacco Abuse during Pregnancy	11
Be Good to Your Baby Before It is Born (Booklet pp 2, 7, 9)	9
Drinking During Pregnancy: Fetal Alcohol Syndrome and Fetal Alcohol Effects	13
Give Your Baby a Healthy Start: Stop Smoking	7
Will My Baby Be All Right? 09-438-00	13
Eating for Two, Nutrition During Pregnancy: 09-219-00	8
Meadjohnson Nutritionals	
Pamphlets	
Jaundice and Your Baby: L-F30-11-90	10
Weaning and Supplementing: A Guidebook for Breastfeeding Mothers (L-F58-11-90)	11
Ohio Neonatal Nutritionists	
Leaflets	
Questions You May Have About Your Child's Special Formula	10
Questions You May Have About Your Child's Tube Feeding	8
Ross Laboratories	
Pamphlets	
WHAT IS WIC?: G374(0.15)/March 1988	5
Your Baby and Crying (includes Coping With Infant Colic): 51226 09899WB(0.25)/ Dec 1991	11
Becoming a Parent Preparing For and Welcoming Your New Baby: G34(1.00) Jan 1991	10
Cooking With Isomil: G714/May 1989	10
Leaflets (adaptation of CDC pamphlet)	
Polio: (10-15-91)	11
Diphtheria, Tetanus, and Pertussis: (DTP 10-15-91)(DTaP 3-25-92)	11
Nutrition Prescriptives, 1988	
Toddler Diet (1-3 years)/Child Diet (3-6 years)	10
Fleischmann's	
Leaflet	
Nutrition Update: The Adolescent Years	12
Nabisco	
Diabetes, Exercise, and You	13
Herbert Laboratories	
Pamphlets	
Understanding and Treating Scabies Patient Instruction Sheet	12
Commercial baby books	
Brazelton TB. *Infants and Mothers: Differences in Development.* New York: Bantam Doubleday Dell Publishing Group, 1983.	11
Carter JM, ed. *The Good Housekeeping Illustrated Book of Pregnancy and Baby Care.* New York: William Morrow, 1990.	11
Christophersen ER. *The Baby Owner's Manual: What to Expect and How to Survive the First Year.* Shawnee Mission, KS: Westport, 1988.	12

Table 1   Reading levels of pediatric patient education materials: A guide for parents—cont'd

TITLE	FOG INDEX GRADE LEVEL
Commercial baby books—cont'd	
Eisenberg A, Murkoff HE, Hathaway SE. *What to Expect the First Year.* New York: Workman, 1989.	14
Eisenberg A, Murkoff HE, Hathaway SE. *What to Expect When You're Expecting.* New York: Workman, 1991.	15
Ferber R. *Solve Your Child's Sleep Problems.* New York: Simon and Schuster, 1985.	14
Greenspan SI. *The Essential Partnership: How Parents and Children Can Meet the Emotional Challenges of Infancy and Childhood.* New York: Penguin, 1989.	15
Hull KH. *The Mommy Book.* New York: Harper Collins, 1986.	10
Leach P. *Babyhood: Stage by Stage, From Birth to Age Two.* New York: Random House, 1983.	14
Leach P. *Your Baby and Child from Birth to Age Five.* 2nd rev ed. New York: Random House, 1989.	11
Olds SW. *The Complete Book of Breastfeeding.* New York: Workman, 1987.	16
Popper A. *Parents' Book for the Toddler Years.* New York: Ballantine, 1986.	11
Princeton Center for Infancy & Early Childhood. *The First Twelve Months of Life.* New York: Putnam Publishing Group, 1982.	11
Samuels M, Samuels N. *The Well Pregnancy Book.* New York: Simon and Schuster, 1986.	16
Shapiro HI. *The Pregnancy Book for Today's Woman.* New York: Harper and Row, 1983.	19
Spock B, Rothenberg M. *Dr. Spock's Baby and Child Care.* 6th ed. New York: Pocket Books, 1992.	10

Table 2 Readability of selected patient education materials

TOPICS	TITLES	SOURCES	READABILITY GRADE LEVEL		
			FOG	FRY	SMOG
AIDS	Mommy-Daddy, What's AIDS?	NAPNAP (National Association of Pediatric Nurse Associates and Practitioners)	12.5	10	11.5
	What Is Safer Sex?	Network Publications	8.0	7	8.1
Allergy	Allergies in Children, Plain Talk for Parents	AAP (American Academy of Pediatrics)	13.6	14	12.3
	Is It a Cold or Allergy?	Sandoz Pharmaceuticals	12.3	11	11.4
Asthma	So You Have Asthma TOO!	Nancy Sander, Provided by Glaxo, Allen & Hanburys	6.3	5	6.7
Behavior	Toilet Training: A Parent's Guide	AAP (American Academy of Pediatrics)	9.0	8	9.0
	Temper Tantrums	Barton Schmitt, Instructions for Pediatric Patients (WB Saunders)	8.9	7	8.8
	Your Child's Fears	Ross Laboratories	9.1	7	8.6
	Your Growing Child from 3 to 6 Months	Ross Laboratories	10.0	7	9.5
Birth Control	Talking With Your Parents About Birth Control	Network Publications	9.8	7	9.6
Dental	Care of Children's Teeth: A Guide from Crest	Procter & Gamble	7.8	7	8.0
Drug Use	Cocaine: Your Child and Drugs	AAP (American Academy of Pediatrics)	9.5	9	9.5
	A Parent's Guide to Prevention: Growing up Drug Free	U.S. Dept. of Education	15.2	13	13.4
Fever Care	Kidcare	McNeil	11.4	9	10.6
Hypertension	About High Blood Pressure in Children	American Heart Association	10.6	10	10.2
Immunizations	What You Should Know—and What You Can Do About Hemophilus B Disease	Lederle-Praxis Biologicals	12.8	13	11.8
	Kindergarten to College . . . Your children may need a second measles vaccination	Merck & Co.	11.8	10	11.1
	Important Information about Hepatitis B, Hepatitis B Vaccine and Hepatitis B Immune Globulin	CDC (Centers for Disease Control)	11.0	9	10.3
	VIP: Measles, Mumps and Rubella: What You Need to Know	CDC (Centers for Disease Control)	10.9	9	10.2

From Klingbeil C, Speece MW, Schubiner H: *Clin Pediatr* 34:96-102, 1995.

Table 2   Readability of selected patient education materials—cont'd

TOPICS	TITLES	SOURCES	READABILITY GRADE LEVEL		
			FOG	FRY	SMOG
Nutrition	Starting Right With the Bottle and Taking the Bottle Away	Health Education Associates, Inc.	6.7	5	7.3
	A Food Guide for the First Five Years	Education Department, National Livestock and Meat Board	11.8	9	11.1
	Starting Solids: A Guide for Parents and Childcare Providers	NAPNAP (National Association of Pediatric Nurse Associates and Practitioners)	10.4	9	10.1
	Breastfeeding: Feeding Your Baby the Natural Way	Ross Laboratories	12.7	10	4.6
Parenting	What Every Parent Should Know	Thomas Gordon, National Committee for Prevention of Child Abuse	15.3	15	13.5
Puberty	The Perils of Puberty	RAJ Publications	8.2	6	8.0
	The Problem with Puberty...	RAJ Publications	9.3	8	9.1
	Talking to Your Child About Growing Up	Parenting Advisor Series-Whittle Communications	12.1	10	11.3
Rash	Guidelines for Parents: Diaper Rash	AAP (American Academy of Pediatrics)	11.5	9	10.7
Safety	Emergency Choking Aid for Infants	Mead Johnson Nutritionals	10.4	8	10.0
	Safe Kids Are No Accident! How to Protect Your Child From Injury	National Safe Kids Campaign	9.4	7	9.3
	10 Years: Safety in a Kid's World	AAP (American Academy of Pediatrics)	6.6	4	7.1
	TIPP—Early Childhood Years: Birth to 6 Months	AAP (American Academy of Pediatrics)	8.5	7	8.4
Sex	Teen Sex: It's Okay to Say: NO WAY!	Planned Parenthood	7.2	6	7.9

Table 3 Reading levels of standard patient education materials for cancer

PAMPHLET NAME	TARGET AUDIENCE	FLESCH GRADE LEVEL
American Cancer Society Materials		
At Your Service	Patients with cancer and their families	15
Cancer Word Book	People interested in the scientific and medical terms used in oncology	8
Cancer: Your Job, Insurance and the Law	Patients with cancer	15
Caring for the Patient at Home: A Guide for Patients and Families	Patients with complex needs who are discharged to the home	13
Chemotherapy: What it is, How it Helps	Patients with cancer who are receiving chemotherapy and who are considering treatment with chemotherapy	8
Choice or Chance: Taking Control	Individuals who want information about cancer prevention; targets lower-literate population	6
Facts on Lung Cancer	Individuals who want information regarding lung cancer and its detection and treatment	12.5
Helping Children Understand: A Guide for a Parent With Cancer	All parents with cancer	8
The Hopeful Side of Cancer	Individuals interested in prevention and early detection of cancer	12
Sexuality and Cancer: For the Female and Her Partner	Women with cancer who are concerned about the impact of cancer on their sexuality	8
Sexuality and Cancer: For the Man Who Has Cancer and His Partner	Men with cancer who are concerned about the impact of cancer on their sexuality	9
Smart Move	Individuals interested in smoking cessation	6
Questions and Answers About Pain Control	Patients who are experiencing chronic pain associated with cancer	12
You Can Protect Yourself	Spanish-speaking individuals who are interested in cancer prevention and early detection activities	6.8
National Cancer Institute Materials		
Advanced Cancer: Living Each Day	Patients who have advanced disease and are ready to discuss loss and death	12
Cancer Prevention: Good News, Better News, and Best News	Individuals interested in prevention and early detection of cancer	8
Chemotherapy and You: A Guide to Seek Help During Treatment	Patients undergoing initial courses of chemotherapy	6
Clearing the Air	Individuals interested in smoking cessation	16
Diet, Nutrition and Cancer Prevention: A Guide to Food Choices	Individuals interested in dietary prevention of cancer	8
Diet, Nutrition and Cancer Prevention: The Good News	Patients and family members interested in learning more about healthy dietary habits and strategies for cancer prevention	8

From Cooley ME and others: *Oncol Nurs Forum* 22:1345-1351, 1995.

Table 3 Reading levels of standard patient education materials—cont'd

PAMPHLET NAME	TARGET AUDIENCE	FLESCH GRADE LEVEL
National Cancer Institute Materials—cont'd		
Eating Hints: Recipes and Tips for Better Nutrition During Cancer Treatment	Patients with cancer who are experiencing difficulties with nutrition	8
Facing Forward	Individuals who have successfully completed cancer treatment	7
Prostate Cancer: Some Good News Men Can Live With	Men over the age of 40	15
Radiation Therapy and You: A Guide to Self Help During Treatment	Patients undergoing initial courses of radiotherapy	14
Taking Time: Support for People With Cancer and the People Who Care About Them	Patients who have recently been diagnosed with cancer and patients who have experienced a recent recurrence	9
What Are Clinical Trials About?	Patients with cancer and family members who are interested in discovering what clinical trials are all about	10
What You Need to Know About . . . Cancer	Patients who are newly diagnosed with cancer and desire information about their type of cancer	13
What You Need to Know About . . . Lung Cancer	Patients who are newly diagnosed with lung cancer	9
When Cancer Recurs: Meeting the Challenge Again	Patients who have recently been diagnosed with recurrent cancer	9
When Someone in Your Family Has Cancer	Patients with newly diagnosed, early stage cancer who have school-age children	7

Table 4 Sample glossary of difficult terms

DIFFICULT WORDS/TERMS	POSSIBLE SUBSTITUTIONS
chemotherapeutic agent	anticancer drug
clinical trial	research study
concomitant	given at the same time
determine	find out or see if
difficulties	problems
granulocytopenia	drop in white blood cell count
intradermally	given under the skin
investigation	study
nausea	sick to the stomach
oncology	cancer
opportunity	chance
participate	take part
venipuncture	draw blood
withdraw/discontinue	stop taking part

From Meade CD, Howser DM: *Oncol Nurs Forum* 19:1523-1528, 1992.

Table 5   Emergency department discharge instructions

ORIGINAL INSTRUCTION SETS	SIMPLIFIED INSTRUCTION SETS
Wound instructions	
Keep wound(s) clean and dry.	Keep wound clean and dry.
Elevate wound(s) above the level of the heart to reduce swelling.	Keep the wound above your heart to keep swelling down.
Watch for the common signs of infection: pain, pus, swelling, redness, fever, and red streaks. If any of these signs are seen return to the Emergency Room IMMEDIATELY.	Look for signs of infection: pain, pus, swelling, redness, fever and red streaks. If you see any of these come back here IMMEDIATELY.
If you have received a tetanus booster, be aware that some people experience pain and mild swelling at the site of the injection. Local heat may reduce the swelling and aspirin or acetaminophen can relieve the pain. Allergic reactions to the tetanus immunizations are rare. However, if you develop shortness of breath, a rash or itching over the body, return to the Emergency Room at once. You will need a booster in 10 years, or in 5 years if you receive a severe injury or laceration.	If you have had a tetanus shot today: —You will need a booster in 5-10 years. —Some people have pain and swelling at the site of the shot. Heat can help with the swelling and Tylenol can help with the pain. —Allergic reactions to tetanus shots are rare. The signs of a reaction are trouble breathing, a rash, or itching. If any of these happen come back here IMMEDIATELY.
Sprains and bruises	
To reduce swelling: —Keep the affected extremity elevated above the level of your heart as much as possible. —Use ice compresses over the affected area for 20 minutes every 2 to 4 hours for the next 24 hours, then use heat for 20 minutes every 4 hours.	You will have pain and swelling. To keep swelling down: —Keep the injured part above your heart as much as you can. —For the next 24 hours, put ice on the injured part for 20 minutes every 2 to 4 hours.
To reduce pain: —Take the pain medication as prescribed or aspirin or acetaminophen. —Keep the affected extremity at rest as much as possible while it still hurts. —If given crutches, do not bear weight on the affected leg until it is comfortable to walk.	For pain: —Take the pain medicine you were given or Tylenol or Advil. —Rest the injured part while it still hurts.
If the pain persists or if you are not healing as expected, see your personal physician or contact the doctor to whom you were referred.	If you are not getting better as fast as you think you should, see your doctor or the doctor whose name we gave you.

From Jolly BT, Scott JL, Sanford SM: *Ann Emerg Med* 26:443-446, 1995.

■ COMMONLY OCCURRING HEALTH-RELATED WORDS (*n* = 345) AND THEIR FREQUENCIES, GROUPED BY GRADE LEVELS

Grade 4							
Ability	28	Eat	32	Meal	41	Temperature	29
Accident	41	Examination	10	Medical	61	Test	42
Acid	20	Exercise	59	Medicine	20	Thermometer	29
Adult	42	Experience	24	Milk	85	Training	10
Age	142	Eye	65	Mother	30	Treatment	116
Air	11	Face	11	Mouth	14	Tube	34
Animal	18	Failure	14	Muscle	55	Type	50
Appetite	16	Family	93	Neck	17	Vision	17
Arm	15	Fat	127	Needle	13	Weight	52
Baby	151	Female	17	Nerve	11		
Back	47	Fever	47	Normal	63	Grade 6	
Balance	10	Food	159	Nurse	10	Abdomen	10
Bed	17	Foot	42	Oil	30	Abdominal	17
Birth	10	Germ	25	Pain	70	Absorb	21
Bite	10	Glasses	19	Patient	68	Abuse	17
Blood	78	Grain	26	Period	34	Alcohol	33
Blood (pressure)	76	Group	51	Physician	68	Allergic	23
Body	124	Growth	37	Pill	31	Allergy	30
Bone	66	Gum	15	Poison	25	Area	38
Brain	21	Habit	11	Prescription	19	Artery	12
Breast	34	Hair	10	Pressure	24	Attitude	10
Burn	80	Hand	13	Protection	11	Bacteria	20
Butter	19	Head	37	Rate	23	Barrier	10
Caffeine	10	Headache	63	Reduce	34	Bladder	31
Care	46	Health	106	Repair	21	Calorie	41
Cause	180	Healthy	72	Rest	14	Complaint	13
Cell	32	Hearing	21	Salt	36	Condition	48
Cereal	13	Heart	50	Seed	10	Confusion	12
Change	28	Heat	11	Sex	21	Content	16
Chemical	30	Hospital	25	Skin	58	Control	54
Childbirth	10	Ice	20	Sleep	54	Definition	14
Childhood	15	Idea	17	Sound	17	Degree	40
Cold	10	Infection	105	Speech	10	Delivery	10
Combination	13	Injure	14	Spine	11	Dental	20
Community	16	Injury	124	State	15	Depressed	17
Cream	16	Juice	27	Step	10	Development	23
Curve	10	Kidney	23	Stomach	10	Diet	38
Dead	25	Knee	19	Strength	15	Dietary	23
Death	18	Learning	12	Stroke	11	Disturbance	12
Disease	128	Leg	38	Sugar	29	Dosage	16
Dizziness	11	Level	17	Support	26	Dose	13
Doctor	150	Life	41	Surface	10	Energy	14
Drug	108	Liquid	21	Swelling	10	Environment	13
Ear	37	Liver	21	Tea	12	Expose	14
		Lung	10	Teeth	22	Feelings	34

■ COMMONLY OCCURRING HEALTH-RELATED WORDS (*n*= 345) AND THEIR FREQUENCIES, GROUPED BY GRADE LEVELS—cont'd

Word	Freq	Word	Freq	Word	Freq	Word	Freq
Fiber	47	Symptom	12	Sperm	25	Hypertension	12
Fluid	49	System	25	Study	40	Tract	10
Formula	10	Technique	29	Therapy	27		
Function	37	Term	22	Treat	48	**Grade 16**	
Gain	17	Tissue	17	Urine	53	Contraceptive	14
Illness	47	Vaccine	10	Virus	40	Dementia	15
Increase	55			Vitamin	99	Syndrome	22
Infant	36	**Grade 8**					
Infect	10	Absorption	12	**Grade 10**		**Not Graded**	
Joint	13	Anemia	13	Agent	14	Allergen	13
Laxative	44	Antihistamine	41	Alignment	12	Antidepressant	27
Limit	19	Birth control	35	Antibiotic	24	Awareness	18
Mental	12	Bowel	31	Antibody	12	Bleeding	10
Method	58	Cholesterol	43	Carbohydrate	16	Breathing	15
Mood	38	Complication	12	Constipation	15	Congestion	11
Oral	19	Cycle	27	Cope	15	Contraception	19
Organ	13	Dehydration	12	Deficiency	15	Fallopian	13
Oxygen	13	Diabetes	20	Depression	96	Feeding	26
Pharmacist	12	Diarrhea	49	Fetus	11	Fetal	16
Physical	47	Diet	38	Preparation	15	Guideline	14
Population	19	Dietary	23	Rule	10	Hormone	22
Position	20	Disturbance	12	Stimulant	10	Impotence	12
Pregnancy	85	Dressing	26	Uterus	22	Infertility	17
Pregnant	17	Effect (result)	15	Yogurt	22	Ingestion	14
Prescribe	13	Emotional	11			Iron	35
Problem	197	Excess	10	**Grade 12**		Ligation	13
Process	22	Exposure	22	Calcium	44	Medication	11
Product	60	Fatigue	18	Condom	15	Menstrual	22
Protein	23	Impact	10	Disorder	28	Monitor	12
Range	12	Intercourse	15	Factor	49	Nursing	13
Rash	11	Internal	10	Fluoride	10	Occupational	17
Reaction	12	Intestinal	12	Impairment	12	Osteoporosis	35
Reduction	12	Labour*	14	Incontinence	23	Ovulation	14
Relationship	12	Major	20	Lethal	30	Poisoning	16
Relief	15	Nausea	16	Menopause	15	Postpartum	44
Relieve	20	Nutrition	33	Movement	19	Premenstrual	11
Sense	21	Pattern	11	Multiple	12	Saturated	10
Sexual	43	Potential	11	Nutrient	39	Sexuality	14
Sign	28	Procedure	16	Plaque	15	Sexually	46
Simple	29	Response	14	Rhinitis	12	Sterilization	19
Situation	20	Side effect	51	Stool	32	Tubal	16
Sodium	36	Significant	19	Stress	30	Ultrasound	23
Stage	12	Soluble	12			Urinary	11
Substance	29	Solution	15	**Grade 13**		Vaginal	14
Surgery	13	Specific	15	Estrogen	14	Vomiting	24

*English spelling.

EXAMPLES OF ENHANCING READING EASE*

Original text

You are being asked to participate in a study to determine if your urine and blood contain measurable quantities of autocrine motility factor (AMF), a protein secreted by tumors, which acts on tumor cells to stimulate tumor cell movement; and under circumstances in which you may have abnormal collections of fluid under your lung (pleural fluid) or in your abdomen (ascites), samples of that fluid will be tested as well. (one sentence, 70 words, 12 polysyllabic words)

Revised simplified version

You are being asked to take part in a study to see if we can measure AMF (autocrine motility factor) in your blood or urine. AMF is a protein that comes from tumors. In some cases, samples of fluids from your lung (pleural fluid) and from your stomach (ascites) will be taken. The amount of AMF will be checked. *(four sentences, 59 words, three polysyllabic words)*

Original text: passive voice

Nausea and vomiting have also been reported as well as interference with kidney function.

Revised text: active voice

You may have nausea (feeling sick to your stomach) and vomiting (throwing up) with this drug. You may have changes in how your kidneys work.

From Meade CD, Howser DM: *Oncol Nurs Forum* 19:1523-1528, 1992.
*Heads and text for original passages are 9-point Avant-Garde. Heads for revised passages are 14-point Times, and text is 12-point Times.

RESOURCE LIST: PATIENT EDUCATION MATERIALS

Patient education materials are available from a myriad of sources. The listings in the boxes on pp. 274-281 are from nonprofit and government agencies; thus the bias that one might expect from commercial sources is avoided.

■ ARTHRITIS FOUNDATION: EDUCATIONAL MATERIALS

General information
- Arthritis: Do You know? #5786 (fact sheet)
- Arthritis Answers: Basic Information about Arthritis #4001
- Health, Life and Disability Insurance for People with Arthritis #9332

Self-management
- Managing Your Activities #9329
- Managing your Fatigue #9336
- Managing Your Pain #9333
- Managing Your Stress #9326

Daily living
- Arthritis and Employment: You Can Get the Job You Want #9070
- Arthritis on the Job: You Can Work with It #9073
- Diet and Arthritis #4280
- Exercise and Your Arthritis #9704
- Thinking about Tomorrow: A Career Guide for Teens with Arthritis #9074

Family life
- Arthritis and Pregnancy #9331
- The Family: Making the Difference #9334
- Living and Loving: Information about Sexuality and Intimacy #9190

Children
- AJAO (American Juvenile Arthritis Organization) #8001
- Arthritis in Children #4160
- Arthritis Information: Children #4141 (information list)
- When Your Student Has Arthritis: A Guide for Teachers #9560

Advocacy
- Americans with Disabilities Act (ADA) Resource Manual #4014
- Arthritis and Vocational Rehabilitation #2250
- Arthritis Information: Advocacy and Government Affairs #4142 (information list)
- Guide to Effective Volunteer Lobbying #4012

Treatments
- Managing Your Health Care #9325
- Surgery: Information to Consider #4230

Medications
Information about medications, uses and potential side effects.
- Aspirin and Other Nonsteroidal Anti-Inflammatory Drugs (NSAIDs) #9041
- Corticosteroid Medications #9220
- Gold Treatment #4120
- Hydroxychloroquine (Plaquenil) #9200
- Methotrexate #9040
- Penicillamine (Cuprimine, Depen) #9300

Types of arthritis
Information about causes, symptoms, diagnosis and treatments.
- Ankylosing Spondylitis #9050
- Arthritis and Inflammatory Bowel Disease #9062 (fact sheet)
- Back Pain #4370
- Behcet's Disease #9065 (fact sheet)
- Bursitis, Tendinitis and Other Soft Tissue Rheumatic Syndromes #9055
- Carpal Tunnel Syndrome #9728
- CPPD Crystal Deposition Disease #9054 (fact sheet)
- Ehlers-Danlos Syndrome (EDS) #3428 (fact sheet)
- Fibromyalgia #4340
- Gout #4180
- Infectious Arthritis #4360 (fact sheet)
- Juvenile Dermatomyositis #9535
- Lyme Disease #4275
- The Marfan Syndrome #9338 (fact sheet)
- Myositis #4390
- Osteoarthritis #4040
- Osteogenesis Imperfecta #9075 (fact sheet)
- Osteonecrosis #9337 (fact sheet)
- Osteoporosis #4191
- Paget's Disease #9064 (fact sheet)
- Polyarteritis Nodosa (PAN) and Wegener's Granulomatosis #9056 (fact sheet)
- Polymyalgia Rheumatica (PMR) and Giant Cell Arteritis #4330

■ ARTHRITIS FOUNDATION: EDUCATIONAL MATERIALS—cont'd

Types of arthritis—cont'd

- Pseudoxanthoma Elasticum #4080 (fact sheet)
- Psoriatic Arthritis #9053
- Raynaud's Phenomenon #9324
- Reflex Sympathetic Dystrophy Syndrome #9061 (fact sheet)
- Reiter's Syndrome #4350 (fact sheet)
- Rheumatoid Arthritis #4020
- Sarcoidosis #9057 (fact sheet)
- Scleroderma #9051
- Sjögren's Syndrome #9328
- Systemic Lupus Erythematosus #9052

- In Control #9035: Videotape on effective ways to manage arthritis; optional book and audio-cassettes.
- Living with Arthritis #9037: Videotape on positive ways to cope with arthritis.

Materials in Spanish

- Artritis Reumatoide #4021
- Fibromialgia #4341
- Guia de Medicinas #9063
- La Artritis Infantojuvenile #4165
- Osteoartritis #4041

■ AMERICAN HEART ASSOCIATION OR STATE HEART ASSOCIATION AFFILIATES: EDUCATIONAL MATERIALS

Item number	Title

Blood pressure

50-1055	About High Blood Pressure
50-1105	About High Blood Pressure in African Americans
50-045A	About High Blood Pressure in Children, What Parents Should Know
50-049A	About High Blood Pressure in Teenagers
50-073A	Buying and Caring for Home Blood Pressure Equipment
51-0001	High Blood Pressure
51-1086	High Blood Pressure Fact Sheet
50-065B	Salt, Sodium and Blood Pressure
58-005C	Ten Commandments for High Blood Pressure (Wallet Card)
52-0002	What Every Woman Should Know About High Blood Pressure

Children with heart problems

50-1107	Dental Care for Children with Heart Disease
50-1109	If Your Child Has a Congenital Heart Defect
50-1037	Feeding Infants With Congenital Heart Disease
51-1005	Innocent Heart Murmurs
71-025A	Kawasaki Disease
50-1066	You, Your Child, and Rheumatic Fever

Diet/nutrition

58-006B	Add More Potassium to Your Diet (Wallet Card)
51-1031	American Heart Association Diet, An Eating Plan for Healthy Americans
50-1059	Cholesterol and Your Heart
64-9611	Cholesterol and Blood Pressure Tracking Record
50-067A	Dining Out—A Guide To Restaurant Dining
51-1090	Easy Food Tips for Heart Healthy Eating
50-1006	Facts About Potassium
51-1058	Facts About the New Food Label
50-1035	Guide to Losing Weight
54-9536	How to Have Your Cake and Eat It Too
51-1075	How to Read the New Food Label
64-8075	Making Mexican Food "Heart Healthy"
50-1050	Now You're Cookin'
51-1046	Nutrition for Fitness
51-054A	Nutritious Nibbles, A Guide to Healthy Snacking
50-1126	Reading Food Labels: A Handbook for People With Diabetes
50-1042	Recipes for Low-Fat Low-Cholesterol Meals
50-065B	Salt, Sodium and Blood Pressure
50-1048	Save Food Dollars and Help Your Heart
50-079A	Taking It Off

■ AMERICAN HEART ASSOCIATION OR STATE HEART ASSOCIATION AFFILIATES: EDUCATIONAL MATERIALS—cont'd

Item number	Title
Exercise	
51-1039	E is for Exercise
51-1048	Exercise and Your Heart
51-1060	Exercise Diary
51-1046	Nutrition for Fitness
50-1056	Walking for a Healthy Heart
50-1044	Walking . . . Natural Fun, Natural Fitness
General information	
50-1047	An Older Person's Guide to Cardiovascular Health
50-1062	Controlling Your Risk Factor for Heart Attack
58-1004	Emergency Action Wallet Card
51-1089	Fact Sheet on Heart Attack, Stroke and Risk Factors
51-1062	Heart Attack
50-1053	Heart Attack and Stroke: Signals and Action
51-012A	Heart Quiz
51-1002	How to Make Your Heart Last a Lifetime
58:002B	Medicine Cabinet Sticker
51-1049	RISKO: A Heart Health Appraisal
50-1029	Safeguarding Your Heart During Pregnancy
64-9573	Silent Epidemic: The Truth About Women and Heart Disease
51-030A	Six Important Facts for Healthier Heart
51-1050	What's Your Risk of Heart Attack
Heart disease	
50-1114	About Heart Transplants
50-1058	After a Heart Attack
64-9609	Aspirin and Cardiovascular Disease
50-1045	Coronary Artery Bypass Graft Surgery
50-1002	Dental Care for Adults With Heart Disease
51-1061	Congestive Heart Failure: What You Should Know
50-1030	Heart Valve Surgery
50-1040	Living With Your Pacemaker
71-1020	Marfan Syndrome
51-1035	Mitral Valve Prolapse
78-1003	Bacterial Endocarditis Wallet Card
50-074A	Questions and Answers About Chelation Therapy
50-1020	Sex and Heart Disease
50-1064	Understanding Angina
50-054A	What You Should Know About Coronary Arteriography
70-064A	What You Should Know About Percutaneous Transluminal Coronary Angioplasty

Continued.

AMERICAN HEART ASSOCIATION OR STATE HEART ASSOCIATION AFFILIATES: EDUCATIONAL MATERIALS—cont'd

Item number	Title
Smoking	
51-050A	Calling It Quits
51-1059	Children and Smoking: A Message to Parents
51-1057	Smoking and Heart Disease
51-1051	How to Avoid Weight Gain When Quitting Smoking
Stroke	
50-1127	Caring for the Person with Aphasia
50-1123	How Stroke Affects Behavior
50-1124	Recovering From a Stroke
51-1078	What You Should Know About Stroke
50-1129	Sex After Stroke
51-1082	Good News About Stroke
50-1072	Brain Attack: The Family's Role in Caregiving
Posters	
Exercise	
62-1010	Love Your Heart
62-1008	Target Heart Rate
High blood pressure	
62-019B	Keep Fit and Trim
64-201B	Heart at Work: Take the Pressure Off Yourself
Nutrition	
64-201E	Heart at Work: Eat to Your Heart's Content
62-023A	If You Have to Eat Fast—Eat Smart
64-2015	Another Sign of Heart Disease
Smoking	
62-009E	Are You Sending Smoke Signals
64-201D	Heart at Work: Quitting Leaves a Good Taste in Your Mouth
65-7012	White Liar
Warning signs	
62-1009	Learn How to Recognize a Stroke

Special populations
Mature audience
The following materials have been modified with larger type for the mature audience.

50-1047	An Older Person's Guide to Cardiovascular Health
50-1045	Coronary Artery Bypass Graft Surgery
50-1060	Cholesterol and Your Heart (55+)
50-1049	Medicine Cabinet Sticker (55+)

■ AMERICAN HEART ASSOCIATION OR STATE HEART ASSOCIATION AFFILIATES: EDUCATIONAL MATERIALS—cont'd

Item number	Title
Special populations—cont'd	
Spanish materials	
51-1008	About High Blood Pressure
50-1009	After a Heart Attack
51-1009	Children and Smoking: A Message to Parents
51-0003	Eat Well But Wisely
51-1092	Easy Food Tips for Heart Healthy Eating
51-1079	E is for Exercise
58-1006	Emergency Action Wallet Card
50-1039	Family Learns About Cholesterol
50-1036	Guide to Losing Weight
50-1063	Heart Attack and Stroke: Signals and Actions
51-1054	How to Read the New Food Label
64-8075	Making Mexican Food "Heart Healthy"
51-1063	Six Hopeful Facts About Stroke
50-1103	Smoking and Heart Disease
58-1005	Ten Commandments for the Patient With High Blood Pressure
50-1061	Salvar Vidas!
Easy readability	
64-1025	Doctors Answer Your Questions About High Blood Pressure
64-1021	Signs of a Heart Attack
64-1023	Signs of a Stroke
51-1057	Smoking and Heart Disease
64-1020	Why Exercise?
64-1026	Your Heart and Cholesterol
Prescription pamphlets	
(Available to Patients on Physician's Prescription Only)	
64-9588	Dietary Treatment of High Blood Pressure and High Blood Cholesterol
64-9545	Dietary Treatment of Hypercholesteremia
51-1080	Your Heart and Anticoagulants
64-4001	Step by Step to Lower Your High Blood Cholesterol

ASSOCIATION FOR THE CARE OF CHILDREN'S HEALTH: EDUCATIONAL MATERIALS (SELECTED PUBLICATIONS)

To Tame the Hurt (5055)
Videotape, audiotape, and parent booklet to teach children, adolescents, and their parents how to use simple relaxation, distraction, and imagery techniques to cope with pain

Pain, Pain, Go Away: Helping Children With Pain (1032)
Booklet written to teach parents about pain in children and to help them to ask for better care

A Child Dies: A Portrait of Family Grief (5315)
Book for families, giving practical advice and understanding of the suffering and despair of the death of a child

Children and the AIDS Virus: A Book for Children, Parents and Teachers (5805)
Book for children to read alone or with an adult, helping them understand HIV infection

You and HIV: A Day at a Time (5225)
Illustrated book for children and adolescents with HIV, and their family members; deals with transmission, diagnosis, treatment, home care, and emotional responses

I Will Sing Life: Voices From the Hole in the Wall Gang Camp (5083)
Book written by children who attended Paul Newman's Hole in the Wall Gang Camp

My Hair's Falling Out . . . Am I Still Pretty? (7316)
Video story about two children who are hospital roommates with cancer; explains diagnostic tests, chemotherapy, and hair loss

The Shattered Sugar Bowl (7345)
Video featuring adolescents with diabetes, demonstrating how they can lead active and vital lives while maintaining consistent control of their condition

Introduction to the NICU (7250)
Video to help parents cope with the stress of having a baby in the neonatal intensive care unit, introducing them to equipment and procedures used in infant care and to various people who staff the NICU; emphasizes importance of parents being involved in their baby's care and techniques for safely touching, holding, and repositioning NICU infants

Breathe Easy (5050)
Guide for children up to age 13 with asthma, with illustrations and self-quizzes

What About Me? When Brothers and Sisters Get Sick (5031)
Story for children whose siblings are sick

Association for the Care of Children's Health, Bethesda, Md (1-800-808-ACCH).

■ U.S. Government: Health Publications

One of the most valuable sources of authoritative, concise and current information is the United States federal government. The National Institutes of Health and the Public Health Service in particular produce a vast quantity of information of interest to consumers. This information, in effect, represents a condensation and digest of the findings of the national medical research investment. In this manner, the National Cancer Institute offers information to consumers concerning most types of cancer, current treatments, clinical trials, and research, while the Agency for Health Care Policy and Research translates the current state of the art in many areas of clinical practice into patient versions of practice guidelines. Patient versions of clinical practice guidelines are now available on topics such as treatment of unstable angina, depression, acute pain management, prostate enlargement, sickle cell disease, heart failure, cataracts, urinary incontinence, and early HIV infection. The High Blood Pressure Education Program and the National Cholesterol Education Program produce pamphlets and booklets with the specific intention of educating the general public.

The publications are carefully edited and screened by government researchers for scientific accuracy. Many contain helpful charts and diagrams. Often, they include lists of resources, phone numbers, and addresses of support groups. Few would argue with either the quality or value of these publications.

From Rees AM, editor: *Consumer Health USA: essential information from the federal health network*, Phoenix, Ariz, 1995, Oryx Press.
NOTE: Consumer Health USA is a compendium of consumer health information documents currently available from government sources on topics of concern to the general public.

REFERENCES

1. Bernier MJ, Yasko J: Designing and evaluating printed education materials: model and instrument development, *Patient Educ Counsel* 18:253-263, 1991.
2. Cooley ME and others: Patient literacy and the readability of written cancer educational materials, *Oncol Nurs Forum* 22:1345-1351, 1995.
3. Davis TC and others: Reading ability of parents compared with reading level of pediatric patient education materials, *Pediatrics* 93:460-468, 1994.
4. Hopkinson JH: Frequency of use and comprehensibility of health related words in health education literature, *Patient Educ Counsel* 21:125-133, 1993.
5. Jolly BT, Scott JL, Sanford SM: Simplification of emergency department discharge instructions improves patient comprehension, *Ann Emerg Med* 26:443-446, 1995.
6. Klingbeil C, Speece MW, Schubiner H: Readability of pediatric patient education materials, *Clin Pediatr* 34:96-102, 1995.
7. Meade CD, Howser DM: Consent forms: how to determine and improve their readability, *Oncol Nurs Forum* 19:1523-1528, 1992.
8. Rees AM, editor: *Consumer Health USA: essential information from the federal health network*, Phoenix, Ariz, 1995, Oryx Press.

Index

A

Abstract-concrete continuum, instructional materials and, *41*
Accreditation, patient education and, 226-256
Action, motivation and, 9
Acute lymphoblastic leukemia (ALL), 161
Acute myocardial infarction (AMI), 120
Adapting to illness, motivation and, 14-16, *15t*
Adolescents, learning in, 25-26, *27t-30t*
Adults
  learning in, 24
  older, educational materials for, *278*
Advanced directives (ADs), 195-197
Affective domain, taxonomy of, *38*, *41t*
Agency for Health Care Policy and Research (AHCPR), 94
AIDS; *see* HIV-AIDS patient education
Allergy, patient education materials for, *266t*
Alzheimer's disease (AD), 59, 178
American Academy of Family Physicians Foundation, 210
American Academy of Pediatrics, *261t-262t*
American Cancer Society, 115, *268t*
American Diabetes Association, 146, 147, 228-238
American Dietetic Association, *263t*
American Heart Association, *276-279*
American Hospital Association, 226-256
American Lung Association, *57-58*
Analgesia, patient-controlled, 182, *183t*
Arthritis
  patient education and, *176t*
  patient education standards for, 235-238
  self-efficacy scale for, *85*
  types of, *274*
Arthritis Foundation, 173, *274-275*
Arthritis Self-Efficacy Scale, *85*, 172
Arthritis Self-Management Program (ASMP), 170-172, 173
Artificial nutrition and hydration (ANH), 195, *196*
Association for the Care of Children's Health, *280*
Asthma, 126-128, *131-132*
  mortality from, 128
  patient education and, *176t*

Asthma—cont'd
  patient education materials for, *266t*
Attitude learning, 23
Attribution, motivation and, 7
Autism, 31

B

Behavior
  adherence-enhancing, *181*
  measurement of, 69-81
  patient education materials for, *266t*
  personal health, socioeconomic status and, *199*
Behavioral learning theory, 20
Bill of Rights
  Ostomate, 239
  Patient's, 226-228
Birth control, patient education materials for, *266t*
Blood-glucose awareness training (BGAT), 137
Blood pressure, educational materials on, *276*, *278*
"Bone up on Arthritis" (BUOA), 173
Breast cancer information test, *114*
Breast self-examination (BSE), 8-9, *10-11*, 106-107, 116-117
Bristol Patient Education Programme, *170*
BSE; *see* Breast self-examination

C

Cancer Information Service of National Cancer Institute, 106
Cancer patient education, 106-118, *187t-188t*
  community-based education and, 115-117
  education of special populations and, 115-117
  educational approaches and research base and, 106-115
  Fredette model for improving, *15t*
  general approach to, 106
  national standards and tested programs and, *116t*, 117
  reading levels and, *268t-269t*
Cardiac catheterization, *184t*, 184-185, *185*, *186t*
Cardiopulmonary resuscitation (CPR), 123, 195, *196*
Cardiovascular patient education, 119-126
  community-based, 123-126
  educational approaches and research base and, 119-123, *124t*, *125t*

Page numbers in *italics* indicate boxes and illustrations; page numbers followed by *t* indicate tables.